Prescription
Alternatives

Hundreds of Safe, Natural, Prescription-Free Remedies
to Restore & Maintain Your Health

EARL L. MINDELL, R.Ph., Ph.D.
AND VIRGINIA HOPKINS, M.A.

New York   Chicago   San Francisco   Lisbon   London   Madrid   Mexico City
Milan   New Delhi   San Juan   Seoul   Singapore   Sydney   Toronto

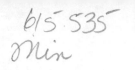

615.535
Min

Library of Congress Cataloging-in-Publication Data

Mindell, Earl.
    Prescription alternatives : hundreds of safe, natural, prescription-free remedies to restore and maintain your health / Earl Mindell and Virginia Hopkins. — 4th ed.
        p.   cm.
    Includes bibliographical references and index.
    ISBN–13: 978-0-07-160031-6 (alk. paper)
    ISBN–10: 0-07-160031-0
    1. Naturopathy.   2. Alternative medicine.   3. Drugs—Side effects.   4. Drug interactions.   I. Hopkins, Virginia.   II. Title.

RZ440.M54   2009
615.5'35—dc22   2008054329

1 2 3 4 5 6 7 8 9 10 11 12 13 14 15 16 17 18 19 20 21   DOC/DOC   0 9

ISBN 978-0-07-160031-6
MHID   0-07-160031-0

Interior design by Scott Rattray

McGraw-Hill books are available at special quantity discounts to use as premiums and sales promotions, or for use in corporate training programs. To contact a representative, please e-mail us at bulksales@mcgraw-hill.com.

The information contained in this book is intended to provide helpful and informative material on the subjects addressed. It is not intended to serve as a replacement for professional medical advice. Any use of the information in this book is at the reader's discretion. The authors and publisher specifically disclaim any and all liability arising directly or indirectly from the use or application of any information contained in this book. A health care professional should be consulted regarding your specific situation.

This book is printed on acid-free paper.

7/09
Bd

CONTENTS

INTRODUCTION

If you have this book, you're probably taking at least two prescription drugs or you know somebody who is. If you or someone you love is taking any type of medication, from an allergy medicine to a beta-blocker, you'll want to know how the medicine affects the body and how to stay healthy while on it. We'll give you that information in this book, but we're also going to tell you how you can solve your health problems without the drugs. Ultimately we hope that this book inspires you to get off your prescription drugs and keep yourself healthy primarily through lifestyle, wholesome foods, and natural remedies. We have found that almost everyone taking a long-term prescription drug can wean him- or herself off drugs and create good health—often vibrant, radiant good health—using simple, safe, natural remedies with no side effects.

As a general rule, prescription drugs cause imbalances in the body, ranging from depletion of vitamins and minerals to constipation and lowered immune function. They can also cause more serious problems, including death. *Prescription Alternatives* gives you a tool for easily and immediately accessing information about how the drugs you are taking affect your body, the steps you can take to counteract these imbalances, and what alternative treatments are available.

Most books sell well for a few years and then decline in sales. Sales of this book have *increased* over the years, as more and more people realize the need to find better ways to stay healthy. In this fourth edition we have added new drugs and their side effects, new research about drugs and natural remedies, and new natural remedies that have proven themselves over time. In particular you'll find a lot of helpful new information in the chapter on heart disease, as research on the underlying causes of heart disease has expanded greatly over the past few years. There is also a good deal of new information about prostate health and impotence drugs, as well as important new research about conventional hormone replacement therapy, which has sent millions of women to their doctors looking for natural alternatives. We'll give valuable insights for both men and women on how to achieve hormone balance.

There is no possible way we could cover every drug available or every problem with every drug. We have tried to cover the most commonly used drugs in detail, but we also urge you to take responsibility for any drug use by consulting with your pharmacist and reading the drug insert. Knowledge of the side effects and interactions of drugs is changing every day. It is our goal to teach you how to be a knowledgeable and discriminating drug consumer who knows how to ask the right questions and get the necessary information to stay healthy.

The United States and New Zealand are currently the only countries in the world that allow drug companies to advertise prescription drugs directly to the consumer. It used to be that prescription drugs could be touted only to physicians. But now consumer ads on TV tantalize you with great promises of health and well-being, skim through the side effects as quickly as possible, and then suggest you contact your physician or a drug company hotline for more information. The drug companies are also responsible for the expensive, slick, four-color ads you now see in consumer magazines and newspapers. You are bombarded with more than $3 billion worth of advertising for prescription and over-the-counter drugs every year. That should give you an idea of how valuable you are as a drug consumer and how staggering the profits are that drug companies rake in every year.

For every dollar that drug companies spend on research and development, they spend 50 cents on advertisements and promotions. The most heavily promoted drugs are not those that represent great breakthroughs in improving your health, but the ones that drug companies stand to profit from the most. You're not the only target of expensive drug company promotions, either: the doctors who prescribe drugs to you are strongly pressured by drug sales reps to prescribe their latest products. It's estimated that drug companies spend approximately $9,000 per physician per year on these promotional efforts. These efforts are working, too. According to the National Institute for Health Care Management, 40 percent of the recent increase in drug sales can be attributed to 25 of the most heavily promoted drugs.

Drugs have powerful effects on the body, so please don't abruptly stop taking any prescription medication. It's best to work with a health care professional to monitor your health as you switch from drugs to natural alternatives.

This book is not intended to convey the message that all prescription drugs are bad. Used conservatively—with great care and only when necessary—they can be lifesavers for some people. On the other hand, prescription drugs are grossly overprescribed and misprescribed in the United States, resulting in the death of at least 160,000 people a year in hospitals alone and in injury to nearly a million.

The other bad habit that this book may help you avoid is what we call the "drug treadmill."

People over the age of 50 are the most familiar with this scenario. Here's how it works: Let's say a fairly healthy 50-year-old named Bob visits his doctor for an annual checkup and is prescribed the seemingly harmless drug Tagamet (cimetidine) for indigestion. The Tagamet causes joint pain, but Bob doesn't know this. So he starts to take Tylenol (acetaminophen) to treat the pain. Bob likes to have a few cocktails before dinner, but he doesn't know that combining alcohol and Tylenol can cause serious liver damage. (Liver damage caused by acetaminophen is one of the leading causes of emergency room visits in the United States.) In addition, the Tagamet is already putting stress on Bob's liver, which is being chronically damaged by the combination of drugs and alcohol. Because of the constant stress, his liver is unable to keep up with the job of detoxifying his body, and soon he is coming down with colds and getting infections. So his doctor prescribes antibiotics, which further compromise his immune system and cause damage to his intestines. Furthermore, Bob now has a chronic sinus infection, for which he takes allergy drugs that make him irritable. This is one example of the drug treadmill, and this book is about how to avoid it.

A Word About Alternatives

Just because a health remedy is found in a health food store or on a website with a lot of green, leafy graphics doesn't mean it's necessarily safe or effective. There are plenty of schemes, scams, and frauds to go around in the world of natural remedies and alternative medicines, not to mention well-meaning but misguided advice from people who haven't done their homework.

One of the most common deceptions in alternative medicine is the practice of claiming that a substance has an effect on the body based on test tube research or a theory that's backed up by a lot of biochemistry babble. These types of medicines are usually associated with a lot of fanfare, exclamation points, extra-bold headlines, and grand claims about how they will cure everything from hangnails to cancer. Just because a medicine comes from the jungle, a tropical island, or the mountains of Nepal does not mean it works. It often just means it's dirt cheap and enormous profits are being made. We have seen dozens of so-called miracle cures come and go over the years, and we suggest having a wait-and-watch attitude toward them.

The remedies we recommend in this book are backed up by generations of use, as in folk medicine, by research, or by both. How do you know whether it's worth trying the latest, greatest natural remedy? Look for human studies published in peer-reviewed journals or opinions from experts in the field who don't have a financial stake in the product. In the Resources and Recommended Reading section at the back of this book, you'll find a list of health newsletters, websites, and books by experts whose opinions we respect.

PART 1

LAYING THE FOUNDATION FOR GOOD HEALTH

Chapter 1 Changing the Pill-Popping Mind-Set

W hat do you want when you go to an M.D.? Most of us, if we're being honest, would say we want the doctor to give us a name for our disease and a pill to make it go away. We call this the pill-popping mind-set, and it has become a deadly habit.

We have been convinced, through multimillion-dollar advertising and marketing campaigns on TV and in popular magazines and newspapers, that everything "wrong" with us is a result of genetics or our biochemistry and that we should look for a pill to fix the "mistake" that nature made. But only a fraction of a percent of what is wrong with us is attributable to genetics and biochemistry. For most of us, what's wrong is a consequence of an unhealthy lifestyle: for example, poor nutrition, overeating, lack of exercise, chronic stress, not enough sleep, and exposure to toxins such as pesticides. These all involve choices we make, which we can do something about. Taking drugs to solve health problems caused by an unhealthy lifestyle is not a good strategy for a high-quality life or even for a long and healthy life.

In articles published in the *Journal of the American Medical Association* (JAMA), government-funded researchers studying adverse drug events (ADEs) in people admitted to big city hospitals found that 701,547 people were treated for ADEs in emergency rooms and 117,318 of those were admitted to the hospital each year in 2004 and 2005. If these numbers reflect big city hospitals, what are the numbers for the entire United States? A report titled *Death by Medicine*, available on the Life Extension website, written by a group headed by Drs. Gary Null and Carolyn Dean states, "This fully referenced report shows the number of people [in the United States] having *in-hospital*, adverse reactions to prescribed drugs to be 2.2 million per year." The Food and Drug Administration (FDA) itself estimates that only 1 to 10 percent of ADEs are reported.

If millions of people are injured each year from ADEs, how many are killed by ADEs? The *Journal of the American Medical Association* reports estimate that over 140,000 Americans die every year from ADEs. This is surely a conservative figure, and it only accounts for those who died in hospitals. Undoubtedly tens of thousands more people die at home or in nursing homes from prescription-drug-related complications but aren't counted in these statistics.

If a disease were injuring and killing that many people every year, we would have millions of dollars mobilized to study it and we would be wearing ribbons on our lapels to increase awareness of the problem. To put this in perspective, ADEs kill *at least* 140,000 people in the United States every year, breast cancer kills about 46,000 American women each year, and according to the Centers for Disease Control and Prevention

(CDC), about 40,000 Americans die from AIDS every year. The elderly and women are the two groups most likely to be victims of an ADE.

As you'll read later, at least 11 million people are abusing prescription drugs, resulting not only in a drop in quality of life but a huge cost to the taxpayer in the form of an increase in accidents, workers' compensation claims, in days of work missed, hospitalizations due to drug overdoses, and drug treatment centers.

Prescription Drug Categories Most Commonly Associated with Preventable Adverse Drug Reactions

Cardiovascular medications: 24.5%
Diuretics (for high blood pressure): 22.1%
Nonopioid analgesics (painkillers): 15.4%
Hypoglycemics (diabetes drugs): 10.9%
Anticoagulants (e.g., Coumadin): 10.2%

Source: *Journal of the American Medical Association (JAMA)* 289 (2003): 1107–16.

If we look at the overall prescription drug problem in dollars, according to studies published in the *Journal of the American Medical Association*, mistakes in prescribing drugs and the treatment of drug side effects costs about $76 *billion* every year. Other studies put the number as high as $136 billion. What's even more outrageous is that American taxpayers are footing the bill for the drugs prescribed to Medicare patients, not to mention ever-higher insurance rates as health care costs soar. The taxpayer pays for the drugs, and then pays for the ADEs associated with those drugs. Considering that the vast majority of drugs are prescribed to the elderly, that means the taxpayer keeps the drug companies in business, while the companies keep peddling dangerous and improperly studied drugs and take no responsibility for the consequences. Drug companies reap profits at a terrible cost to their victims and the average taxpayer.

According to a study published in the *Western Journal of Medicine*, some \$20 billion could be saved each year in hospital costs if people simply took supplemental folic acid and vitamin E. This is based on the well-studied fact that folic acid deficiencies contribute to neural tube birth defects and low-birth-weight premature babies, and that just 100 international units (IU) of vitamin E daily reduces the risk of heart disease. Imagine the billions that could be saved both in drug sales and overall health costs if everyone took a good multivitamin.

Tragically, avoiding prescription drugs isn't quite as easy as asking your M.D. for alternatives. The powerful international drug companies have wormed their way into the very heart of medicine like insidious parasites, controlling what's taught in medical schools, the continuing medical education courses physicians take to keep their medical license, and what research is funded. In fact, the FDA now has drug companies funding their own research, so the concept of independent research has all but vanished in the United States, and smaller companies that may have breakthrough drugs or natural remedies aren't able to compete for FDA approval.

This is no secret. The following quote is from an article in the January 2009 *New York Review of Books* entitled "Drug Companies and Doctors: A Story of Corruption," by Marcia Angell:

> It is simply no longer possible to believe much of the clinical research that is published, or to rely on the judgment of trusted physicians or authoritative medical guidelines. I take no

pleasure in this conclusion, which I reached slowly and reluctantly over my two decades as an editor of *The New England Journal of Medicine*.

The Myth of the FDA as Our Protector

Not long ago there was a television news program about a controversial fake fat that is FDA approved. A woman in a grocery store was asked by the TV commentator what she thought about the new product. Her response was, "Well, if the FDA has approved it, it must be safe."

Nothing could be further from reality. Although the FDA is supposed to be an impartial government watchdog organization protecting consumers from greedy corporations who are looking to make a buck at the expense of our health, in truth it is a politically driven machine largely controlled by food and drug manufacturers. FDA drug approval has much more to do with political maneuvering and who's throwing around the most money and power, and very little to do with how safe and effective a food or drug is. You absolutely cannot assume that just because a food or drug carries the label "FDA Approved" you can take it without concern.

Remember, those FDA-approved drugs are injuring over 2 million people a year and killing at least 140,000 people a year in hospitals alone. That's an epidemic! And yet, how many people have been killed by nutritional supplements and herbs prescribed by alternative practitioners? Zero. That's right. Zero.

Now let's look again at the minimum number of people who have died because they took FDA-approved drugs: about 384 every day just in hospitals in the United States. Next time you're about to walk out of your physician's office with a prescription in your hand, remember that number and think again about whether FDA approval should give you confidence. Contemplate whether it might be worthwhile to take that daily walk and forego that dessert to avoid taking a prescription drug.

If the ADE statistics aren't enough to convince you to kick the prescription drug habit, think about the thousands of women whose children have reproductive cancers because the women took the drug DES (diethylstilbestrol) when they were pregnant. How about all the children with missing limbs whose mothers took thalidomide? Or all the women who took estrogen in the fifties and sixties, thinking they would be forever young, when in truth the grim reaper was about to knock on the door with reproductive cancers.

FDA analysts estimate that the pain drug Vioxx (rofecoxib) caused between 88,000 and 139,000 heart attacks. It was finally pulled from the market, but not before it brought Merck an estimated $2.5 billion in sales. The diabetes drug Avandia (rosiglitazone) is another case in point. According to an article in the *New England Journal of Medicine*, the use of rosiglitazone was associated with a 43 percent higher risk of heart attack and a 64 percent higher risk of death from all cardiovascular diseases. However, at this writing it is still on the market because the FDA found that these dangers were no worse than those incurred by taking other popular diabetes drugs.

There's more. Baycol (cerivastatin), a popular statin drug used for cholesterol control, was recalled in 2001 because it caused at least 31 cases of a deadly muscle-wasting disease. Lotronex (alosetron), a drug prescribed for the relief of diarrhea-predominant irritable bowel syndrome, was linked to several deaths and hospitalizations due to severe constipation. It was recalled in 2000, but the FDA then agreed to put it back on the market—a move that astonished those who recognize its dangers. The heartburn drug Propulsid (cisapride) was recalled in 2000 after being linked to 80 deaths due to heart rhythm irregularities.

Your best bet is not to use any drug unless it's been on the market for at least 10 years. Otherwise, you're just a drug company guinea pig.

On a similar note, it's important to keep in mind that just because something shows up in your health food store or is "natural," it doesn't necessarily mean that it's safe or effective. Plenty of bogus products are labeled natural or alternative. Before you take any type of medication, natural or otherwise, do some research and find out more about it. There's plenty of good information on the Internet, but there's also plenty of bad information out there. Be suspicious of any product that claims to cure everything, especially without any research, history of use in other cultures, or biochemistry to back it up. A typical ploy for unethical marketing of natural products is to cite studies as evidence, which, when examined more closely, are found to have little or nothing to do with the product being sold.

Be aware that with all recommendations of herbs, vitamins, minerals, and other types of natural supplements, including those mentioned in this book, what works for one person or even for most people might not work for you. If you take something and feel worse or have some type of negative side effect, stop taking it and consult a health care professional. Each of us is unique in our biochemistry, and your best guide to what works best for you is attention to how your body responds.

The Pressures of Being an M.D.

A friend of ours named Shirley wrote to us about a visit she had from her elderly father.

She hadn't seen him for a year and was shocked to see how thin and frail he was. He had always been healthy and eager to go on walks, but not anymore. He complained of dizziness, weakness, and sleepiness. He also said his mouth was dry all the time. He seemed mentally foggy and depressed. He had always avoided prescription drugs, but she asked him if he was taking any, and he showed her a bottle of pills prescribed for high blood pressure. She looked the drug up and found he was on the highest dose for that drug. Then she pulled out a copy of this book and looked up his drug—she handed the book to her father and pointed to the paragraph describing the side effects for the drug he was taking. He read it and then sat there silently shaking his head. "That describes me perfectly," he finally said. Shirley's father promised to visit his doctor when he returned home and to ask for a lower dose or a different drug. When she called him to find out what the doctor said, her father explained that the doctor said his symptoms weren't from the drug—they were just caused by old age. Moreover, the doctor told him if he stopped taking the drugs, he would probably have a stroke. Her father had always been afraid of being debilitated by a stroke, so he kept taking the drug as directed. Less than a year later Shirley's father fell, hit his head, and died a short time later.

If you have a typical M.D., he has probably scared you half to death with threats and warnings about what will happen if you go off your drugs, but that's only because he doesn't know any other way. He has been taught that it's too difficult to help a patient make lifestyle and diet changes, and he is at risk of losing his job and medical license if he doesn't conform. He doesn't want to discuss drug side effects, because he's been taught that if you tell patients what the side effects are, then they'll "get" them.

Helping the whole patient, not just a set of symptoms, takes time and thoughtfulness. Physicians are not trained to help you as a whole person. They are trained to diagnose a disease, find a pill or surgery to treat it, and send you on your way. If typical doctors take more than 10 or 15 minutes with a patient, they start to lose money because their malpractice insurance is so high or somebody else is dictating the amount of time they are allowed to spend with a patient.

Being an M.D. at this time in history is fraught with problems. In medical school and during residency, physicians-in-training are given an inhuman workload, putting them in a state of chronic stress and sleep deprivation that makes them particularly susceptible to brainwashing. This is not to say that medical students are consciously being brainwashed, but the effect is similar. What they are taught in medical school becomes a mind-set, a sort of gospel, and they are taught that deviating from the gospel can mean the death of a patient, a lawsuit, or the loss of a medical license. This is a very compelling set of circumstances for toeing the party line, even if it's clearly not working.

The drug companies have a powerful presence from the beginning of the medical student's education. Did you know that drug companies court medical students with free meals and medical supplies and often sponsor talks in medical schools? Why do the medical schools allow this clearly unethical practice? Who do you think is funding the majority of the schools' research and studies? Right, the drug companies. The result is that drug companies are dictating what is taught in our medical schools.

Once an M.D. has a practice, he or she is courted by drug companies with free samples, and if the M.D. prescribes enough of their product, he or she gets offers of free vacations or other perks. Knickknacks, often with drug names emblazoned on them, as you've probably noticed in your own doctor's office, are common currency between drug salespeople and doctors, as are lunches and dinners in upscale restaurants. Drug companies also sponsor continuing medical education (CME) courses, which are required for keeping a medical license. The ultimate bribery by drug companies is sending an M.D. on an exotic vacation and including CME courses along with it. The physician spends a few hours a day listening to lectures on how to prescribe the company's drugs and the rest of his or her time on the beach or golf course.

In 1996, 41,000 drug salespeople were peddling their wares directly to U.S. physicians; by 2005, that number skyrocketed to 100,000. Meanwhile, in the United States alone, drug companies in 2000 spent more than $15.7 *billion* dollars promoting their products.

In their fervor over this or that new (and very expensive) wonder drug, these reps press physicians to bypass lifestyle changes, which might help relieve symptoms, and instead go straight into a course of prescription medication. The practice of prescribing new and more costly medicines over lifestyle changes or older, tried-and-true, less pricey drugs is a major reason why medicine is going bankrupt so quickly and adverse effects are on the rise.

In some instances, a brand-new drug will be sold aggressively to doctors before any substantial, science-based information is available to them. The drug Celebrex (celecoxib) is a good example. By the time *Journal of the American Medical Association* published the results of the first clinical trial that compared it with another similar drug, the maker of celecoxib had already sold a billion dollars' worth of the drug—based only on the word of drug reps, which as you can imagine can be far from scientific, reliable, or impartial. Drug companies are frequently cited by the FDA because their reps make inaccurate or improper statements about the safety and effectiveness of the medicines they are promoting. The companies cited may be slapped on the wrist with fines, but what's a few hundred thousand dollars when your sales figures are in the billions?

Perks from drug salespeople have finally come under FDA scrutiny, and the more outrageous perks have been prohibited. Still, we're sure that the drug companies will come up with new, creative ways to persuade physicians to use their hottest new products. A small organization of physicians that calls itself No Free Lunch has signed an agreement not to take any gifts from drug firms. If your doctor has joined, you're ahead of the game.

Medical research—which doctors rely upon for current information about drugs—is also largely controlled by drug companies. They're the ones with the big bucks to fund large-scale studies, so their products get much more attention in research circles than do less extravagant, nonpatentable medicines such as supplements, herbs, and natural hormones. Researchers often must sign contracts stating that the sponsoring drug company has control over what is done with the results of the research; if the results are not favorable, the company can quash the research and never publish it. Every few years the FDA makes a little noise about this unethical practice, and there are a few exposés in the media, but ultimately nothing is done to stop it. The ultimate consequence is the tens of thousands of patients who are injured or die every year from taking poorly or dishonestly researched drugs.

Pressure to conform also comes from the physician's state medical board, which has the power to take away his or her license. Physicians are subject to having their medical license taken away if they fail to conform to the "standard of care" dictated by the board. Thus physicians who fail to prescribe the "right" class of drugs for a common problem, such as high blood pressure, can be threatened with the loss of their license.

The typical physician leaves medical school half a million dollars in debt and is eager to begin a lucrative practice to pay off the loans. He or she may be starting a family and paying a mortgage. The last thing in the world the physician needs is any type of threat to his or her medical license. The pressure to conform and go along with the status quo is tremendous.

Now the physician's job has been reduced to seeing a patient for 10 to 15 minutes, making a diagnosis, and finding out which drug the physician's health maintenance organization (HMO) requires him or her to prescribe for that disease. How long has it been since you have met a physician who is happy with his or her job? It's easy to see why there is such widespread dissatisfaction in the profession. Being a physician no longer has much to do with healing.

Intelligent, well-intentioned, and courageous physicians who genuinely want to heal their patients must struggle to break free of the "diagnose and prescribe a pill" mind-set. It takes time, perseverance, and a willingness to venture into the brand-new territory of preventive, natural, and holistic approaches to healing. It takes a willingness to be challenged by the state medical board and to be fired by an HMO. Be sympathetic to the pressures brought to bear on your physician, but don't ever be pressured or bullied into taking drugs you don't need.

Portrait of a Conventional Medicine Approach

What's the difference between a conventional medicine approach to a health problem and an alternative approach to a health problem? Let's say a woman in her fifties named Pam goes to her physician for an annual checkup, and he finds that her blood sugar levels are high. In spite of the fact that she is at least 50 pounds overweight, he never questions her about her eating habits. Rather, he tells her she is prediabetic and prescribes an oral diabetes drug to control the problem.

Pam dutifully and unquestioningly takes the drug, while continuing her habit of eating pastries for breakfast along with three or four cups of sugar-laden coffee, drinking soda pop all day, snacking on candy bars and chips in the afternoon, and having pudding or pie for dessert. Her idea of a vegetable is ketchup or peas from a can, and her carbohydrates are all refined white rice, white bread, and pasta. She gets virtually no exercise and never drinks any water.

The drug Pam is taking for her prediabetic condition gives her chronic indigestion, so she starts taking an H2 blocker called Tagamet, which reduces her digestive symptoms. But now her stomach acid, which was low to begin with, is practically nonexistent, so she's not digesting her food and is not getting many nutrients from her food. The drug is also putting stress on her kidneys, and it happens that her estrogen is low, too, so she starts getting chronic urinary tract infections.

Pam is put on antibiotics for her urinary tract infection, but that lowers her immune system defenses and kills all the beneficial bacteria in her colon. So she gets a bad case of the flu that just won't go away, and she has constant gas from the colon imbalance. She starts taking antihistamines for the chronic sinus infection she's developed, and her physician tells her he thinks a hysterectomy will solve her urinary tract problems. She gets the hysterectomy and is put on synthetic hormones, which make her feel depressed and weepy, so the physician gives her some Prozac (fluoxetine).

Do you get the picture? This is an extremely common scenario. We'll bet that nearly every family physician in the United States has been through either this exact scenario or a variation on the theme. The woman is now taking a diabetes drug, an H2 blocker (Tagamet), antihistamines, synthetic hormones, and Prozac. She's exhausted all the time, she's mentally flaky and emotionally withdrawn, and she's just waiting for her next health problem to hit, which it will. She's on the royal road to heart disease or a stroke and is likely to begin losing her eyesight soon. She's got arthritis and chronic headaches.

What is the future of someone like this? Her quality of life is horrible, she's no fun to be around anymore, she'll cost the medical system and taxpayers hundreds of thousands of dollars before she dies, and she feels helpless. She's doing everything the physician tells her to do, like a good girl, and she's still sick and getting sicker by the day. Her future will be more drugs, more drug side effects, more disease, more surgeries, and more pain. This is no way to live, and yet this is how millions of Americans, caught in the insidious web of an unhealthy lifestyle, conventional medicine, and drugs, will live out their so-called golden years.

Now let's take a look at a different scenario.

Portrait of an Alternative Approach

Now let's say Pam is wary of taking pills and goes to a naturopathic doctor referred to her by a friend. This doctor looks at her blood and urine tests and talks to her about her eating and exercise habits. He asks her if she's willing to make some changes in her diet and to start getting some exercise, and she agrees to do that if it's not too hard. She has tried diets before, she says, and they never work. The doctor tells her that

he's asking for a permanent lifestyle change, not a temporary diet, and she agrees to try it out for six months.

The doctor asks her to make an appointment with his staff nutritionist to create a diet and supplement program that's manageable for her, gives her the phone number of a support group of other people in a similar position, and recommends an exercise program especially designed for older women at the local YMCA. The staff nutritionist asks Pam to restrict her sugar to one small treat a day, encourages her to substitute fruit when she gets serious sugar cravings, recommends some cookbooks that will teach her how to prepare whole grains and fresh vegetables, and asks her to drink four to six glasses of water every day in place of the soda. She gives Pam some sample meal plans and encourages her to ask the women in her support group for ideas about shopping and preparing these new foods. The nutritionist also recommends a multivitamin, as well as a vitamin and mineral formula for stabilizing blood sugar, which contains chromium, zinc, vanadyl sulfate, and some herbs.

The doctor asks Pam to come back in a month to have her blood sugar checked again and encourages her to call if she's having problems with any part of the new lifestyle. A month later Pam returns, delighted to report that she's lost five pounds, has much more energy, and has made wonderful new friends both in her support group and in her exercise group. Her blood sugar test comes out normal, and her blood pressure has dropped a few points. She's complaining about indigestion on the new diet, so the doctor asks her to try taking betaine hydrochloride before meals to supplement what may be low stomach acid and to notice whether any particular food is bothering her. The nutritionist asks her to keep taking the formula for blood sugar for another two months and asks her to now cut her sugar treats down to three times a week.

Pam returns in three months and her blood sugar is still normal, she has lost 10 more pounds, her digestion is fine, and she has joined a synchronized swimming group. She reports that she hasn't felt better in years, and she loves her new lifestyle.

What is the future of someone like this? She's happy, she's healthy, she's physically fit, she's emotionally and mentally stable, she's not taking any drugs, and her golden years are likely to be truly golden. Her medical costs are minimal, and her enjoyment of life is maximal. This scenario is just as real as the one before it. What a dramatic difference!

Modern medicine is wonderful if you have a life-threatening infection that requires antibiotics, if you need surgery, if you have a broken bone, or if you need a diagnosis for a disease, but for nearly all other health problems, you're better off working with alternative medicine. By now there are many thousands of physicians who are combining safe, effective alternative medicine with what they learned in medical school and giving excellent health care. Unfortunately, you are unlikely to find them at your HMO, which is the height of irony, since HMOs could save millions of dollars a year simply by introducing preventive and alternative medicine into their organizations.

Taking Back the Power to Stay Healthy

Too many of us have put our health into the hands of our physicians. We have a philosophy that says, "I should be able to eat as much sugar and fat as I want; drink as much coffee, soda pop, and alcohol as I want; overwork; undersleep; and underexercise and not suffer any conse-

quences." After all, with the miracle of modern medicine, you can just go to the physician and you will receive a pill or have surgery to fix your problem, and insurance will pay for 80 percent of it. Such a deal!

The truth is that we begin suffering from our bad habits in our forties, and for too many people, life from about age 50 on is one round after another of physicians, surgeries, and drug side effects. We may be kept alive, but what is our quality of life?

This is not to suggest that you need to eat nothing but brown rice and tofu and run five miles a day, but it is to suggest that if you're hooked on sugar or fat, you scale back, and if you're a couch potato, you get up and move your body. (You'll get more specifics in the next chapter.) When your physician offers you a drug, don't just take it, find out whether there are lifestyle changes and/or natural alternatives that might work just as well.

The Bottom Line

Clearly Americans are at great risk of being injured or killed by prescription drugs. The FDA is not going to protect you from unsafe drugs—they're too busy protecting the interests of the drug companies. You cannot count on your doctor to prescribe drugs to you in a conscientious way or to recognize side effects when they occur. You may be at greatest risk from drug injury or death when you're hospitalized. This puts the burden of responsibility squarely on the shoulders of each one of us to live a healthy lifestyle in order to avoid prescription drugs, to become thoroughly educated about safer alternatives, and to educate ourselves about any drug that we do choose to take. We hope this book will help you achieve your goals of optimal health.

Chapter **2** # How to Avoid Prescription Drug Abuse

W hen you think of a person who abuses drugs, you probably have in mind a gang member in the inner city, a troubled teen, or a Hollywood celebrity who let fame and riches get out of hand. But some of the world's most-prescribed medications are being abused on a par with street drugs—at an equal cost in lives ruined and ended and at a far greater cost to the taxpayer.

A 2006 survey by the National Institute on Drug Abuse (NIDA) confirms that prescription drug abuse is a serious issue. Even as statistics show a decline in the use of illicit drugs like heroin and cocaine, the rate at which Americans are using prescription medicines for nonmedical purposes—the NIDA's definition of drug abuse—has risen astronomically since the early 1990s. The 2006 survey found that about 48 million people, or 20 percent of the U.S. population, have abused prescription drugs at least once. Our guess is that the numbers for prescription drug abuse are much higher, but most of it goes unreported.

Those most at risk for prescription drug abuse are people with a history of drug or alcohol abuse or addiction, teens, and those in the medical profession—who have far easier access to drugs than the general population. The elderly are vulnerable, too, but their prescription-related mishaps are more likely to be accidental.

Prescription Drug Abuse in Teens

To find out how bad the prescription-drug-abuse problem has become for teens, the Partnership for a Drug-Free America surveyed about 7,300 kids from ages 12 to 19, publishing its results in early 2008. They found that one in five teens had abused Vicodin, a powerful prescription painkiller; one in five had abused stimulants like Ritalin or Adderall, or benzodiazepine tranquilizers like Xanax or Valium.

Marijuana, cocaine, and heroin were once the drugs parents worried most about. Today, increasing numbers of teens are turning to prescription drugs, which are easily accessed through classmates who swipe them from parents' medicine cabinets. Some teens and young adults have figured out how to get these medicines prescribed by fibbing to doctors and then act as "candy men" who pass the medications out to classmates. Just imagine: when your teen walks out the door to go to a party with friends, he or she may actually be heading for a so-called pharm party, where a bowl of prescription drugs is passed around and each kid picks a few pills from the "trail mix."

Adults often get into a cycle of prescription drug abuse because they are in pain or are struggling with anxiety, lack of sleep, or difficulty focusing or staying alert. They think—often based on ads for the drugs in question—that specific pharmaceuticals will help, and they get the medications either through their doctor or on

their own. Then they end up needing more and more or continue to want to use the drug after their symptoms have resolved. In the teen set, however, it's sometimes just about getting high, and for those who get hooked, it's about staying high, no matter what the cost.

Other kids who have been steeped in the "Generation Rx" culture from toddlerhood think there's nothing wrong with taking a Ritalin when they need to stay up late studying or with taking a Valium when they have the jitters before an exam. This type of abuse is sometimes called self-medication.

For that matter, plenty of young adults, college-aged and through their thirties, medicate themselves with prescription drugs without assistance from a physician. A story published in the *New York Times* in 2005 described twenty- and thirty-somethings who illegally get or give out medications and take them to try to modulate mood, self-treat depression or anxiety, combat insomnia, or stay awake later at night. This practice is illegal but not often prosecuted.

Painkillers are the most common prescription drug abused by younger teens; stimulants are more commonly abused by older teens and college students. Girls are at greater risk than boys for prescription drug abuse.

This problem of prescription drug abuse in teens has heads shaking and tongues clucking. The experts ask, "How could they not know any better?" What did we expect when we started saturating the media with direct-to-consumer ads, proffering a pill for every ill? The truth is that most of the time, teens who want to try these pills can easily find them in their parents' medicine cabinets. What kind of example are adults setting as they increasingly bring home bottles of painkillers, antidepressants, stimulants, and sedatives? What kind of messages are doctors sending when they so quickly jot off a prescription for one of these drugs to someone as a first resort? This seems to be a terrible double standard, one that teaches children that pharmaceuticals are the answer to every problem but expects them not to see pharmaceuticals as the answer to every problem.

Most of the drugs being abused are addictive and dangerous, particularly when combined with alcohol and with one another. According to Westley Clark, M.D., M.Ph., J.D., the director for substance abuse therapy at the Substance Abuse and Mental Health Services Administration, "Young adults, even teens . . . do not seem to realize that this misuse can lead to serious problems and addiction." Some kids even end up dying because they don't understand that even FDA-approved prescription drugs can kill when misused or used in combination with each other or with alcohol.

Parents: don't think a 10-year-old is too young to hear about this! Let them know that these drugs are probably going to be available to them and that they will encounter considerable pressure to try these drugs. Also tell them that prescription and over-the-counter (OTC) drugs can be very dangerous or deadly when misused. Narcotics like Percocet or OxyContin, for example, can slow the heart to dangerously low rates if taken in overdose or in combination with alcohol or benzodiazepines. Point out that stimulants like Ritalin have been known to cause death when abused, particularly when they are crushed and snorted or injected. And if you happen to have any of these medications in your house, monitor them carefully and be sure to dispose of unused pills in a place where your child won't find them.

Prescription Abuse in the Elderly

The kind of prescription drug abuse that usually affects elderly people has more to do with what's prescribed to them than with efforts to get high. One might look at it as drug abuse inflicted *upon* the unwitting person, rather than the person inflicting it upon him- or herself. Older folks are vulnerable because they tend to be much more sensitive to the effects of a drug and they take the lion's share of prescription drugs in the United States. Forty percent of seniors take 5 or more prescription drugs weekly; 12 percent take more than 10. Many also combine their drugs with over-the-counter medications. Adverse reactions to drugs are now the fifth leading cause of death among seniors. According to gerontologist Jerry Gurwitz, M.D., drug-related injuries to seniors number at around 2.3 million per year, with 200,000 of them qualifying as dangerous enough to kill.

A slight overdose or negative side effect has a much greater potential to cause illness and even death in an elderly person. Many medicines are simply unsafe for seniors, but a report by the government's General Accounting Office, an investigative branch of Congress, found that more than 17 percent of noninstitutionalized elderly Americans were receiving at least one of those 20 drugs considered inappropriate for the elderly.

How many elderly people end up in nursing homes and hospitals due to symptoms caused by dangerous combinations of drugs? How many of these unfortunate folks are then given *more drugs* to treat these side effects?

What are the worst culprits for dangerous side effects in seniors? Sedatives, antidepressants, pain medications, and antipsychotics, all of which can cause dizziness, falling, and problems with thinking and memory. Doctors may believe that these symptoms are caused by aging rather than by the drugs they are prescribing. Because of the requirements of managed care, many seniors receive prescriptions from several different doctors, and it's rare that these doctors ever confer about the patients they share. Patients may also use different pharmacies for different prescriptions.

If someone you care about is aging, is taking more than three prescriptions on a regular basis, and seems to be in declining health, take the initiative to make a list of the drugs he or she is using, along with any vitamins, herbs, and other supplements. Use this book to find out everything you can about the side effects and interactions. Speak with the doctor to be sure that the patient is receiving the minimum effective dose. A pharmacist can be a great resource, especially if you can find one who specializes in geriatrics. Anytime a doctor suggests a new drug, research it carefully and do your best to find natural alternatives. If the person you are advocating for takes a sudden turn for the worst, keep in mind that the drugs could be to blame.

The rapid growth of the world's elderly population represents a potentially huge financial windfall for the drug companies. If you are over the age of 50 and your blood pressure or cholesterol reading is even slightly above the so-called normal level for your age, you will automatically be put on a drug to get those numbers back within those limits. Most of the time, the drug—even when it's effective at reducing blood pressure or cholesterol count—will also end up *causing* ill health and side effects, for which your physician will prescribe more drugs, which will cause more side effects, and so on. The result might be a set of lab tests that look terrific to your doctor and chronic drug-related symptoms that drastically reduce your quality of life. Please read the sections in this book on drugs for high blood pressure and cholesterol and their natural alternatives very carefully before agreeing to take a blood pressure or cholesterol medication.

How Prescription Drug Abuse Begins

You don't have to be an impressionable teen, a feeble elderly person, or an addict or alcoholic to become hooked on prescription drugs; anybody can fall into this trap. People who have never used street drugs, tobacco, or alcohol are just as susceptible to prescription drug abuse as those who have. Those who abuse prescription drugs usually start out rationalizing their problem as OK because a physician wrote out the prescription. This is a dangerous assumption.

A tragic prescription drug-abuse scenario is the recovering alcoholic who breaks a bone or has surgery and is given a potent narcotic pain reliever such as Vicodin or Demerol. Despite the well-known risk of addiction and abuse with these medications, the prescribing physician fails to ask whether the patient has a drug-abuse problem. The patient trustingly takes the drug with the intention of using it only for a week or two but gets hooked into that familiar downward spiral of addiction and dependence. Doctors are all too willing to continue to write prescriptions for patients who insist they need the drugs for their pain. In a perfect example of an unexpected side effect, Vicodin abuse has been linked with 48 cases of complete and sudden hearing loss, a consequence no one anticipated.

More than 20 million people over the age of 12 have used one or more psychotherapeutic drugs for nonmedical purposes at some point in time. Other surveys estimate that as many as 50 percent of the drug overdoses treated in hospitals are a result of prescription drug abuse.

The Twenty Most Abused Drugs

Legalized drug abuse is common in America, mostly in the form of physicians writing out prescriptions for medications that are addictive or consciousness altering. Of course, the pharmaceutical companies are making a bundle. Are the physicians who write out these prescriptions and the companies that sell the drugs any better than the drug lords and street pushers our society despises so much?

On the Drug Enforcement Agency's (DEA) list of the top 20 most-abused controlled substances, 12—or more than half—are prescription drugs. Here is the DEA's list of the 20 most-abused drugs in America. All the boldface drug names on this list are prescription drugs.

The drugs with an asterisk (*) after them are in the benzodiazepine family. Codeine (8) and hydrocodone (13) are addictive narcotics used as cough suppressants and painkillers. Propoxyphene (9) is another addictive narcotic used for pain, despite a lack of evidence that it is any more effective than a placebo; aspirin works as well. Oxycodone (17) is combined with acetaminophen (Tylenol) in the widely used drugs Percocet and Tylox or with aspirin in Percodan. Oxycodone is similar to a narcotic and is addictive. Try acetaminophen or aspirin alone first, and use these drugs only as a last resort. Methadone (20) is a synthetic narcotic used to replace heroin. Reportedly, addicts who use methadone don't get the same high as on heroin but avoid the withdrawal. Nevertheless, this is a highly addictive substance with a wide range of side effects.

1. Cocaine	11. **Misc.**
2. Heroin	**benzodiazepines***
3. Marijuana	12. PCP
4. **Alprazolam***	13. **Hydrocodone**
(Xanax)	(Tussionex)
5. **Diazepam***	14. Amphetamine
(Valium)	15. Hashish
6. **Clonazepam***	16. **Chlordiazepoxide***
(Klonopin)	(Librium)
7. **Lorazepam*** (Ativan)	17. **Oxycodone**
8. **Codeine**	18. **Temazepam***
9. **D-propoxyphene**	(Restoril)
(Darvon)	19. LSD
10. Methamphetamine	20. **Methadone**

The drugs most likely to be abused are painkillers (especially opioids and narcotic analgesics), sedatives, tranquilizers, and stimulants. Of the top 10 prescribed drugs in the United States, 3 are narcotic painkillers. We obviously have a huge problem in the United States with addiction to narcotic painkillers. Shouldn't somebody at the FDA, our government watchdog agency that we pay for with our taxes, be taking a hint from this statistic and taking some action?

Painkillers

Addiction to painkilling drugs is not the same as the use of these drugs by people with cancer or other illnesses who take them for legitimate pain. If anything, legitimate pain is undertreated in the United States because of the stigma and fear of drug addiction. This type of pain is what the drugs are made for in the first place, and they should be used accordingly. Nobody should have

Painkillers with Potential for Abuse

Buprenorphine (Buprenex)	Butorphanol (Stadol)
Butalbital	Codeine (often mixed with other painkillers such as acetaminophen)
Darvocet	
Demerol	Darvon
Dilaudid	Dezocine (Dalgan)
Fioricet	Ergotamine
Hydrocodone	Fiorinal
Meperidine	Levorfanol
Methotrimeprazine (Levoprome)	Methadone
	Morphine
Nalbuphine (Nubain)	Oxycodone
Pentazocine (Talwin)	Percocet
Percodan	Propoxyphene
Roxicet	Roxiprin
Sumatriptan (Imitrex)	Talwin
Tramadol (Ultram)	Tussionex
Tylox	Vicodin

to suffer pain unnecessarily. There is no gain or heroism in this type of preventable suffering.

If you have a legitimate need for painkilling drugs and have to take them for more than a week or two, you will eventually have to go through physical withdrawal from them. If this is done very gradually, it doesn't need to be traumatic or painful. The people who get in trouble with these drugs are those who deny that they're physically dependent on them. This denial is generally the strongest indicator that they've become physically and emotionally dependent.

For most abusers, the first introduction to painkillers is after surgery, a broken bone, a back injury, or treatment for headaches. If the drugs are taken for more than a week or two, physical dependence will begin and withdrawing from the drug becomes increasingly difficult as each day passes.

Every time the person tries to stop taking the drug, the discomfort of withdrawal becomes confused with the original pain. Complicating the picture even more, the painkiller will dull emotional pain long after the physical pain has worn off. People will convince themselves, their families, and their physicians that the physical pain is still present, but it is really the withdrawal symptoms and emotional pain that are being treated.

Stimulants

Stimulant drugs prescribed under the guise of antidepressants or appetite suppressants are the next most commonly abused prescription drugs. These are sold on the street as uppers; most of the so-called legitimate drugs are variations of the street drug called speed or methamphetamine. These drugs create a false sense of confidence and energy, speed up the metabolism, increase the heart rate, and raise blood pressure. They can also cause irritability. Typically the abuser of these drugs is a woman who goes to her physician for anxiety, depression, or some other emotional problem. If she is overweight, lethargic, depressed, or diagnosed with adult attention deficit/hyperactivity disorder (AADHD), there's a good chance that a stimulant will be prescribed.

Abuse of stimulants is common in college students and young adults who want to achieve in school or at work. It's all too easy to get some Adderall or Ritalin from unethical Internet pharmacies, relatives, or friends. Both physical and psychological addiction is a common outcome. While the abuser may be amazed at his or her ability to go without sleep, read boring books, pay attention in class, and keep up with homework or work assignments, he or she may not know that these drugs can be damaging to the heart, brain, and nervous system.

What goes up must come down, and withdrawing from stimulant drugs can be extremely difficult, with severe rebound depression and weight gain.

Stimulants with Potential for Abuse

Amphetamines

Antidepressants

Caffeine

Dexedrine (dextroamphetamine)

Diethylpropion

Mazindol

Methamphetamines

Methylphenidate (Ritalin)

Phenmetrazine

Phenylpropanolamine (nonprescription, i.e., Dexatrim, Acutrim)

Stimulants such as Ritalin (methylphenidate), Adderall (d-amphetamine), Desoxyn (methamphetamine), and Focalin (dexmethylphenidate HCl) are being prescribed left and right to treat so-called ADHD in children. If some of the names of these medications sound like street drugs to you, you're not mistaken—many are identical to highly addictive street drugs. No long-term studies on the safety of these drugs for the developing nervous systems of young people have been completed, and evidence of their effectiveness at improving a child's ability to learn or enjoy life is virtually nonexistent. There is strong anecdotal evidence that treatment with Ritalin can cause disfiguring tics—in fact, such strong evidence that in the small print of the prescribing information, doctors are warned not to prescribe the drug to children who have a family history of Tourette's syndrome, a disorder that includes tics.

In our "pill for every ill" culture, children are being taught to take drugs instead of learning to ride out the normal ups and downs of life. What will the long-term effects be on the growing, changing, evolving brain chemistry of a child? We don't know, and we may never know. What we do know is that antidepressants are no substitute for love, affection, a supportive and communicative family atmosphere, a good diet, and exercise.

Benzodiazepines

The benzodiazepines are a class of drugs widely used to treat anxiety, depression related to anxiety, and insomnia, and are generally used as tranquilizers. Most nonbarbiturate sleeping pills are benzodiazepines. There are other sedatives and tranquilizers not in this class, all of which are addictive, but for the most part they have been replaced by the benzodiazepines. You can pretty much assume that if you're taking a drug for anxiety; to ease tension, nervousness, or stress; or to help you sleep, it has the potential for abuse. The barbiturates are another story, which will be covered next.

During the 1970s, hundreds of thousands of women became hooked on the trendy antianxiety drug Valium, which is a benzodiazepine. Their physicians reassured them that the drug wasn't addictive, because the medical literature claimed it was only habit-forming in some people who were "prone to addiction." Physicians also reassured women that the drug created a physical dependence only if it was taken in very high doses for a long period of time. Nothing could be further from the truth, but this ignorance sold millions of dollars worth of drugs to unsuspecting women who thought they were temporarily being helped through a hard time.

Possible Withdrawal Symptoms from Antianxiety Drugs

Anxiety	Confusion
Fatigue	Fear
Hallucinations	Headache
Insomnia	Loss of appetite
Mental fogginess	Seizures
Shakiness	Sweatiness

Antianxiety Drugs with Potential for Abuse

Alprazolam (Xanax)

Chlorazepate (Tranxene)

Chlordiazepoxide (Librium, Mitran)

Clonazepam (Klonopin)

Diazepam (Valium, Zetran, Dizac)

Flurazepam (Dalmane)

Halazepam (Paxipam)

Lorazepam (Ativan)

Meprobamate (not a benzodiazepine) (Equanil, Miltown)

Oxazepam (Serax)

Prazepam

Quazepam (Doral)

Temazepam (Restoril)

Triazolam (Halcion)

Let's talk about the phrase "prone to addiction." Although some people do tend to more easily become addicted than others, nearly any human being who is going through a hard time physically, emotionally, mentally, or spiritually is prone to addiction. It is human nature to try to correct an imbalance in the body or the psyche, and if a drug gives the illusion that balance has been achieved, it has the potential for abuse. When the physician in the white coat, that authority figure whom we have been trained not to question, tells us the pill will be good for us and solve our problem, few have the wherewithal to say, "No thanks."

Drug addiction can begin as innocently as taking something to help you sleep or to help you through a difficult time in your life. Insomnia is a very common symptom of stress and anxiety. Physicians tend to regard the benzodiazepines as harmless temporary aids for people who are stressed, anxious, and not sleeping, but they are in fact quite addictive, interact dangerously with alcohol and many other drugs, and have lists of side effects as long as your arm. Please don't ever be fooled into thinking these are benign, harmless drugs. There may be a time in your life when you need to take them for some reason, but be vigilant and be aware that you *will* go through withdrawal when you stop taking them.

All of the so-called antianxiety drugs have the potential for abuse. When the short-acting benzodiazepines such as lorazepam (Ativan) came out, they were applauded for their diminished potential for abuse. Experience has shown us that the short-acting versions did, in fact, create physical dependence and withdrawal symptoms—right away, instead of over time.

Barbiturates

The barbiturates are a class of drugs widely acknowledged to be addictive but still occasionally prescribed. They were much more widely prescribed before the benzodiazepines came along. Their withdrawal symptoms can be severe enough to be fatal, and they deplete folic acid, a nutrient important for heart health and preventing birth defects. At this point, virtually no good reason exists for taking a barbiturate drug, though they are still prescribed, on occasion, for insomnia or as anticonvulsants. Some of the names of the barbiturates are phenobarbital (Solfoton, Bellergal), mephobarbital (Mebaral), amobarbital (Amytal), butabarbital (Butisol), secobarbital (Seconal), and pentobarbital (Nembutal).

Antidepressants

If you are prescribed an antidepressant, you are likely to get a selective serotonin reuptake inhibitor (SSRI) such as Prozac, Paxil, or Zoloft, or a serotonin/norepinephrine reuptake inhibitor (SNRI) such as Celexa or Effexor. These uppers raise levels of the feel-good brain chemicals serotonin and norepinephrine. They give some users increased energy and almost always create a sense of emotional detachment that makes coping with life's stresses a little easier.

When taken by mouth, SSRIs and SNRIs can take days to weeks to kick in, so they aren't often used by people who are looking to get high. Young people have been known, however, to grind the pills and snort them, which does produce a quick high. Only in recent years have these medications become affordable, since some have lost their patent protection and are no longer more costly than street drugs.

Those who end up with an addiction to these medications are usually those who are initially prescribed the drug for mild anxiety or depression, or even just to get them through a life stress or period of mourning. They take the medicine for a period of time, and when they try to stop, they may find themselves in the throes of terrifying, severe withdrawal.

Some people who take SSRI or SNRI drugs begin to escalate dosage on their own or with a doctor's help when the old dose stops working—which is not an unusual circumstance. Others engage in a practice known as "chipping," where they begin taking extra, unprescribed doses, often late in the day or in the early evening to rev up their energy or boost their spirits.

As might be expected, drug manufacturers claim that these drugs are not addictive, but hundreds of thousands of people who have had to withdraw from them might disagree. According to Dr. Joseph Glenmullen, a Harvard Medical School professor of psychiatry and author of *Prozac Backlash* (Simon & Schuster, 2000) and *The Antidepressant Solution* (Simon & Schuster, 2006), these drugs *do* meet the relevant criteria for addiction: the need for escalating doses, debilitating withdrawal, and cravings for the drug after stopping. These issues are far more common than the drugmakers would like to admit.

The long-term side effects of these medications can include visual hallucinations, sensations like electric shocks to the brain, nausea, dizziness, and anxiety. We have no idea what the long-term effect is of fiddling around with the brain chemistry this way, and there is mounting evidence that these drugs may be causing permanent changes in the brain. One in every 10 Americans has taken one of the SSRIs or SNRIs at some point. Many continue to use them for years on end, convinced that they have some sort of "biochemical imbalance" that requires the medication—a theory that has never been proven nor even given any significant scientific weight. When they stop taking it, they mistake withdrawal symptoms for a relapse into depression or anxiety and think they can't be without the drug. This is a form of addiction.

I Don't Know How to Heal You, So Take This Drug

Ironically, the prescription drugs most likely to be abused are those most likely to be prescribed when your physician doesn't know how to treat your problem.

For example, conventional medicine is notoriously unable to help back pain. If you go to your physician with back pain, chances are you'll be given painkilling drugs or undergo surgery, neither of which will heal the back. But since your physician doesn't know what else to do and you are in terrible pain, he or she will keep prescribing the drugs for you. Every year thousands of people become hooked on painkillers that they first took for back pain. (If you have chronic back pain, we recommend that you read the book *Healing Back Pain* by John Sarno, M.D., Warner Books, 1991, before you do anything else.)

Chronic headaches are another source of pain that conventional medicine is often unable to heal effectively. The medical solution tends to be a potent painkiller when the cause is usually a hormonal imbalance, a food sensitivity, or chronic stress and tension.

Women who visit a physician's office complaining of nervousness, lethargy, or depression are likely to be prescribed drugs. However, a conscientious physician will rule out physical causes such as nutritional deficiencies or hormone imbalances before pulling out the prescription pad. If no physical problem presents itself, a woman will likely benefit far more from a referral to a good counselor than she will from antidepressants or antianxiety drugs.

When your physician prescribes a drug for an illness he or she doesn't know how to treat, try an alternative health care professional such as a naturopathic doctor, an acupuncturist, or a chiropractor.

When Are You Addicted?

If your physician prescribed it, the drug must be OK, right? When your physician prescribes drugs for a real medical need, such as for pain after surgery, that's a legitimate use. But if you're still taking the drug every day six weeks, six months, or six years later, you have a problem.

In spite of their extensive training in prescribing drugs, physicians are ill equipped to recognize the symptoms of drug addiction and even less well equipped to help a patient withdraw from drugs. Your physician is just as afraid of the stigma of having a drug-addicted patient as you are of being one. It's much easier to write you another prescription than to take the time and trouble to help you through drug withdrawal—a painful, complicated, and emotionally wrenching process. To help you withdraw from a drug, find a different physician from the one who has been prescribing you drugs. Beware of physicians who insist that addictive drugs won't hurt you; that's their own form of denial, and it's no help to you.

Keep in mind that two of the primary symptoms of addiction (versus a purely physical dependence) are (1) denial that there is a problem and (2) repeated attempts to stop taking the drug, followed by a relapse. One of the requirements for getting unhooked from a drug is having the personal honesty to admit there is a problem and the courage to follow through and take action.

In our culture of instant gratification, we tend to forget that qualities such as contentedness, inner calm, inner peace, and emotional balance are won through the accumulation of wisdom, experience, and introspection. The truth is that the vast majority of people prescribed a benzodiazepine, an antidepressant, or some other type of drug that affects the mind and emotions simply need some help making it over a rough spot in their lives. They need a sympathetic ear, somebody who will listen objectively and caringly.

The distinctions made by drug manufacturers and the medical profession between drugs that are "habit forming" and those that are "addictive" are strictly academic and seem to have been created largely to justify prescribing dangerous drugs. If you are hooked on a drug, the difference between one that is addictive and one that is habit forming is academic. Our defi-

Guidelines for Safe Use of Medications

Patients are rarely given enough information about how to safely and effectively use their medication to avoid addiction. Here are some guidelines.

1. If you have abused any type of drug in the past, including alcohol, or even if you haven't abused drugs but you know you have an addictive personality, tell your physician and your pharmacist and ask directly if the prescribed drug is likely to cause you a problem.
2. Ask your M.D. and your pharmacist if the drug you are being prescribed is addictive or habit forming, or if it could create a dependence. If the answer is yes, ask for detailed information, such as:
   - Does this drug create a physical dependence?
   - How long does it take to create a physical dependence on this drug?
   - Will I have to go through physical withdrawal when I stop taking this drug? (If the answer is yes, ask your M.D. how he or she plans to help you do that.)
   - Is there a drug I could take that is not addictive?
3. Ask your M.D. or pharmacist to explain precisely how you should take your medi-

cine. Be sure the following information is on the container:
   - How often to take it
   - Whether it should be taken with or without food
   - What it is for—for example, pain or indigestion
   Examples:
   Take one capsule 3 times daily with food for stomach upset.
   Take one capsule ½ hour before bedtime with juice for sleep.
   Take one capsule every 4 hours between meals for infection until gone.
4. Have your physician put on the label the number of refills you have.
5. When you receive your prescription, read the label out loud to the pharmacist. Make sure you understand how, when, for how long, and why you are supposed to be taking the drug. If you have any questions, ask your pharmacist. The container may also contain an expiration date and tell how it should be stored.
6. Tell your physician and your pharmacist about any other drugs (prescription or over-the-counter) you are taking. If you drink a lot of alcohol, coffee, or soft drinks or if you smoke, be sure to mention it.

continued

Guidelines for Safe Use of Medications *(continued)*

7. If you are allergic to any foods or drugs, tell your physician and your pharmacist. If you are pregnant, lactating, or trying to become pregnant, tell your physician and your pharmacist.

8. If you notice any side effects after taking a medication such as dizziness, light-headedness, nausea, vomiting, diarrhea, skin rash, or any other out-of-the-ordinary symptom, call your physician or pharmacist immediately. You may experience these side effects right away or in a few days or weeks. You can literally be taking a drug for years without any side effects but then have them suddenly appear.

9. Throw away any medications you are no longer using. Look through your sup-ply of medications, check the expiration dates, and throw any old medications in the trash. If you have kids or teens in the house, or anyone prone to drug addiction or abuse, empty the pills from the container and dispose of them separately, putting the drug into a trash receptacle where you are sure it won't be found. If there are refills left, remove the label from the bottle.

10. Keep all of your medicines out of the reach of children, and never give your prescription drugs to anyone else, even friends or family.

11. Read the labels on all your over-the-counter medicines. Look for cautions or contraindications.

---

nition of an addictive drug is one that creates a dependence that falls outside of a legitimate medical need. If you have been using a drug for so long that you find you can't stop, you are addicted, regardless of what the drug is.

How you answer the following questions may give you some indication of whether you are inappropriately dependent on your medication:

1. Do I need to take my medicine more often than it was prescribed?

2. Do I become tense, nervous, or anxious if I don't take the medicine for more than one day?

3. Can I sleep without it?

4. Do I have to have extra supplies because I am afraid I will run out?

5. Do I have two M.D.s writing prescriptions for the same drug, in case one cuts me off?

6. Do I feel in a fog mentally when I take the drug?

7. Do I feel more alert when I take the drug?

8. Do I talk about the drug a lot to my friends and family?

9. If a pill breaks, do I save the bits and pieces?

10. Have I tried to stop taking the drug without success?

11. Do I want to stop taking the drug?

12. Have I tried to stop taking the drug and experienced such bad withdrawal symptoms that I went back on it?

If you answered yes to any of these questions, please consider the possibility that you are abusing the drug or drugs you are taking and get some help. Resources for prevention and recovery are listed in "Resources and Recommended Reading" at the back of the book.

Can Your Children and Grandchildren Get into Your Drugs?

Just because you can't open that childproof cap on your medication bottle, don't assume that your grandchild can't. It's a fact that more kids get into medicines at their grandparents' homes than at their own homes. Grandparents are more likely to be taking medication and are less likely to be vigilant about keeping it away from curious youngsters. If you have children in your house, even for just a few hours, be sure all your medications are out of reach or inaccessible. This also applies when you're visiting someone who has children—you have to assume they will wander into your room, open your bags, and act accordingly. Many pills come in attractive colors and are small enough to be easily swallowed. Some new pills look like little jelly beans and smell like candy.

Prescription drug abuse is a growing problem. Most addiction is created out of ignorance of the dangers of drugs. The key to preventing and avoiding addiction to prescription drugs is awareness, both for yourself and loved ones.

Chapter 3 Drug Interactions and How Your Body Processes Drugs

M ost drug testing is done on adult men between the ages of 25 and 50, but this is insufficient since drugs may act and interact very differently in children, teenagers, women, pregnant and nursing women, menopausal women, and particularly the elderly, where nutrient absorption and liver function is an issue. Your physician's only way of gauging your tolerance to a drug is to begin with the standard dose for an adult male and see what happens. If you don't complain of side effects or that there is no effect, chances are the dose will never be changed.

Dozens and dozens of factors can influence what effect a drug has on you, from how much sleep you got last night and what you had for breakfast to the condition of your liver and your blood pressure. For example, alcohol abuse can greatly increase or

Drugs That Are Metabolized Differently in Women Than in Men

Probably many more drugs than just these are metabolized differently in women than in men, but these are the ones we currently know about. If you are given a drug and experience negative side effects, ask your physician to try changing the dosage.

Acetaminophen	Amitriptyline	Benzodiazepines
Beta-blockers	Chlordiazepoxide	Diflunisal
Erythromycin	Imipramine	Methylprednisolone
Oxyzepam	Piroxicam	Prednisolone
SSRIs	Trazodone	

decrease tolerance to a drug, as can obesity, exercise, stress levels, and exposure to pollutants such as car exhaust, pesticides, or industrial chemicals. The elderly are far more sensitive to most drugs because their liver and kidney function is diminished; yet they are the population most likely to be taking handfuls of drugs each day. Entire medical journals are devoted to the metabolism of drugs, and new discoveries are made daily about how drugs interact with each other and in different people. For that reason, anytime you want to start taking a new drug— prescription or over-the-counter—we encourage you to talk to your pharmacist or go online and read the prescribing information sheet for that drug. If you're taking other drugs, find out if they might interact with the new one. In the section "Resources and Recommended Reading" at the back of this book, you'll find suggested online resources for checking drug interactions and side effects.

Biorhythms and Time of Day

One factor that's rarely taken into account in drug studies is the time of day, yet it can have a profound effect on how your body processes drugs. For example, the adrenal hormone corti- sol tends to be highest in the morning and low before bedtime. The worst asthma attacks tend to occur between 2 A.M. and 6 A.M. when cortisol is at its lowest. Your stomach lining is more susceptible to damage from drugs such as aspirin in the morning, and aspirin reduces blood pressure more effectively when taken at night. Some types of chemotherapy are more or less effective at certain times of day or night.

Drugs and nutrients can affect each other in your digestive system, in your bloodstream, in your liver and kidneys, or at the cell level where

Factors That Can Increase Drug Levels

Sex	Kidney or liver
Age	damage
Race	Nutritional deficiencies
Overweight or	Supplements
underweight	Exposure to toxins
Pregnancy and nursing	such as paint fumes,
Illness	solvents, pesticides
Over- or underexercise	Alcohol abuse
Food	Smoking
Other drugs	Stress
Digestion	Time of day

the drug or nutrient receptor is. Just as it takes a variety of vitamins, minerals, amino acids, and enzymes to process food so that your cells can use it, drugs also go through changes as the body uses them. They are changed as they are made useful, as they are being used, and as they are being excreted from the body. Any interference in this process caused by nutritional deficiencies or interference from other drugs, food, or alcohol can raise or lower drug levels.

Drugs and Their Potential Side Effects

Common Drugs That Can Cause Breast Enlargement in Men

ACE inhibitors	Indomethacin
Amitriptyline (Elavil)	Ketoconazole
Cimetidine (Tagamet)	Ketoprofen
Digoxin (Lanoxin)	Methyldopa
Famotidine (Pepcid)	Naproxen
Ibuprofen and related NSAIDs (non-steroidal anti-inflammatory drugs)	Spironolactone

Drugs That Can Cause Diarrhea

Antibiotics
Antidepressant/antianxiety drugs (benzodiazepines, lithium, valproic acid)
Antihypertensives (reserpine, guanethidine, methyldopa)
Cholesterol-lowering drugs (clofibrate, gemfibrozil, the statins)
Cholinergic drugs (metoclopramide)
Gastrointestinal drugs (laxatives, antacids)
Heart drugs (digitalis drugs, quinidine, hydralazine, beta-blockers, ACE inhibitors, diuretics)

Common Drugs That Can Decrease the Effectiveness of Oral Contraceptives

Antibiotics	Griseofulvin
Anticonvulsants	Rifampin
Azole antifungals	Ritonavir

If you're taking oral contraceptives and are prescribed one of these drugs, be sure to use an alternative form of birth control during the time you're taking these drugs and for at least two weeks afterward. If you get pregnant while on the pill, you may not realize it until the progestins it contains have put the fetus at significant risk of birth defects.

Drugs That Can Cause Weight Gain

Anafranil	Lithium
Antidepressants (Wellbutrin)	NSAIDs (ibuprofen, naproxen)
Antihistamines	Oral contraceptives
Corticosteroids (prednisone)	SSRIs (Prozac, Zoloft, etc.)

If You're Pregnant or Breast-Feeding, Don't Take It

There are virtually no drugs that have no effect on a developing fetus, and the effects are nearly always negative. Unless you are in a life-threatening situation, it's just not worth it.

Drug effects are poorly studied in pregnant animals, and for all practical purposes they are unstudied in humans. An indication on the drug package insert that no negative effects have been found does not mean there aren't any. It may just mean it hasn't been studied. You have to assume that any drug you take will hurt your baby.

The same goes for breast-feeding. There are few drugs that don't end up in breast milk. Those that don't may end up there eventually or affect it in other ways. Something as seemingly harmless as an aluminum-containing antacid taken when a woman is breast-feeding can cause developmental retardation.

Pregnancy and breast-feeding are wonderful opportunities to use nutrition as your medicine and to explore safe, gentle alternative approaches such as acupuncture and acupressure, massage, chiropractic, and meditation.

If you absolutely must use a medication while breast-feeding, refer to the online information offered by Thomas Hale, R.Ph., Ph.D.,

Potentially Dangerous Drugs to Avoid

The following drugs are included on the FDA watch list because of concerns about serious side effects. There are actually many more drugs on the list. Please visit the FDA website and its MedWatch section for a more detailed list. Notice that some of the medications are as seemingly simple as an eczema cream (elidel), shampoo for lice (lindane), or heartburn drug (prevacid), yet could have serious side effects. The FDA's MedWatch list changes frequently, so it's worth checking it against any new medications you may be taking.

Accutane	Ketek
Adderall XR	Lindane lotion and shampoo
Advair	Lotronex
Ambien	Mifeprex
Avandia	Nolvadex
Chantix	Palladone
Concerta	Prevacid NapraPac
Cordarone	Protopic ointment
Coumadin	Remicade
Dexedrine	Ritalin
Duragesic	Serevent diskus
Elidel cream	Strattera
Fentora	Symbicort
Focalin	Symlin
Forteo	Wellbutrin

at ibreastfeeding.com. That's also the best place to find the latest edition of his book, *Medications and Mother's Milk*. Dr. Hale is the world's foremost expert on mixing drugs with breastfeeding. He catalogs hundreds of drugs and gives detailed information about whether they can be used at all by nursing mothers and how to use them to minimize their effects on the baby.

Your Body's Drug Disposal Systems

The four major routes for excreting a drug from the body are the kidneys, liver, skin, and lungs. Most drugs are processed out through the liver and then the kidneys.

If you have kidney or liver disease, how your body handles drugs is profoundly affected. Food, drink, or lifestyle habits that stress and damage your kidneys or liver, such as alcohol abuse or chronic exposure to toxins such as solvents and paint fumes, can also affect how you process drugs. Even taking as seemingly harmless a drug as Tylenol (acetaminophen), which is hard on the liver, can affect drug levels. Kidney or liver stress or damage usually raises drug levels higher than normal by slowing down the excretion process. Smoking can cause drugs to leave the body more quickly than usual.

The aminoglycoside antibiotics such as streptomycin, kanamycin, and gentamicin cause kidney damage in as many as 15 percent of patients treated with them, but thousands of other drugs cause less obvious stress on your kidneys. When your drug information insert indicates renal (kidney) problems, you should be aware that the drug is probably going to be hard on your kidneys.

Drugs That Can Stress or Damage the Kidneys

ACE inhibitors	Methysergide
Acyclovir	Mitomycin
Allopurinol	Morphine
Aminoglycosides	NSAIDs
Amphotericin	(acetaminophen,
Beta-blockers	aspirin, ibuprofen,
Captopril	celecoxib, rofecoxib)
Cephalothin	Penicillins
Chemotherapy drugs	Phenylbutazone
Chlorothiazide	Phenytoin
Chlorpropamide	Piperidine
Clofibrate	Probenecid
Cyclosporine	Procaine
Diuretics	Quinidine
Furosemide	Salicylate
Isoproterenol	Streptozotocin
Lithium	Sulfonamides
Macanylamine	Tolazoline
Methotrexate	

Keeping Your P-450 Pathways Clear

Many types of drugs are prepared for clearance out of the body through the liver using the cytochrome P-450 enzymes, also known as the cytochrome P-450 pathways.

In a drug free body or in the presence of only one drug, the P-450 pathways can handle the load. When you have more than one drug cleared through the same pathway, the system quickly gets overloaded, stalling the removal of the drugs from the system. The result is an overdose that can be life threatening.

Some examples of drugs that either use the P-450 pathways or block their action are

Cimetidine (Tagamet)

Cholesterol-lowering drugs in the statin family

Macrolide antibiotics such as erythromycin and clarithromycin

Most antifungal drugs such as ketoconazole and miconazole

Antiarrhythmic drugs such as disopyramide (Norpace)

Phenytoin (Dilantin), used to treat seizures

Bromocriptine (Parlodel), used to treat Parkinson's

Benzodiazepine antianxiety drugs such as diazepam (Valium) and nefazodone (Serzone)

Calcium channel blockers such as nifedipine (Procardia)

Theophyllines used to treat asthma

Tricyclic antidepressants such as Elavil (amitriptyline)

Blood thinner warfarin (Coumadin)

Tacrine (Cognex), used to treat Alzheimer's

Caffeine

These are just the most commonly used drugs. Grapefruit juice also uses this pathway, which is why drinking it is contraindicated with some drugs.

Are you getting the picture? This is a very popular pathway through the liver for clearing certain types of waste matter from the body.

How many people do you suppose have been killed in a scenario similar to this one: Joe is taking a calcium channel blocker long-term, is temporarily put on a macrolide antibiotic to treat chronic bronchitis, and then has a glass of grapefruit juice and a cup of coffee with breakfast. This raises his levels of the calcium channel blocker so high that his blood pressure drops precipitously, causing heart failure. It's not an unlikely scenario. Or let's say it's the evening, and he takes some Tagamet (which is available over-the-counter) for heartburn and a Valium to help him sleep. Our guess is that this type of mismatching harms or kills hundreds of people every day.

Since it's unlikely that the package insert on the drug you're taking will tell you it's cleared through the P-450 pathways, your best bet is to check with your pharmacist before mixing any drugs, even over-the-counter drugs. Labels that warn of such things as hepatic (liver) toxicity, injury, dysfunction, or function impairment, which is medicalese for liver poisoning, should flash a red light in your head. This doesn't necessarily mean that it's a P-450 drug, since most prescription drugs are hard on the liver in some way, but it should make you very wary if you're taking other drugs.

Taking Care of Your Liver When You Take Drugs

The liver is one of the busiest organs of the body, working constantly to process food for transport through the bloodstream and to metabolize waste matter for excretion through urine or feces. The list of prescription drugs that stress or damage the liver is probably longer than those

If the Drug You're Taking Causes Drowsiness, Don't Drive!

According to an organization called Citizens Against Drug-Impaired Drivers (CANDID), prescription and over-the-counter medications that cause drowsiness contribute to more than 100,000 car crashes a year. If your drug insert warns against driving while under the influence of the drug, please take that warning seriously!

that don't. If you drink alcohol in excess and take liver-stressing drugs, you could be doing substantial damage to your liver.

Some symptoms of liver toxicity are swelling and redness in the palms of the hands, yellowish skin and whites of eyes, itching, small benign fatty tumors and reddish spots on the skin, or lumps under the skin of damaged blood vessels.

Drugs That Are Hard on the Liver

Nearly all prescription drugs are hard on your liver, but these are at the top of the list:

Acetaminophen
Analgesic painkillers
Anesthetics (given during surgery)
Antibiotics
Anticoagulants
Antihistamines
Anti-inflammatory drugs
Blood-pressure-lowering drugs
Chemotherapy drugs
Cholesterol-lowering drugs
Diabetes drugs (oral)
Heart disease drugs
Oral contraceptives
Parkinson's drugs
Tuberculosis drugs

Use Caution with Acetaminophen

One of the most commonly used drugs that damages the liver is acetaminophen (Tylenol), which is loudly touted in advertising for pain relief because it doesn't upset the stomach the way aspirin and ibuprofen do. What those ads neglect to tell you is that acetaminophen is very hard on the liver.

Recent research has shown that acetaminophen may inflict most of its damage on the liver by blocking the production of the important antioxidant glutathione. Without glutathione, the liver's ability to break down toxins for elimination is impaired. According to a study published in the journal *Free Radical Biology and Medicine*, one hour after an injection of acetaminophen, glutathione levels decrease by as much as 83 percent! That is a vulnerable liver. If some type of stress is placed on the liver (i.e., alcohol, pesticides) at the same time the acetaminophen hits it, the damage could be considerable.

If you're in pain, you may be in the position of having to pick your poisons, so here's a health-protecting strategy: if you're going to take acetaminophen, take the liver-protective herb milk thistle beforehand (follow the directions on the bottle) and add 500 mg of N-acetyl cysteine to

Drugs That Can Impair Athletic Performance

If you're taking a prescription drug, be aware that it might impair your ability to get a good workout. It may cause drowsiness, impair reaction time, upset the stomach, decrease endurance, or cause low blood sugar or muscle cramps.

Antianxiety drugs (alprazolam, diazepam, lorazepam)
Antibiotics
Antidepressants (amitriptyline, desipramine, imipramine, nortriptyline)
Beta-blockers (atenolol, metoprolol, propanolol)
Diabetes drugs (insulin, glipizide, glyburide, tolazamide, tolbutamide)
Diuretics (bumetanide, furosemide, hydrochlorothiazide)

your daily vitamins. Cysteine is the precursor to glutathione. Also be sure to avoid alcohol when you're taking acetaminophen.

Because drugs have potent and specific actions, they can easily become toxic in excess. One of the biggest reasons that natural remedies are preferable to use over prescription drugs whenever possible is that the natural remedies tend to be much gentler and safer if you take too much.

Drugs That Can Sink Your Sex Life

If you're a guy, you may think that your sex drive has dropped just because you've passed the age of 50. Not necessarily so! Although a man of 50 doesn't have the energy of an 18-year-old, most male impotence after the age of 50 has to do either with clogged arteries or with the drugs physicians love to hand out to men at that age.

If you're suffering from impotence and are taking a prescription drug, call your pharmacist or your physician and ask if one of the side effects of the drug is impotence. If you're taking more than one drug, including over-the-counter drugs, it could be causing your impotence even if it is not listed as a side effect.

Common Drugs That Can Deplete Nutrients

There are many more drugs that deplete nutrients, which you'll read more about later in the drug lists, but this list gives you some of the more common drugs that deplete important nutrients.

The consequences of chronic nutrient depletion caused by taking a drug long-term are serious and include, for example, senile dementia (B_{12}), birth defects (folic acid), osteoporosis

Drugs That Can Sink Your Sex Life

Antibiotics

Anticholinergics (used for ulcers and other gastrointestinal disorders, for nausea, for tremors caused by Parkinson's and psychiatric drugs, and sometimes for asthma)

Anticonvulsants

Antidepressants

Antihistamines (for allergies and sinus congestion)

Antihypertensives (drugs that lower blood pressure)

Antipsychotics

Appetite suppressants

H2 blockers such as Tagamet, Pepcid, and Zantac

Heart disease medications (many), including beta-blockers, calcium channel blockers, ACE inhibitors, and antiangina drugs

Painkillers such as indomethacin, naproxen, and naltrexone

Prostate drugs such as Proscar

Sedatives, tranquilizers, sleeping pills

(minerals), chronic muscle pain (CoQ10), and liver damage (acetaminophen).

Again, if you're considering taking a new drug, please check carefully to find out what other drugs, foods, or supplements may interact with it. The best source of information is a face-to-face visit with a good pharmacist. Compounding pharmacies are often a good place to go for detailed information. Otherwise, do an online search for the drug and read the prescribing information sheet. Check the section "Resources and Recommended Reading" at the end of this book for more recommendations.

Drugs That Can Deplete Nutrients

Drug	Nutrient Depleted
Acetaminophen	Glutathione
Ace inhibitors	Zinc
Acid or H2 blockers	Minerals, B vitamins, vitamin D
Antibiotics	B vitamins and probiotics
Antacids	Calcium and vitamin D
Beta-blockers	CoQ10
Bisphosphonates for osteoporosis	Calcium and vitamin D
Celebrex	Folic acid
Diabetes drugs	B vitamins
Digoxin	Calcium, magnesium, vitamin B_1, phosphorus
Diuretics	Minerals, B vitamins, vitamin C
Laxatives	Minerals
NSAIDS (ibuprofen, naproxen, aspirin)	Folic acid, vitamin C
Statins	CoQ10
Steroids	Minerals

Chapter 4 How Drugs Interact with Food, Drink, and Supplements

Everything you put in your mouth has some effect on your body, so it makes sense that drugs would have an effect on what you eat, and what you eat would have an effect on how your body processes drugs. Although the possible interactions and effects of drugs, food, drink, and supplements on your unique biochemistry are nearly infinite, we can make some generalizations and watch for some dangerous combinations.

A nutrient can increase the effect of a drug, decrease its effect, or delay its action, and a drug can interfere with the absorption of nutrients. Deficiencies in a vitamin, mineral, or other nutrient such as protein can increase or decrease a drug's action.

Taking Medication with or Without Food

When you fill a prescription, it should always say either, "Take with food," or "Take between meals" (without food). Some drugs will be virtually ineffective if you take them with food, and others will give you an upset stomach unless you take them with food. Most drug absorption takes place in your small intestine, and how your digestion is working will have a major impact on how the drug is absorbed. If you take a medication with a very fatty meal, it will take your stomach longer to empty and that will delay the action of the drug. If you eat a small, acidic meal with very little fat, your stomach may empty very quickly and the drug may take effect more quickly than usual. Some drugs will bind to your food, others will compete with nutrients for receptor sites, and others will stimulate digestion.

The following lists identify drugs that react with food. Some drugs are absorbed more quickly when you take them with food, mainly because they increase the production of bile, which speeds up digestion, or because they change the pH of the stomach, again speeding or slowing digestion. If you have been taking a

Drugs That Are Absorbed More Quickly When Taken with Food

Carbamazepine	Diazepam
Dicumarol	Erythromycin
Griseofulvin	Hydralazine
Hydrochlorothiazide	Labetalol
Lithium citrate	Metoprolol
Nitrofurantoin	Phenytoin
Propoxyphene	Propranolol
Spironolactone	

Drugs That Are Not Absorbed as Well When Taken with Food

Ampicillin

Atenolol

Captopril

Chlorpromazine

Erythromycin

Isoniazid

Levodopa (Don't take with high-protein foods, because it competes with amino acids for absorption.)

Lincomycin

Methyldopa (Don't take with high-protein foods, because it competes with amino acids for absorption.)

Nafcillin

Penicillamine (Don't take with dairy products, iron-rich foods, or vitamins, because it binds with some minerals, including calcium.)

Penicillin G

Penicillin VK

Propantheline

Rifampin

Tetracyclines (Don't take with dairy products, iron-rich foods, or vitamins, because they bind with some minerals, including calcium.)

drug between meals and then suddenly take it with food, or vice versa, you could get an overdose or not enough.

Drugs and Nutrients

Although not many nutrients such as vitamins, minerals, and amino acids, taken in normal doses such as in a daily multivitamin, will adversely affect drugs, many drugs can cause nutritional deficiencies. Antacids deplete calcium; aspirin depletes vitamin C and folic acid; diuretics deplete minerals (especially calcium, magnesium, potassium, and zinc); some cholesterol-lowering drugs interfere with the absorption of fat-soluble vitamins such as A, D, and E; corticosteroids such as prednisone deplete vitamin D, potassium, and some of the B vitamins; some cholesterol-lowering drugs deplete coenzyme Q10 and vitamin E; and conventional hormone replacement therapy and birth control with progestins deplete magnesium, the B vitamins, and folic acid.

Drugs that block folic acid production or absorption include the arthritis and chemotherapy drug methotrexate, anticonvulsants such as phenytoin and carbamazepine, nonsteroidal anti-inflammatory drugs (NSAIDs, including ibuprofen, aspirin, and indomethacin), some antiulcer drugs (the H2-receptor antagonists, such as cimetidine and ranitidine), and bile acid sequestrants for lowering cholesterol levels, cholestipol and cholestyramine.

Both excess potassium (such as is caused by ACE inhibitors) and cimetidine (Tagamet) and proton pump inhibitors such as omeprazole can interfere with the absorption of vitamin B_{12}. A deficiency of B_{12} can cause symptoms of senility. How many older people have been put into nursing homes because they were taking cimetidine long-term, which blocked B_{12} absorption? We see ads on TV for these drugs over and over and over again, and eventually, even though we know better, we think the drugs are harmless because that's how they're portrayed in the advertising.

The tuberculosis drug isoniazid depletes vitamin B_6, as do the yellow dyes called tartrazines found in 60 percent of all prescription drugs and in many processed foods. Among the many symptoms of a B_6 deficiency are hormonal imbalances and carpal tunnel syndrome.

Grapefruit juice can increase the strength of many drugs by blocking the liver enzymes that are used to clear the drug out of the body. The following drugs can all interact dangerously with grapefruit juice: the calcium channel blockers (including felodipine, nicardipine, nifedipine, nimodipine, and isradipine); the statin drugs (lovastatin, simvastatin); the antianxiety drug buspirone; the benzodiazepine tranquilizers; the psychotropic drugs carbamazepine, nefazodone, and quetiapine; the antihistamine loratadine (Claritin); ethinyl estradiol (the main ingredient in oral contraceptives); the heart drug amiodarone; the impotence aid sildenafil (Viagra); and the steroid methylprednisone.

Many, many drugs will increase the strength of alcohol and vice versa. Always use caution when combining any drug with alcohol.

Fiber can block absorption of a drug and may even carry most of it right through the digestive tract. If you're taking any type of fiber such as psyllium (e.g., Metamucil) to treat constipation and irregularity, take medications at least an hour before or two hours after you take the fiber.

Drugs That Interact with Minerals

Drugs can have a profound effect on how the body handles nutrients. Some reduce mineral absorption, others cause minerals to be excreted in the urine in higher than normal quantities, and others interfere with how the body processes minerals.

• Antibiotics: The antibiotic Neomycin interferes with the absorption of iron. Tetracycline blocks the absorption of dietary minerals; conversely, taking minerals with an antibiotic will also block the action of the antibiotic. The quinolones (Noroxin, Penetrex, Cipro) block the absorption of iron and zinc.

• Anticonvulsants such as carbamazepine, phenobarbital, phenytoin (Dilantin), or primidone lower levels of copper and zinc.

• Magnesium and aluminum antacids deplete calcium and phosphate. Sodium bicarbonate, also used as an antacid, depletes magnesium and potassium.

• Arthritis medications such as D-penicillamine (Cuprimine) can reduce absorption of zinc, iron, and probably other minerals as well.

• Aspirin and indomethacin (Indocin) can cause enough blood loss through the stomach over time to cause an iron deficiency. Aspirin can also cause potassium depletion.

• Cholesterol-lowering drugs such as cholestyramine (Questran) and colestipol (Colestid) can lower the body's stores of iron.

• Corticosteroids such as cortisone and prednisone can deplete zinc, calcium, chromium, magnesium, potassium, and selenium.

• Diuretics, frequently used in the treatment of high blood pressure and heart failure, can cause minerals to be lost in urine.

• Conventional HRT (versus natural) can deplete magnesium.

• H2 blockers such as Tagamet and Zantac can deplete calcium, iron, and zinc.

• Laxatives reduce absorption of minerals.

• Oral contraceptives tend to increase levels of copper, which in excess can cause a decrease in blood levels of iron and zinc; they also reduce levels of magnesium and selenium.

• Alcohol depletes iron, selenium, zinc, and magnesium, in addition to many other important nutrients. Alcoholic drinks like wine and whiskey are also relatively high in the toxic element cadmium, which is taken up in greater quantities when zinc levels are low.

Never Mix Drugs and Alcohol

As much as we might like to think alcohol is simply a social lubricant or pleasant accompaniment to dinner, it is a drug and has profound effects on the body. When you mix alcohol with any drug, prescription or over-the-counter, you are entering into the no man's land of drug-drug interactions. If you use alcohol, even just a glass of wine with dinner, always ask your physician or pharmacist how a drug interacts with alcohol. If they don't know, ask them to look it up for you.

The drugs listed here are known to either increase the effects of alcohol, are increased themselves by alcohol, or have the potential to cause liver damage when combined with alcohol.

Acetaminophen may cause liver damage.
Antidepressants
Antifungal drugs such as ketoconazole (Nizoral) may cause liver damage.
Antihistamines
Aspirin
Barbiturates
Benzodiazepines and other antianxiety drugs
Bromocriptine (Parlodel)
Calcium channel blockers such as verapamil (Verelan, Calan, Isoptin)
Cephalosporin antibiotics—don't drink alcohol for at least three days after taking these drugs
Diabetes drugs (oral)
H2 blockers such as cimetidine (Tagamet) and ranitidine (Zantac)

Indomethacin and other anti-inflammatory
drugs (Indocin)
Methotrexate may cause liver damage.

Narcotics (Darvon, Empirin, Talwin)
Nitroglycerin
Tranquilizers and sleeping pills

Drugs That Interact Dangerously with Alcohol

If the drug you're taking isn't on this list, don't assume it doesn't interact with alcohol.

Drug	Effect
Acetaminophen	Can cause liver damage
SSRI antidepressants	Can increase effects of alcohol
Aspirin	Stomach bleeding
Barbiturates	Can cause extreme sedation
Benzodiazepines	Can cause extreme sedation
Bupropion	Increased risk of seizures
Cimetidine	Increases effects of alcohol
Codeine	Low blood pressure, slowed breathing
Diabetes drugs	Upset stomach, hypoglycemia, headache
Ibuprofen	Internal bleeding
Phenytoin	Can cause extreme sedation
Reserpine	Increases effects of drug and alcohol
Tetracycline	Reduces the effect of the tetracycline
Tricyclic antidepressants	Can cause extreme sedation

Chapter 5

How Drugs Interact with Other Drugs

O nce you reach the age of 50, you are almost guaranteed to walk out of a physician's appointment with a prescription for a drug. At the very least, you may be told to take an aspirin every day, and if your blood pressure or cholesterol counts are even a hair above "normal," you'll be given prescriptions for blood pressure and cholesterol-lowering drugs.

When you start taking any type of drug, you are heading down a long road full of potentially dangerous drug interactions and side effects. Some 36 percent of all hospitalizations are due to drug reactions, and of those, at least 25 percent are caused by adverse drug interactions. There are approximately 13,000 prescription drugs available in the United States, and yet the FDA does not require drug interaction studies as part of its drug approval process. New drugs have been studied by themselves but not necessarily in combination with other drugs.

When you take a new drug in combination with another drug, you're a guinea pig for the drug companies and the FDA. Thousands of people die each year in these hidden human experiments. Our educated guess is that tens of thousands of deaths in older people attributed to "natural causes" or heart failure are actually caused by drug reactions or interactions. Even when a physician becomes aware that a hospitalization or death is the result of a drug reaction, he or she will probably not report it.

If you have any new health complaints, be suspicious of the drugs you're taking. Ask your pharmacist to inform you of any known interactions when you are taking a new drug or experiencing new symptoms, and carefully read the patient insert that should come with every new medication (you may have to use a magnifying glass and a medical dictionary to do this).

Be extremely conservative and cautious about taking prescription drugs. It is not just a matter of life and death, it is also a matter of quality of life. One of the most common side effects of a drug-drug interaction is mental fogginess or confusion. Tragically, many older people are put on as many as eight or a dozen drugs, and when they become lethargic and confused, they are diagnosed as senile and stuck in a nursing home, when a simple change of medication could have remedied the problem and kept them independent.

The other very common scenario is the drug treadmill, where you are given two or more drugs and when you have side effects from them, you are given more drugs to treat the side effects, which creates more side effects, and so on.

Not Only Prescription Drugs

It's not just prescription drugs that can dangerously interact with each other. Over-the-counter drugs can react with prescription drugs, causing them to be stronger, be weaker, or produce a new symptom. For example, if you're taking the corticosteroid prednisone and you start taking

Most Prescribed Drugs in America 2006

1. Lipitor
2. Hydrocodone APAP
3. Toprol-XL
4. Norvascs
5. Amoxicillin
6. Hydrocodone APAP
7. Synthroid
8. Nexium
9. Lexapro
10. Albuterol
11. Singulair
12. Levothyroxine sodium
13. Lisinopril
14. Ambien
15. Zyrtec
16. Prevacid
17. Zoloft
18. Warfarin sodium
19. Advair Diskus
20. Furosemide

Source: *Pharmacy Times*, 2007, pharmacytimes.com/issues/articles/2008-05_003.asp.

ibuprofen or aspirin every day to treat chronic headaches, the combination could cause gastric (stomach) bleeding. Combining ACE inhibitors with ibuprofen can increase potassium to dangerous levels, causing side effects such as muscular weakness, numbness, and an irregular heartbeat.

If you suddenly find yourself suffering from urinary retention or incontinence, it may be because you're combining an antihistamine such as Benadryl that you bought in the drugstore for your allergies with an anticholinergic drug to treat Parkinson's disease.

If the drug you have been taking is no longer working, it may have to do with using an H2 blocker such as cimetidine (Tagamet), sold over-the-counter for heartburn. Cimetidine interacts with dozens of drugs, either increasing or decreasing their action.

If you're taking an asthma drug such as theophylline, watch your caffeine consumption; caffeine can cause an overdose of theophylline, with symptoms of a rapid or irregular heartbeat, nausea, dizziness, headache, and shakiness. Caffeine is present in coffee, most soft drinks, many over-the-counter headache remedies, and Midol. Theophylline levels in the body can also be increased by capsaicin, which is found in Tabasco sauce, chili peppers, and often in natural arthritis formulas. Theophylline levels can be decreased by eating charbroiled meats. Many, many common drugs increase or decrease levels of theophylline.

Most Common Drug Offenders

Because of the thousands of drugs on the market, it is impossible for any physician to know all of the possible drug-drug interactions that could threaten your health and even your life. That doesn't count the interactions with food, over-the-counter drugs, and supplements. It means it's up to you to minimize your drug intake and keep close track of what you are taking. Any drug combination can cause a new interaction, because your body and your biochemistry are unique.

Drug Interactions Involving Commonly Used Nonprescription Medications

Drug Interactions with Aspirin and Other Salicylates

Drug/Drug Class	Potential Effect
ACE inhibitors	Worsening hypertension or congestive heart failure
Anticoagulants	Increased risk of gastrointestinal bleeding
Alcohol	Risk of enhanced gastrointestinal bleeding
Methotrexate	Increased risk of methotrexate toxicity
Sulfonylureas (for diabetes)	Amplified drop in blood sugars
Probenecid, sulfinpyrazone	Worsening of high uric acid levels and gout
Valproic acid	Drowsiness, behavioral disturbances

Drug Interactions with Nonsteroidal Anti-Inflammatory Drugs (NSAIDs)

Drug/Drug Class	Potential Effect
Anticoagulants	Increased risk of bleeding
Blood pressure drugs	Increased blood pressure
Digoxin	Increased blood digoxin concentrations and toxicity
Alcohol	Increased risk of bleeding
Lithium	Increased blood lithium concentrations and toxicity
Methotrexate	Increased risk of methotrexate toxicity

continued

Drug Interactions Involving Commonly Used Nonprescription Medications (continued)

Important Drug Interactions Involving Cough and Cold Medicines

Drug/Drug Class	Potential Effect
Antihistamines plus depressants (depressants may include alcohol, benzodiazepines, opiate painkillers, barbiturates, phenothiazines)	Increased depressant effects
Antihistamines plus thioridazine	Increased levels of thioridazine, resulting in abnormal heart rhythm and increased risk of possibly fatal arrhythmia
Monoamine oxidase inhibitors (MAOIs) plus sedating antihistamines	Increased and prolonged sedative effects
Decongestants containing phenylpropanolamine (PPA), phenylephrine, and pseudoephedrine plus blood pressure drugs	May counteract effects of blood pressure drugs
Phenylephrine/pseudoephedrine plus MAOIs	Severe hypertensive reaction, possibly including headache, vomiting, visual disturbances
Dextromethorphan (over-the-counter cough medications) and MAOIs	Additive effects on serotonin levels may lead to "serotonin storm"

Drug Interactions Involving H2-Receptor Antagonists (Stomach Acid Blockers)

Drug/Drug Class	Potential Effect
Benzodiazepines	Increased risk of benzodiazepine toxicity
Dofetilide	Increased risk of dofetilide toxicity
Antifungals	Reduced bioavailability of anti-infective agent
Phenytoin	Increased risk of phenytoin toxicity
Procainamide	Increased risk of procainamide toxicity
Propanolol	Increased risk of propanolol toxicity
Theophylline	Increased risk of theophylline toxicity
Warfarin	Increased risk of bleeding

When prescribing a drug, your physician should take into account not only interactions between drugs but also how various drugs are going to interact with your unique health profile. If you have an irregular heartbeat and high blood pressure and your physician prescribes a diuretic that depletes magnesium, it will only make the irregular heartbeat worse. If you have asthma and high blood pressure and your physician prescribes an inhaler for the asthma, it could raise your blood pressure even more.

Here are the classes of drugs most often associated with serious interactions with other drugs, foods, and supplements:

- Benzodiazepines such as Ativan and Valium used as antidepressants

- Ephedrine and pseudoephedrine, found in many allergy, cough, cold, and decongestant medicines

- Heart drugs, including digoxin, calcium channel blockers, beta-blockers, and diuretics (especially the "loop" diuretics such as furosemide and the thiazide diuretics)

- H2 blockers such as cimetidine (Tagamet)

- MAOIs such as Marplan and Nardil used as antidepressants

- NSAIDs (nonsteroidal anti-inflammatory drugs, such as ibuprofen)

- Steroids (such as prednisone)

- Theophylline, an asthma drug

- Warfarin (Coumadin), a blood thinner

If you are taking any of these types of drugs, it is extremely important to be watchful at all times for drug interactions. For example, if you're taking an MAOI and eat foods that are high in the amino acid tyrosine (i.e., avocados, aged cheese, not-quite-fresh liver or pâté, nuts, pickled foods, processed meats such as salami and bologna, wine, yogurt, soy sauce, and bananas), the inter-

action could cause life-threatening high blood pressure, severe headaches, dizziness, mental confusion, visual disturbances, and fever. MAOIs are outdated drugs that also react with dozens of over-the-counter drugs. These drugs should be taken only as a very last resort.

Top Drugs Implicated in Emergency Room Visits

Warfarin (blood thinner)
Insulin (diabetes)
Aspirin (heart/pain)
Clopidogrel (blood thinner/antiplatelet)
Digoxin (heart)
Metformin (diabetes)
Glyburide (diabetes)
Acetaminophen-hydrocodone (pain, e.g., Lorcet, Lortab, Vicodin, Zydone)
Phenytoin (seizures)
Glipizide (diabetes)
Levofloxacin (antibiotic)
Lisinopril (heart/ACE inhibitor)
Trimethoprim-sulfamethoxazole (antibiotic)
Furosemide (heart/loop diuretic)

Source: Budnitz, D. S., "Medication Use Leading to Emergency Department Visits for Adverse Drug Events in Older Adults," *Annals of Internal Medicine* 147 (2007): 755–65.

Chapter 6

How to Read Drug Labels and Information Inserts

Every prescription drug comes with what is called a drug information insert or package insert. You will rarely see this when you fill a prescription at a pharmacy, but you should never take a drug without reading it first. Ask your pharmacist for a copy. The drug companies don't really want you or the physician to read these inserts, because no drug looks good after you've read all its possible side effects and adverse reactions (so it is printed in extremely tiny, hard-to-read type). At the same pharmacy where you fill your prescriptions, you can buy a magnifying glass for a few dollars so you can read your drug insert. It will be one of the best investments you've ever made in your health.

You absolutely cannot count on the U.S. Food and Drug Administration (FDA), the drug company, your physician, or your pharmacist to keep you safe from dangerous drugs and their interactions. Your pharmacist is your greatest ally when it comes to protecting you from drugs, but ultimately it's up to you to stay informed and to make decisions about your health. Your physician doesn't want to tell you about possible drug side effects, because he or she has been programmed in medical school to believe that if you're told about side effects, you'll become a hypochondriac and get them. Unfortunately, that attitude is unlikely to change anytime soon. You are the best judge of whether you are having a bad reaction to a drug. Please trust your body's feedback and pay attention to it.

Every year tens of thousands of people take home a prescription drug for a minor ailment and end up very ill, sometimes permanently, or even dead, because they weren't aware of the risks associated with the drug. A dangerous side effect or adverse reaction may have happened in less than 1 percent of the people who took the drug in testing, but if you happen to be in that 1 percent, it could save your life to be informed.

For new drugs, the information listed on the package insert comes primarily from FDA-required studies on the drug. But don't think that just because the drug company has spent tens of millions of dollars jumping through FDA-required hoops that means that the drug is well studied. In fact, many studies use patients in mental institutions, nursing homes, homeless shelters, universities, and other places with untypical test subjects. Anyone in a mental institution is already going to be thoroughly drugged, making any study results virtually useless because of drug interactions. Those in homeless shelters are often abusing street drugs or alcohol, again creating unpredictable reactions, not to mention a population impossible to follow up on. University students may or may not be taking drugs and using alcohol, but in any case they are generally young and healthy, unlike the majority of people who take prescrip-

tion drugs. Another factor making drug studies less than meaningful is that few drugs are studied for more than three months, making long-term side effects unpredictable.

The Public Citizen Health Research Group, which publishes the book and newsletter *Worst Pills, Best Pills*, suggests avoiding any drug that hasn't been on the market for at least seven years. Before that time, you are, in effect, a guinea pig for the FDA and the drug company.

Deciphering Your Drug Insert

The *Physicians' Desk Reference* (PDR) is a large red volume that you've probably seen on the shelf in your physician's office. It is updated every year, and in it is printed the drug information insert for nearly every prescription drug on the market. Thanks to the Internet, you now have free access to the same information. Simply put the name of your drug into a search engine, and you'll find numerous listings for it. If the drug you're researching has its own website, be sure to read the physician information, which is much more thorough than the patient information. In the Resources and Recommended Reading section at the back of this book you'll find some suggestions for websites that list drug information and online medical dictionaries.

Here are the categories of information provided in the PDR and a translation of some of the medical terms that make the PDR difficult to understand without a medical dictionary.

• **Brand name.** Once the patent runs out on a drug it can be sold by almost anyone. The brand name of a drug is specific to the company that is packaging and selling it. For example, pseudoephedrine is the generic name of an antihistamine, but it is sold under the brand names Sudafed, Chlor Trimeton, Dimetapp, and others.

• **Generic name.** This is the name a drug is called regardless of its brand or trade name. For example, acetaminophen is the generic name for Tylenol, and ibuprofen is the generic name for Advil and Motrin.

• **Form.** How the drug is taken. Most drugs are taken as capsules, pills, tablets, or liquids. In the hospital, many drugs are delivered as liquids through an injection or IV.

• **Description.** This describes the drug in chemical terms, often with an accompanying molecular diagram. It also lists fillers, binders, dyes, and other nondrug ingredients in the medication. This is important if you are allergic to food dyes, preservatives, or even ingredients such as corn that may be used as a filler. If you find you are sniffling, sneezing, wheezing, coughing, or experiencing fatigue or puffiness after taking a medication, it could be due to an allergic reaction to a preservative or food dye, especially the yellow and red dyes, which are used in the majority of prescription medications.

• **Clinical pharmacology.** This is a description of what the drug does in the human body. Most of these descriptions conclude with a paragraph stating that the action or mechanism of the drug is not fully understood. Always keep that in mind—even the drug company often doesn't really know how the drug works.

• **Indications and usage.** This tells you what the drug is prescribed for. If your specific ailment isn't listed here, that's called an "unlabeled use," meaning the drug hasn't been studied or approved by the FDA for that use. Once a drug is approved by the FDA for any use, physicians are free to prescribe it for any reason they choose.

Physicians frequently prescribe drugs for unlabeled uses, and drug companies frequently cleverly market drugs for unprescribed uses even though they legally aren't supposed to. For example, the antidepressant Prozac is now approved by the FDA for treating depression, obsessive-compulsive disorder, and bulimia, and it's also now being sold under the name Sarafem for the treatment of premenstrual syndrome. For years before it was approved for anything but depression, it was marketed for obsessive-compulsive disorder and premenstrual syndrome. Currently, Prozac is being used off-label to treat obesity, and it's being given to children without FDA approval. (Since most of the drugs available have not been tested on children, nearly every drug prescribed to a child is being used off-label.)

Another example of off-label drug use is the practice of using the stomach acid blocker Cytotec (misoprostol) for the induction of labor in pregnant women. If an obstetrician wants to hurry a woman's labor along, he or she can insert tablets of Cytotec into her vagina and stimulate very powerful contractions. This practice is common despite the fact that it greatly increases the risk of uterine rupture.

The drug companies spread the word about these unlabeled uses through drug company reps. Another common ploy is to fund a so-called study showing that the drug works for an unlabeled use and then release the results of the study to the media (TV news programs such as "20/20" are favorites for this type of marketing). Another tactic they use is to find a few people who experienced a "cure" for the disease by taking the medication and then take those stories to the media. This type of media coverage, as well as articles that are "planted" in magazines by public relations companies or departments, creates what is known as patient demand. You see a story on a news program about the unlabeled use of the drug, and the next time you go to your physician you mention it. It's a very effective form of marketing. You can pretty much assume that any media coverage a drug gets has been created through manufacturer marketing and public relations. If it's negative coverage, chances are a competitor created it.

Don't be overly concerned if your ailment isn't listed—chances are the labeled use hasn't been very well studied either!

• **Contraindications.** This is where the drugmaker is supposed to say, "If you have _____ (disease), don't take this drug." Most of the time what's listed here is something useless like, "Do not take this drug if you have a known allergy or sensitivity to _____ (drug name)"—as if you would know that ahead of time.

• **Warnings.** This is where you want to pay close attention. This section lists a variety of conditions that might make taking the drug dangerous. For example, the warnings section for the drug Procardia (nifedipine) warns that it can cause "excessive hypotension" (low blood pressure), which can be life-threatening. It also warns of the possibility of increased angina, myocardial infarction (heart attack), a withdrawal syndrome, and congestive heart failure. Our guess is that only a handful of the hundreds of thousands of people taking this drug are ever aware of these *very real* dangers. If they weren't real dangers, they would not be included. This is also the place to look for warnings about using the drug with patients who have renal or hepatic impairment, dysfunction, or disease. *Renal* refers to the kidneys, and *hepatic* refers to the liver. Nearly all prescription drugs are hard on your liver, but this type of warning should alert you to added risk.

• **Precautions.** This is another section of the drug insert where your physician may be warned about prescribing the drug to people with renal or hepatic dysfunction, or it may advise them to frequently monitor kidney and liver function. Again, a red flag should go up—this drug is particularly hard on those organs. This section also lists drug interactions. If you are taking any other type of drug, read this section carefully, and if you find you are already taking a drug on the list, do not take the new drug until you have spoken with your physician or your pharmacist about the interaction.

If the drug you're taking has caused cancer, genetic mutations, or impaired fertility in laboratory animals, this is the place to find it. Physicians like to pooh-pooh this type of research, but we'd like you to take it very seriously. If the cancer, mutation, or impaired fertility wasn't significant, it wouldn't have made it onto the drug information insert. While rodents aren't an ideal model of what happens in a human, it's an accurate enough indicator to cause concern.

This is also where warnings about taking the drug if you're pregnant show up. However, it's safest to consider all drugs unsafe during pregnancy. Drugs should be completely avoided

Drugs That Can Cause Incontinence

Antibiotics	Atropine
Benzodiazepines	Beta-blockers
Bupropion	Diuretics
Doxazosin	Fluoxetine
Isradipine	Levobunolol
Lithium	Misoprostol
Nicardipine	Nifedipine
Prazosin	Sleeping pills
Spironolactone	Terazosin
Tranquilizers	

Medical Terms Frequently Found in Drug Information Inserts

Adenomas: Benign tumors.

Agranulocytosis: A sudden drop in white blood cells called granulocytes, indicating a serious dysfunction of the immune system.

Alopecia: Hair loss.

Amenorrhea: Absence of menstruation.

Anaphylaxis: A severe allergic reaction that can be fatal.

Anemia: Deficiency of red blood cells in the blood.

Angina: Chest pain.

Anorexia: Loss of appetite.

Arrhythmias: Irregular heartbeats.

Arthralgia: Joint pain.

Bradycardia: Slow heartbeat.

Cerebral: Having to do with the brain.

Clinical trials: Drug studies on humans, versus rodents or in a test tube.

CNS: Central nervous system; refers to the nerves of the brain and spinal cord, which is to say those nerves that regulate almost everything in the body.

Dermatitis: Skin rash.

Dys **as a prefix:** Dysfunction, difficult, painful.

Dyspepsia: Indigestion, heartburn, bloating.

Dyspnea: Difficult breathing.

Dysuria: Painful urination.

Edema: Water retention, bloating, swelling due to water retention.

Electrolyte: In the human body, this usually refers to the minerals calcium, potassium, and sodium.

Fibromyositis: Joint or muscle pain and swelling.

Gastrointestinal: Having to do with the digestive system.

Glossitis: Inflammation of the tongue.

Hemorrhage: Uncontrolled bleeding or loss of a large amount of blood.

Hepatic: Having to do with the liver.

Hirsutism: Excessive hair growth.

Hyper **as a prefix:** Too much.

Hypo **as a prefix:** Too little.

Hyper- or hypocalcemia: Too much or too little calcium in the blood.

Hyper- or hypoglycemia: Too much or too little sugar in the blood.

Hyper- or hypokalemia: Too much or too little potassium in the blood.

Hyper- or hypomagnesia: Too much or too little magnesium in the blood.

Hyper- or hyponatremia: Too much or too little sodium in the blood.

Hyper- or hypotension: High or low blood pressure.

Hyperkinesia: Restlessness or jerky, rapid movements.

In vitro: In a test tube.

In vivo: In a body.

IV: Intravenous, usually referring to a drug given through a needle into a vein.

Jaundice: Yellowing of the skin and sometimes the whites of the eyes usually caused by liver or gallbladder dysfunction.

Leukopenia: An abnormal drop in white blood cells, indicating a compromised immune system, often caused by an adverse drug reaction.

Malaise: Weakness, discomfort as in feeling a flu or fever coming on.

Myocardial infarction: Heart attack caused by blockage of an artery.

Orthostatic hypotension: Dizziness when standing from a sitting or lying position.

Neuritis: Swelling of a nerve.

Neuropathy: Nerve pain, swelling, degeneration.

Neutropenia: An abnormal drop in white blood cells called neutrophils.

continued

Medical Terms Frequently Found in Drug Information Inserts (continued)

Pallor: Pale skin.

Palpitations: Pounding or racing heart.

Parenteral: Substances going into the body other than via the mouth and digestive system. It usually refers to drugs or nutrients given intravenously, through a vein.

Paresthesia: Numbness, tingling.

Photosensitivity: Sensitivity to sunlight, which can cause a rash, hives, or swelling.

Porphyria: Abnormal pigmentation of the skin.

Pruritus: Itching.

Pulmonary: Having to do with the lungs.

Renal: Having to do with the kidneys.

Stomatitis: Inflammation in the mouth.

Syncope: Fainting.

Tachycardia: Rapid heartbeat.

Thrombophlebitis: Swelling of a vein, often associated with the formation of a blood clot.

Thrombosis: Blood clot.

Tremor: Shakiness or quivering, often seen in the hands of older people.

Urticaria: A skin rash usually caused by an allergic reaction.

Vertigo: Dizziness.

---

during pregnancy unless the mother's or child's life is at risk.

• **Adverse reactions.** When a drug company is testing a drug on humans, it is required to record all the adverse reactions or side effects a patient has to it. The adverse reactions may have nothing to do with the drug, but there is no way of separating an authentic adverse reaction from a coincidental reaction. On the other hand, adverse reactions are notoriously underreported. For example, if a drug is reported to cause dizziness in 13 percent of the people taking it, it's likely to be much higher than that.

The bottom line is that if you experience any of the side effects or adverse reactions listed on the drug insert, you should tell your physician. If the side effect is even remotely life threatening, get medical attention right away.

M.D.s have a way of making patients feel as if they are responsible for drug side effects and minimizing the discomfort they can cause. If this happens to you, please either stand up for yourself, have someone such as a spouse do it for you, or find another doctor. You should never have to suffer from drug side effects, nor should you ever allow your physician to get you onto the drug treadmill by prescribing new drugs to treat the side effects of the first or second one.

Drugs That Can Cause Photosensitivity

Amantadine	Antibiotics
Antidepressants	Antifungals
Antihistamines	Antihypertensives
Antipsychotics	Benzocaine
Benzodiazepines	Carbamazepine
Chemotherapy drugs	Clofibrate
Disopyramide	Diuretics
Etretinate	Isotretinoin
NSAIDs	Oils and chemicals used
Oral contraceptives	in perfumes and
Quinidine	cosmetics
Trimeprazine	Oral diabetes drugs
Tretinoin	Promethazine

• **Overdosage.** This section gives the symptoms of an overdose of the drug and if available, an antidote to an overdose. Many heart drugs, such as ACE inhibitors, beta-blockers, digitalis drugs, and the blood-thinning drugs, can be fatal if levels are even a little bit too high. There are many factors that can raise levels of these drugs, including drug-drug interactions, drug-food interactions, alcohol consumption, and stress. Knowing the symptoms of an overdose can be lifesaving if you catch it early.

• **Dosage and administration.** This section lists the amounts the drug comes in and in what form it is delivered—for example, capsule, tablet, oral, liquid.

Generic and Brand Names of Commonly Used Drugs

(Not all brand names are listed.)

Acetaminophen (Tylenol)

Albuterol (Ventolin, Proventil)

Amlodipine (Norvase)

Amoxicillin (Amoxil, Trimox, Augmentin)

Ampicillin (Polycillin, Amicillin)

Aspirin (Bayer, Bufferin)

Atenolol (Tenormin)

Bupropion (Wellbutrin, Zyban)

Captopril (Capoten)

Carbamazepine (Tegretol, Atretol)

Cephalosporins (Cefaclor, Cephalexin, Duricef)

Chlorpromazine (Thorazine)

Cimetidine (Tagamet)

Citalopram (Celexa)

Clarithromycin (Biaxin)

Diazepam (Valium)

Digoxin (Lanoxin)

Diltiazem (Cardizem)

Erythromycin (Ery-Tab, E-Mycin)

Fluoxetine (Prozac, Sarafem)

Fluvoxamine (Luvox)

Furosemide (Lasix)

Glipizide (Glucotrol)

Griseofulvin (Fulvicin, Grifulvin)

Hydralazine (Apresoline)

Hydrochlorothiazide (Reserpine)

Labetalol (Normodyne, Trandate

Levodopa (Larodopa, Dopar)

Lisinopril (Prinivil, Zestril

Loratadine (Claritin)

Lovastatin (Mevacor)

Medroxyprogesterone (Provera)

Methyldopa (Aldomet, Amodopa)

Methylphenidate (Ritalin)

Metoprolol (Lopressor, Toprol)

Nifedipine (Procardia)

Omeprazole (Prilosec)

Paroxetine (Paxil)

Phenytoin (Dilantin)

Piroxicam (Feldene)

Pravachol (Pravastatin)

Propoxyphene (Darvon)

Propranolol (Inderal)

Sertraline (Zoloft)

Simvastatin (Zocor)

Spironolactone (Aldactone)

Terazosin (Hytrin)

Triamterene (Dyrenium)

Valproic acid (Depakote)

Warfarin (Coumadin)

Abbreviations on Prescription Slips and Bottles

Abbreviation	Meaning
q.d./QD	Take once a day or take every day
b.i.d./BID	Take twice a day
t.i.d./TID	Take three times a day
q.i.d./QID	Take four times a day
q.h.	Every hour
q.12h.	Take every 12 hours
q.4-6h.	Take every 4 to 6 hours
p.r.n.	As needed or if needed
p.o. or per os	Take by mouth
p.c.	After a meal
a.c.	Before a meal
a.p.	Before dinner
c	With
h.s.	At bedtime
rx	prescription
ut dict.	as directed
tsp.	teaspoon
ml	milliliter
mg	milligram

Other Words You Should Know

It's preferable not to take any prescription drug long-term, but if you do, it's wise to purchase a medical dictionary and use it to look up words in the drug information insert that you don't understand. You can find a paperback medical dictionary in almost any bookstore, and you'll find suggestions for online medical dictionaries in "Resources and Recommended Reading" at the back of this book.

Know Your Generic Names

Throughout Part 2 of this book, you will find hundreds of drug names. Although in some cases both the generic name and the brand name will be listed, often only the generic name will be listed. If you are taking a generic version of your drug, it will often just be called by its generic name. But if not, you can usually find the generic name on your pill bottle or the container it came in. If the generic name is not on the bottle, ask your pharmacist to write it on. The generic name will also be found on the drug insert information, or you can find it online.

Chapter 7

Surgery, Drugs, and Nutrition: Minimizing the Damage and Maximizing Your Recovery

American physicians are generally way too eager to use the surgeon's knife to carve up and cut out whatever they think is ailing you, at great expense to you and great profit to them and the hospitals they work for. Sometimes when you have a chronic illness, it may seem like having surgery will be a quick and easy end to the pain. But if you don't address the problems that caused the pain in the first place, you'll wind up sick again within a few months, with nothing to show for your surgery but a huge medical bill, a scar, and possibly a missing organ.

Of the 750,000 hysterectomies done every year, it is estimated that 650,000 of them are unnecessary. U.S. physicians perform some 300,000 cesareans a year, most of them unnecessary. Carving up men's prostate glands started to be big business, but men caught on that it wasn't necessary and squawked loudly, and the practice has rapidly declined. (Women need to learn to protest louder when mainstream medicine mistreats them.) Other surgeons' favorites that are often unnecessary are procedures for gallstones and heart disease (especially bypass operations).

Having surgery of any kind is not something to take lightly. There is always a risk of dying in surgery, and the risk of a life-threatening infection is also very real. Hospitals are one of the best places to pick up an infection that is resistant to antibiotics. That alone is reason enough to avoid hospitals unless absolutely necessary.

When you see a physician who is recommending surgery, keep in mind that surgeons like to do surgery. That is their business, that is what they are good at. Always get a second opinion from someone not connected to your physician or the same hospital or HMO, and go to a naturopathic doctor or an M.D. who practices alternative medicine to find out if he or she thinks the problem can be solved without surgery. Even if the visit is not covered by insurance, it may be one of the best investments you ever make.

Having given you all the warnings, there are times when surgery is definitely necessary. Dental extraction, appendicitis, and some cancers come to mind. With elective surgeries, only you can make the final decision about whether surgery is truly necessary, and when you do choose to have it, go into it fully prepared and in the best health possible.

In addition to the list of supplements you can take to support your body, it's also important to support yourself emotionally and get plenty of rest before and after surgery. Be sure you have plenty of help at home, and stock the kitchen with nutritious fruit and vegetable drinks and soups. If you are experiencing a lot of anxiety in the week or so prior to surgery, you can use the antianxiety herb St. John's wort or the relaxant herb valerian to help you through. Follow the directions on the container, and don't overdo it, please. Chamomile tea is mild and soothing.

Preparing for Surgery

The two biggest challenges of surgery for your body, besides that of healing the actual wound, are the threat of infection and the stress on your liver. There's no way around it: when you have surgery, you will be given lots of drugs, and most of them are very hard on your liver. This especially applies to anesthesia drugs. Take extra good care of your liver before, during, and after surgery. Your liver is responsible for taking nutrients and farming them out to the rest of the body, and it is also responsible for breaking down or neutralizing toxic waste products such as excess hormones and pesticides. If your liver is busy fighting damage from drugs, it won't be able to heal your body as quickly or effectively.

One of the most irresponsible practices in mainstream medicine is giving people large doses of acetaminophen (i.e., Tylenol) after surgery. This painkiller is notoriously hard on the liver and is the last thing your body needs after surgery. If at all possible, avoid this drug before, during, and after surgery. Make it clear to your physician and your anesthesiologist that you are not interested in being given acetaminophen after surgery unless it is absolutely necessary.

To spare your liver, you should also avoid alcohol for the week before surgery, as well as foods high in fat (especially hydrogenated oils and fried foods). Other factors that can stress the liver include exposure to pesticides, solvents, paints, and gasoline.

Many prescription drugs can harm the liver. These include steroids (prednisone), antifungal drugs such as ketoconazole (Nizoral), and tuberculosis drugs (Laniazid). If you are taking any kind of prescription or over-the-counter drug, get out a magnifying glass and read the package insert for warnings about "hepatic function impairment" or "hepatoxicity." This is medicalese for liver damage.

We recommend that you support your liver by taking some special supplements before and after surgery:

• **Milk thistle (Silybum marianum)** is an herb that is very supportive of the liver. Take it as a tincture, one dropperful three times daily, or as tablets or capsules (follow directions on the container), in a standardized product (meaning that the amount of the active ingredient, silymarin, is guaranteed). Take it between meals for a week before surgery and for two weeks after.

• **Alpha-lipoic acid** (also called thioctic acid) is a substance made by the body that directly supports the detoxifying abilities of the liver. Diabetics should use alpha-lipoic acid with caution as it can cause hypoglycemia. You can take two 100 mg capsules three times a day, with meals, for a week before surgery and for two weeks after.

• **Cysteine** is an amino acid precursor to the important liver antioxidant glutathione. It is commonly used in hospital emergency rooms to treat patients with acetaminophen-induced liver poisoning. It will also help stimulate your immune system. You can take one 500 mg capsule of N-acetyl cysteine three times daily between meals for the week before surgery and for two weeks after.

• **Fiber** is important to good bowel function, which is important to a healthy liver. If your colon is not effectively eliminating toxins, they will be sent back to the liver. Eating plenty of fiber will ensure that your bowels are moving well. This means eating plenty of whole grains, fresh fruits, and fresh vegetables. Having your bowels moving well will also be helpful when you are required to take a laxative the day before surgery.

Avoid Infection, Speed Healing, and Boost the Immune System

Infection is a major risk of surgery. The sooner you get yourself out of the hospital the lower your risk of getting an infection. You can help avoid infection and speed up the healing process by keeping your immune system strong. In addition to the vitamins you're taking as part of the Six Core Principles for Optimal Health (see Chapter 9), you will support your body if you take the following supplements.

• Your biggest ally in fighting infection and speeding healing is vitamin A. Take 15,000 IU of vitamin A (not beta-carotene) daily for a week before surgery, 50,000 IU the 2 days before and after surgery, and then continue with 15,000 IU daily for about 10 days. (If you're pregnant, don't take more than 15,000 IU daily.) If you're having dental surgery, you can rub it on your gums before and after surgery to greatly speed up the healing process.

• Take extra antioxidants, zinc, and a B-complex vitamin for two weeks before and after surgery. They will support your immune system and the healing process. Take an extra 1,000 to 2,000 mg of vitamin C (don't take so much that you get diarrhea), 200 mcg extra of selenium, and 15 mg extra of zinc. Also take a bioflavonoid antioxidant such as grapeseed extract and green tea extract to help speed wound healing.

• Glutamine is a nonessential amino acid that becomes essential when we're under certain types of stress, such as surgery. The immune system can't function without glutamine. It speeds up the healing process, aids in detoxification in the liver and kidneys, and supports the health of the small intestine. Take 500 mg twice daily between meals for a week before and two weeks after surgery.

Homeopathic Remedies for Surgery

Homeopathic remedies are particularly effective for helping cope with surgery, and you can safely take them just before surgery and just after since they are tiny sugar pellets or tablets that dissolve under the tongue.

Homeopath Dana Ullman, author of *The Consumer's Guide to Homeopathy* (Tarcher/Putnam, 1996), recommends arnica in a 30C dose before and after surgery. Take four pellets under the tongue the night before, the morning of the surgery, and just before the surgery.

Homeopathics also work well to treat the nausea that almost always occurs after surgery. Ullman recommends nux vomica in a 6C or 30C dose. You can refer to Ullman's book for homeopathic remedies for specific types of nauseas and treatment for different types of surgery.

Chapter 8

How to Avoid Medical Errors in the Hospital

S tan was a cardiologist for 35 years in a major American city. He was in and out of a large hospital every day looking after his patients and, of course, was intimately familiar with all the goings-on in his medical community. After he retired, Stan was told by his physician that he needed to be hospitalized for some surgery. This normally calm, cool, and collected professional went into a panic. He was terrified at the prospect of being hospitalized. He made his wife promise that either she or his sister would be by his side at all times during his hospital stay, day and night. He conferred with his physician ahead of time about what drugs he would be getting, how often, and in what dosages, and he wrote this all down for his wife and sister. He instructed them to double- and triple-check any medication he was given against what he had written and told them that under no circumstances was he to be given anything else unless he or his physician, in person, specifically approved it.

It may sound to you like Stan was being a bit paranoid, but in reality he was just being smart. After decades of working in a hospital, he was all too aware of how easy it is for patients to be injured and even killed by improper medication. According to a Harvard study done a few years ago, these types of errors result in 200,000 injuries to hospital patients every year.

Have an Advocate

Don't go into a panic if you need to be hospitalized, but do have a friend or relative be your advocate to make sure you're getting the proper care and medication. Stan's concerns were confirmed in a study published in the *Journal of the American Medical Association* in which over a six-month period, 4,000 patients admitted to two Boston hospitals were tracked by Harvard researchers. They found 247 "adverse drug events," meaning medication errors that injured the patient in some way. Of these, 70, or 28 percent, were considered preventable. Of the 70, 56 percent were caused by physician error and 34 percent by improper administration by a nurse.

Watch Closely for Errors: This Is Your Life

To look at the media today, you'd think that medical error would be the least of your worries—but you'd be wrong. You are more likely to die from medical error than from breast cancer, a car crash, or AIDS. The likelihood of being killed by a medical mistake is 80 times greater than being killed in a gun accident. Taking steps to protect yourself may not win you any popularity contests in the hospital ward but could very well save your life.

You can protect yourself by keeping track of what medications you are being given. Before you go into the hospital, ask your physician what medications you will be given; the exact brand name and generic name; what they are being prescribed for; the dosage (how many mg per pill) and how many pills you take each time; how many times in a 24-hour period you will be given them; in what form (i.e., oral, intravenous); and for how many days. Make your own daily chart with these details, and each time you are given a medication by a nurse, double-check what the physician told you against what the nurse is giving you. If anything changes, ask why, and if you don't receive a satisfactory answer, refuse the medication until you can personally check with your physician or with the hospital pharmacist. If you are unable to do this, have a friend or relative do it for you. This may sound like a lot of trouble to go through, and you may get some resistance from the hospital staff, including your physician. On the other hand, it could save your life. These precautions are especially important if you are going into the hospital for an operation.

The most frequent types of medication mistakes are:

- Prescribing the wrong drug, that is, mixing up the names of drugs that sound alike or giving inappropriate drugs to seniors and children
- Giving the wrong dosage of a drug, that is, too much or not enough, or too frequently or not frequently enough
- Mixing drugs without being aware of adverse drug interactions
- Giving a drug via the wrong route, that is, orally instead of intravenously

- More than one physician prescribing drugs without paying attention to what the others are ordering
- The side effects from a drug not being monitored
- Stopping a drug too soon or not continuing it long enough

Before You Go to the Hospital

1. Select the hospital—and surgeon—with the most experience treating your problem. If you have the luxury of choosing between two or more hospitals, choose the one that has done your procedure the most. Practice may not make perfect, but it does reduce the chances of mistakes being made. Choose the surgeon with the most experience in performing the surgery you're going in for, as well.

The more nurses per patient, the better. You're safest in a hospital with a low patient–registered nurse ratio. According to an analysis by the *Chicago Tribune* newspaper, overworked or poorly trained nurses are often to blame for medication errors, delay of needed care, or the improper performance of medical procedures they have not been adequately trained to do. The *Chicago Tribune* report also revealed that at least 119 deaths had occurred while unlicensed nurse's aides making nine dollars an hour were caring for patients. In two of the Chicago-area hospitals included in the analysis, administrators had created cost-saving plans that allowed housekeeping staff to dispense medications to patients!

2. Get a second opinion. Visit a practitioner not connected with the physician who recommended the surgery. An alternative medicine M.D. or naturopath may be able to help you

solve the problem without an operation. Hysterectomies, bypass surgeries, cesarean sections, and gallstone surgeries are often recommended when less extreme, gentler treatments can take care of the problem.

3. Become an expert on your condition and its treatment. This is easier to do than ever before with the resources available on the Internet. If you have trouble understanding the information you find, ask your doctor to explain it to you. You and your advocate should have a good idea of what your hospital stay will be like, such as which tests and other procedures will be performed and when. Medication is often given via IV after a surgery, so be sure to ask about everything that is put in your IV. That way, when your treatment deviates from your expectations, you can ask questions and be sure you're not getting a procedure or a drug meant for the person in the next bed.

In the Hospital

1. Demand that anyone who touches you wash his or her hands or wear new surgical gloves. Virulent, antibiotic-resistant infections abound in modern hospitals, and they can be life threatening for patients whose bodies are weakened by surgery. These infections are most often passed to you via the hands of medical staff. It is required procedure in all U.S. hospitals that medical personnel wash their hands or change gloves in-between patients, and yet it rarely happens.

2. Insist on seeing an attending (senior) physician from time to time. Most teaching hospitals push their interns and residents to the limit, and an exhausted resident who has been working for 24 hours straight is more likely to make a mistake than a senior physician who has had

a good night's sleep. Besides, there's no substitute for the knowledge that attending physicians have gained over years of experience.

3. When you do see an attending physician, take the opportunity to ask any questions that have come up for you during your stay. If you have any doubts about the care being given by nurses or medical students, bring them up with the attending physician.

Stay on Good Terms with the Hospital Staff

Overworked, underpaid, overwrought hospital staffers are likely to take offense if you repeatedly question their judgment. Tell them that it really isn't anything personal, that you know they're being worked too hard, and that human error is inevitable even under the best of circumstances. Let them know that you understand that everyone involved is working toward the same goal: the best possible outcome in your treatment. Tell them that you believe the patient should take on some responsibility to ensure that mistakes don't happen. Make your inquiries and demands nonthreatening; be direct, but don't adopt an adversarial tone if you can avoid it. Keep things as friendly as possible so that no one has to waste energy on unnecessary confrontations.

When you leave the hospital, take home in writing your doctor's instructions for a smooth recovery, including a list of all medications and dosages. Ask friends and family to help you out with nutritious meals and tender loving care during your recovery.

PART 2

PRESCRIPTION DRUGS AND THEIR NATURAL ALTERNATIVES

Chapter 9

Six Core Principles for Optimal Health

The number of ways to stay healthy is at least as great as the number of ways to get sick. Because everyone is unique in their genetic, physical, emotional, mental, and spiritual makeup, no one program will completely cover everyone. You will discover for yourself, through trial and error, what works for you and what doesn't, and hopefully with the help of a competent health care professional you can create a lifestyle that rewards you with vibrant good health and energy.

That being said, there are some guidelines that everyone can use to lay a solid foundation for good health, and they are summarized in the Six Core Principles for Optimal Health. These six core principles are basic and simple, and anybody can follow them.

While this book is not a substitute for the individual medical care your health care professional provides, it can help empower you to become a more active and knowledgeable participant in your own health care.

The Six Core Principles for Optimal Health are simple and effective whether you do one step or all six. The more steps you take, the better you'll feel. Optimal health is like driving a finely tuned automobile instead of an old clunker. Either one might be able to get you from place to place, but what a difference in the drive!

Step 1: Drink Plenty of Clean Water

Two-thirds of the human body is water, yet water is our most neglected nutrient. Of course water is a nutrient. It's more necessary for sustaining life than food. You can survive more than a month without food, but without water, the human body can function for only about a week. You cannot expect to enjoy optimal health if you deprive your body of the water it needs.

If you drink four to eight glasses of clean water daily (more or less depending on your size, lifestyle, and individual biochemistry), your body will thank you in so many ways. For one thing, your skin will be glowing with good health in just a month or so. Constipation will be a thing of the past, especially if you also exercise and eat fiber-containing foods. You will find controlling your weight easier. Many times when you think you're hungry, a glass of water will suffice.

Because water is a solvent, it helps rid your bloodstream of excess fat, which can help reduce your blood serum cholesterol level. It's possible that 99 percent of all kidney stones result from not drinking enough water.

Make It Sparkling Clean

Notice that the recommendation is to drink clean water. In most places in the world these days, including North America, drinking clean water means avoiding tap water. To ensure that your water supply is clean, use a filtration system. You can purchase an inexpensive water filter or a complete household unit, depending on your needs and your budget.

Bottled water is often not much cleaner than tap water, and all those plastic bottles are very hard on the environment. Try using one of the hard plastic or steel water bottles and fill it from your in-home filter—just be sure to keep the water bottle clean.

Recently, some stories in the media proposed to debunk the "myth" that Americans really need to drink up to eight glasses of water a day—that it's just a ploy created by the folks who profit from the sale of expensive bottled water. These stories also announced that juices, milk, sodas, tea, and coffee do in fact count toward daily fluid intake. Although many people who much prefer to drink four cans of soda over four glasses of filtered water likely breathed a sigh of relief when they heard this on the news, they shouldn't switch back to their old ways quite yet. The up-to-eight recommendation is backed up by solid research. For example, research on Seventh-Day Adventists found that those who drank five or more glasses of water daily had only half the risk of heart attack and stroke when compared to those who drank only two glasses a day, and that those who were better hydrated had less viscous, "sticky" blood. Risk of bladder cancer has been found to be significantly lower in men who drink the most water. Exercise-induced asthma is caused in part by water loss from the airways; properly hydrating before workouts can help prevent attacks. The risks of developing kidney stones and constipation are both minimized by adequate water intake.

Some would argue that it's highly unlikely our ancestors drank up to eight glasses of water a day. On the other hand, they may have consumed more water because they were much more physically active. They also didn't live in the highly toxic world we do, and they didn't eat processed food. Drinking water helps your body cleanse itself day in and day out. Sodas, juices, coffee, and tea don't serve this purpose as effectively.

Step 2: Get Back to Basics and Rediscover Delicious Whole Foods

You are what you eat, but if you eat a lot of refined foods, you won't be a more refined person—you will be a drastically less healthy person. Our national health began a dramatic decline when refined and processed foods were introduced. The rise in chronic degenerative diseases such as heart disease and diabetes correlates with the rise in consumption of foods that have all the nutrients stripped out of them and harmful preservatives and additives put in. If you're eating lots of canned, packaged, preserved, and frozen foods, gradually switch to whole foods. Whole foods are essentially as nature made them. Foods packaged by nature come complete with all the nutrients you need. You get enzymes, vitamins, minerals, amino acids, and hundreds of other nutritional substances you need for a healthy, energetic body capable of handling stress and fighting off disease.

Go for Whole Grains and Legumes

Grains such as wheat, corn, millet, barley, oats, quinoa, amaranth, and rice are not only delicious, they contain a wonderful potpourri of nutrients as well as fiber. Get reacquainted with whole grains. Try oatmeal or a whole-grain cereal or bread for breakfast. For lunch, have a salad on a bed of brown rice or millet. Add barley to soups and stews, and try corn tortillas with

your vegetables. If any new grain upsets your digestion, introduce it more gradually or skip it. Please note that "whole wheat" bread is *not* the same as whole grain—it's usually just white bread with some brown coloring and a few flakes of bran added.

Fresh Vegetables and Fruits: Your Ticket to Longevity

People who eat plenty of fresh vegetables and fruits have a lower cancer risk, as well as less heart disease and a lower risk of diabetes. Instead of the canned and frozen varieties, head for the fresh produce section. Treat yourself and your family to daily salads, lightly steamed vegetables seasoned with olive oil and lemon, and a delicious dessert of fresh fruit. Not only will you live longer, you'll feel better along the way.

Healthy Oils

One of the primary causes of heart disease in this country is bad fats. This doesn't just apply to saturated fats (which really aren't bad for you unless you eat too much of them). It applies much more to the trans-fatty acids found in hydrogenated oils and margarine-type products, which, thank goodness, have almost disappeared from store shelves. However, you will still find them soaking fried foods in restaurants.

Most of the unsaturated fats found in vegetable oil are rancid, which is also a major health risk. For cooking, it's best to stick to the monounsaturated fats, olive and canola oil. Olive oil is the best—it's delicious and extra-virgin olive oil is largely unprocessed, so you get all the good nutrients in it. (Use a lighter olive oil for cooking at high heat.) Although canola oil is also processed, it's the best oil for baking and other uses where you want a very light oil. Used in moderate amounts, butter is also a healthy fat.

Many people enjoy coconut oil, which is wonderful for baking. Although it is a saturated fat, research has shown that it can actually help you lose weight.

Meats, Poultry, and Other Protein Foods

The verdict is in: the high-carbohydrate, low-fat, low-cholesterol diet doesn't prevent heart disease, and it has worsened the obesity problem more than it has improved it. Protein, fats, and cholesterol from animal foods and eggs have an important place in a health-promoting diet. These foods provide essential nutrients, satisfy the appetite, and promote better blood sugar balance.

This doesn't mean you're free to eat as many charred spareribs, double cheeseburgers, marbled steaks, or buffalo wings as you like if you want to be in good health. Choose lean meats, ideally from free-range, grass-fed livestock; if possible, buy organically raised poultry and use organic eggs. They are more expensive, but a great investment in your health. Organically raised livestock are not given antibiotics or growth hormones, which collect in the flesh, eggs, and milk of their conventionally farmed counterparts and increase cancer risk and risk of antibiotic resistance in people who consume them. Organic and free-range animals are also fed more wholesome diets, with less contamination by estrogenic chemicals, and so less of these toxic, carcinogenic estrogens collect in the foods that come from them. Wild game, such as venison, buffalo, and pheasant, is a good alternative to conventional store meats; they usually have eaten a more natural diet and their meat has a healthier fatty acid content and higher concentration of nutrients.

Charring creates carcinogens, so char and burn animal foods as little as possible.

Fish

Remember when your mother told you to eat your fish because it was "brain food"? As usual, she was right. Fish is nature's richest source—outside of mother's milk—of an omega-3 fat called docosahexaenoic acid (DHA for short), which has been found to be important for the optimal development of the nervous system. Fish is also loaded with another important fat, eicosapentaenoic acid (EPA for short). EPA has powerful anti-inflammatory qualities that balance the proinflammatory qualities of other fats and oils. High intake of these omega-3 fats has been found to decrease the risk of heart attack and breast cancer, and the evidence that they protect against allergy, asthma, depression, and other diseases is accumulating quickly.

There's a catch, however. The fish we eat has almost all been contaminated by the heavy metal mercury, which is highly toxic to the nervous system—especially in babies in utero and in breast-fed infants (mercury passes readily from mother to child via breast milk). Released by coal-fired power plants into the atmosphere, mercury falls with rain into lakes and streams. Microorganisms consume the mercury, and from that point it moves up the food chain and into ocean waters as fish eat the microorganisms, larger fish eat the smaller fish, and so on. Fish at the top of the marine food chain are the most contaminated, with mercury levels in their flesh that can exceed one part per million (ppm). The Food and Drug Administration (FDA) has recommended that pregnant women completely avoid swordfish, shark, tilefish, and king mackerel. Pregnant women are also warned to avoid eating more than 12 ounces per week of smaller saltwater fish, such as cod and tuna, which can contain between 0.17 and 0.60 ppm of mercury. Shellfish are no exception to mercury contamination, with one delicacy—lobster—leading the FDA's list with an average of 0.31 ppm. Freshwater fish vary in their levels of contamination, but so many of them live in waters polluted with multiple toxic chemicals that they should generally be avoided.

It seems like a cruel catch-22: oils from fish are important for the health and development of babies and children, but the mercury that contaminates them could cause retardation and adversely affect coordination, intelligence, and memory. The anti-inflammatory omega-3 oils are important counterparts to other oils found in the modern diet and appear to prevent the most common causes of death, but at what cost can we get enough of them?

The answer is to play the odds as best you can. Eat only fish from deep, cold waters, such as salmon, cod, bass, halibut, sardines, albacore tuna, and flounder, and eat them only two to three times weekly. Avoid large, predatory fish, especially swordfish, shark, king mackerel, and tilefish. Farmed fish may have less mercury in them, but they also may be lower in the omega-3 fats that make fish so nutritious. Be especially prudent about limiting fish intake if you are pregnant, but be sure to add extra DHA to your diet in the form of supplements. The best of these supplements are carefully processed to remove toxins, including mercury. In fact, just about everyone can benefit from high-quality fish oil supplements. We'll tell you more about these supplements later on.

Nuts and Seeds

Unsalted nuts and seeds are excellent sources of healthy fats, vitamins, and minerals. Walnuts and pumpkin seeds are rich in anti-inflammatory omega-3 fats, which have been found to promote cardiovascular health, temper allergic reactions, improve immune function, and even help prevent cancer. Almonds are rich in calcium and magnesium and make a delicious, protein-rich snack.

Fermented Dairy Products

Throughout history, healers have used fermented milk—what you and I know as yogurt—as a medicinal food. The friendly bacteria that yogurt contains promote good digestion and help improve the balance of good and bad bacteria in the body. Stay away from those colorful little containers of sugary yogurt sold at most supermarkets. Instead, buy a larger container of plain, organic yogurt that contains live cultures, and mix in your own fruit or granola. Whole milk yogurt is especially satisfying and can be used as a substitute for sour cream. If you must have a touch of sweetness, stir in a small amount of maple syrup or all-fruit preserves.

Become a Label Reader

The best way to avoid processed foods and hydrogenated oils is to read labels. Don't be fooled by products that say "all natural," "no cholesterol," or "no sugar added" on the front of the package. These terms are misleading. Checking out the nutrition content label is the only way to really know what you're getting.

Processed foods tend to be high in fat, sodium, or sugar. So you say you'll fix that by purchasing low-fat or low-sodium foods. OK, but watch out for the old shell game. When manufacturers cut down on one of these three, they usually add more of one of the others. For example, nonfat yogurt is usually loaded with sugar or even worse, artificial sweeteners such as aspartame.

If you're eating processed foods, you're not tasting real food. In fact, there's no taste left.

That's why they add all the fat, salt, and sugar. Again, the only way you'll know what you're getting is by reading the label.

Label reading is really like detective work. For example, sugar goes under lots of names. The suffix -ose at the end of a word stands for *sugar*. There's sucrose (common table sugar), dextrose, and fructose (fruit sugar). Watch out for highly refined fructose, which is used in cola drinks and many of the so-called natural soft drinks. Basically, it's so refined that it's no different from regular white sugar. By the way, brown sugar is just good old white sugar with molasses coloring. Of course, it's best to cut down on the sugar in your diet. It's just empty calories; there's no nutrition, plus it zaps your energy.

Simple sugars enter your bloodstream quickly, giving you that much-touted lift. But the catch is that your pancreas is caught off guard by the sugar rush and it releases too much insulin. The result is an in-body processing error that lets you down the hard way: a drop in blood sugar, usually within the hour, that leaves you feeling less energetic, less alert, and more irritable than you were before.

Step 3: Add Movement to Your Life

Movement is essential for optimal health. For some of you, exercise is a four-letter word. But once you start moving, you will get more out of life. You'll notice that your mood is brighter and that life's little annoyances don't get to you the way they once did. You'll have more energy and sleep better than you have in years. Since exercise improves circulation and endurance, you may even find your sex life has renewed vigor—in fact, you may start finding you're getting as much exercise from your midnight aerobics as from your daily walk.

Brisk walking at least five days a week for 30 minutes to an hour (about two to four miles) is all you need to do. If you can take a brisk walk every day, so much the better. The most recent government exercise guidelines recommend an hour of exercise every day, mostly due to the fact that previous guidelines didn't appear to make a dent in the ballooning obesity problem. While an hour of activity a day, if you can fit it in, is better than half an hour, the so-called health authorities are barking up the wrong tree on this one. Even an hour of exercise a day is not going to slim you down if you're living on a diet full of fattening processed foods and mega-sized restaurant entrées! If you have a weight problem and you're committed to getting slim, you'll benefit from trying to work in a full hour a day of exercise in addition to following our dietary recommendations. You can break it up if you like—for example, do 15 minutes in the morning, 30 minutes at lunch, and 15 minutes at night. If you're exercising for health benefits and to maintain your present weight, half an hour a day is just fine.

It's essential for children to have exercise daily, preferably at least two hours and preferably outdoors so they can soak up the sun's rays and get plenty of vitamin D.

If you have any medical condition that might make brisk walking hazardous to your health, consult your doctor first. If you haven't been exercising at all, start slowly until you have increased the distance to at least two miles. As you get into shape and your usual walking course feels easier, push yourself to the next level by increasing your walking speed, the duration of your walk, or changing to a hillier course.

You can walk any time of the day. If you're a morning person, your energy will be high at that time of day, and if you're a city dweller, pollution levels are lowest before rush hour begins.

Movement . . .

Helps Prevent
Arthritis
Back pain and injuries
Heart diseases
Osteoporosis
Stroke
Type 2 diabetes

Decreases
Blood pressure
Body fat
Cholesterol
Rate of cancer

Increases/Improves
Balance
Circulation
Energy
Immune system
Muscular strength and
 flexibility
Reflexes
Self-esteem
Sex life

While you are walking, move your arms in time with your walking pace. Most of you should be perspiring a bit after your walk. Your pace should reach 3 to 4 miles per hour. That means you'll cover a mile every 15 to 20 minutes. Stretching before exercise and cooling down afterward are very important for safe, effective exercise.

Step 4: Maintain a Healthy Weight

You can lose weight and never go hungry when you cut out excess fats, refined carbs, and other processed foods; focus on high-quality proteins and vegetables; and move your body. The goal is to gradually create a new, healthier lifestyle. As you change your eating habits and exercise more, the weight will naturally come off. There is way too much pressure on women in our culture to have the body of a teenager for life. Women and men naturally put on weight as they age, which is fine. What you want to avoid is obesity, and we all know what that is.

Lose the Fat

You don't need to cut fat completely out of your diet; that's not good for you either. But you do need to keep it lower than our national average, which is 40 percent of our daily calories.

Think of it, if you're 15 pounds overweight, you're carrying around a bowling ball with you. Do you have one, two, or three bowling balls? That weight puts extra stress on your heart, plus you're using up precious energy that could be used doing something you really enjoy. If you reduce your intake of processed foods, eat meats and other animal foods in moderate amounts, and follow the general guidelines given earlier in this chapter, it won't be difficult to reduce the fat in your diet to 30 percent of your total calories, and you will probably lose weight. For most Americans, this means cutting fat consumption nearly in half.

Saturated fat has gotten a bad name. It is not bad for you except in excess. In fact, it's necessary for good health. The problem is that most Americans eat way too much of it. Saturated fat is usually solid at room temperature. It includes butter, marbled meat, and tropical oils such as coconut, palm kernel, or palm oil. Use canola oil in your cooking rather than unstable, unsaturated vegetable oils. When you stir-fry vegetables, use water at the beginning at high heat, then throw in a small amount of oil at the last minute. When you cut the fat to about 30 percent of your daily calories, you dramatically decrease your chances of obesity, heart disease, diabetes, high blood pressure, and stroke.

Sugar Is Fat, Too

As far as calories are concerned, sugar that isn't burned off right away might as well be fat. All sugars are turned into fat when they can't be used by your body fairly quickly. That's why it's wise to turn to fresh, raw vegetables when you want to munch on something. Vegetables are nature's perfect source of vitamins, minerals, and fiber. Next time you get a snack attack, try some carrot or celery sticks. Also try jicama (hick-ah-ma) sticks, a starchy Mexican vegetable that looks like a big potato and has a mild, sweet taste. When you cook vegetables, lightly steam or stir-fry them. If you've been used to boiled vegetables, you'll be amazed at how tasty and flavorful lightly cooked vegetables are.

If you have a sweet tooth, switch to fruit. Grapes are especially sweet. Apples and pears make good afternoon snacks. Although the sugars in fruit are still sugar, they aren't absorbed as quickly as refined white sugar, and unlike white sugar, a piece of fruit has vitamins, minerals, and fiber. (If you have a craving for chocolate, you may be deficient in magnesium—try munching on some figs or almonds.) Don't overdo it with the dried fruit; when the water is removed, fruit becomes a highly concentrated source of sugar and calories. When you get an afternoon or evening craving for fat, try a handful of unsalted nuts such as almonds or cashews. If you have problems with fluctuating blood sugar, be sure to eat some protein with your snack. Try chicken or turkey jerky (without too many preservatives), yogurt, cottage cheese, nuts, and seeds.

Make Your Carbs Complex

Complex carbohydrates such as whole grains, brown rice, and legumes (beans) are metabolized much more slowly in your body than refined carbohydrates.

When you eat refined grains such as white flour and white rice, your body treats them as if they're sugar. If you don't burn them off right away, they directly become fat. When you eat complex carbohydrates, your body tends to use them for energy more slowly, so you have a better chance of burning them off. Complex carbohydrates are also much higher in vitamins and minerals. The refining process strips the fiber and nutrients out of grains.

And watch out: *whole wheat* on a label does not necessarily mean "whole grain." Many whole wheat breads are not much better for you than the infamous Wonder Bread. It's easy to find whole-grain cereals in the supermarket these days—just beware of high levels of salt and sugar.

Potatoes and the new types of whole-wheat pasta and Jerusalem artichoke pasta count as complex carbohydrates, but they tend to be broken down into sugars faster than the others mentioned, so eat them in moderation.

Double the Fiber and Absorb Fewer Fats

You've probably heard a lot about how good fiber is for you. It's true! The American Cancer Society recommends 25 to 30 grams of fiber a day, yet most people get only half of that. Aim for 30 to 35 grams, or approximately 1 ounce of fiber every day, and here's why: fiber speeds up the movement of food through the intestinal tract. The faster the food moves through, the less time there is for your body to absorb fats. Fiber also acts as a whisk broom to sweep the small intestine clean, keeping it free of infection. In the large colon, it absorbs the toxins being removed from the body.

The good news is that increasing your fiber is a piece of cake (so to speak). If you're eating whole foods and plenty of fresh vegetables, it's easy to get your fiber every day. If you're over the age of 50 and need a little help, you can add anywhere from 1 teaspoon to 1 tablespoon of psyllium seed or psyllium husk (pronounced silly-um) to your diet daily. You know this fiber as Metamucil, but unfortunately Metamucil contains sugar or artificial sweeteners and food colorings. Pure psyllium is better for you and it's cheaper. You can buy psyllium in health food stores.

Psyllium is easy to use. Just stir it into juice or water, and drink immediately. Then drink a glass of water immediately afterward. Start with a teaspoon of psyllium, and if necessary work your way up gradually to a tablespoon.

If you have a bowel disorder, check with a doctor first before using psyllium or increasing the fiber in your diet. It's important to add fiber to your diet gradually if you're not used to it, or you could experience gas and bloating.

Step 5: Get Acquainted with Natural Healing Remedies

Over the past few decades, it has become clear that prescription and over-the-counter drugs are not the magic bullets we thought they would be. It's true that these drugs have saved many lives, but it's also increasingly true that they are taking a great many lives and ruining even more with debilitating side effects. One quarter of the elderly population, or 6.6 million people, are taking a drug they should never take. There's a good chance that the side effects of prescription drugs cause many so-called symptoms of aging such as fatigue, forgetfulness, and impotence. Take as few prescription drugs as possible, and learn to treat common problems such as indigestion and allergies with common sense and practical, natural alternatives.

You can avoid the vast majority of prescription drugs simply by following the Six Core Principles for Optimal Health. When you do need to treat a cold, allergy, illness, or symptom of aging, you can nearly always use simple, effective natural remedies and herbs. High blood pressure, high cholesterol, diabetes, prostate troubles, menopause symptoms, allergies, arthritis, indigestion, and many of our other common illnesses can all be avoided with a healthy lifestyle or treated very safely and effectively with natural remedies.

Make a list of all the over-the-counter and prescription medications you're taking. Next to each one, write down the reason you're taking it. Next time you visit your physician, bring the list with you and ask your physician to circle the medications that are really necessary and cross off the ones you could do without. You might be surprised at how many you can do without. When you get home, throw away any crossed off medications.

Next, find the drugs you're taking in this book and read that chapter, especially the section on the natural alternatives. If you decide to go off of a prescription drug and try the natural remedies, please work with a health care professional, especially if you want to stop a drug that could be dangerous to go off of suddenly, such as drugs for heart disease.

If you're not taking any prescription drugs, congratulate yourself. If your physician wants to put you on one, go on the defensive. Ask important questions such as, Exactly what will this drug do? How long will I need to take it? Are there any safe, effective ways to treat this problem without drugs? Is this the lowest dose I can take? What are the side effects?

Step 6: Get on the *Prescription Alternatives* Vitamin and Mineral Plan

The first five Core Principles lay the foundation for your optimal health. But optimal health is more than just not being sick. When you are radiantly healthy, your body becomes a finely tuned instrument beautifully designed to fight off just about anything that comes its way. Nutritional supplements such as vitamins and minerals are health insurance. You are making sure your body has everything it needs to stay balanced and tuned.

A lot of people ask, "Why do I need to take vitamins if I eat well?" First, much of the soil our food is grown in is depleted of essential minerals. Second, by the time food gets on your table, sometimes weeks after it has been picked, it has lost many of its important vitamins, such as vitamin C. Third, our bodies are so assaulted these days by environmental pollutants and stress that we need extra vitamins and minerals to boost our immune systems. And realistically, very few of us eat a truly balanced diet.

You would need to eat huge quantities of fresh, organic produce to get the vitamins and minerals present in a few vitamin supplements. For example, you'd have to drink eight glasses of fresh-squeezed orange juice every day to get just 1,000 mg of vitamin C.

The Basic Plan

Here's the basic program: a high-potency multiple vitamin with minerals (minerals also enable your body to use the vitamins). Be sure to read the label—with many multivitamins you would need to take up to 12 a day to get the amounts listed below. Here's what your daily multivitamin intake should contain:

Vitamins

Vitamin A, 1,000 to 5,000 IU
Beta-carotene as mixed carotenoids, 10,000
    to 15,000 IU

The B vitamins, including:
   B_1 (thiamine), 25 to 100 mg
   B_2 (riboflavin), 25 to 100 mg
   B_3 (niacin), 25 to 100 mg
   B_5 (pantothenic acid), 25 to 100 mg
   B_6 (pyridoxine), 50 to 100 mg
   B_{12}, 1,000 mcg
   Biotin, 100 to 300 mcg
   Choline, 25 to 100 mg
   Folic acid, 400 mcg
   Inositol, 100 to 300 mg
Vitamin C, 100 to 300 mg
Vitamin D, 1,000 to 2,000 IU
Vitamin E as mixed tocopherols and
    tocotrienols, at least 400 IU

Minerals

Boron, 1 to 5 mg
Calcium (citrate, lactate, or gluconate), 100
    to 500 mg
Chromium, 200 to 400 mcg
Copper, 1 to 5 mg
Magnesium (citrate or gluconate), 100 to 500
    mg (women should take a total of 300
    to 400 mg daily)
Manganese (citrate or chelate), 10 mg
Selenium, 200 mcg
Vanadium (sulfate), 25 to 200 mcg
Zinc, 10 to 15 mg

Too Much of a Good Thing?

While taking nutritional supplements is a great form of health insurance, there is such a thing as overdoing it. Nutritional supplements are very concentrated, and as such they put your liver to a lot of work to process them. In nature, nutrients are packaged with protein, starches, fiber, and thousands of phytochemicals, and our bodies have evolved over eons to process nutrients in this form. Taking handfuls of nutritional supplements every day may be counterproductive if it stresses your liver, which is already hard at work processing your food and cleaning toxins from your body. If you feel nauseous or tired after taking vitamins, there's a good chance you're overdoing it. Step back and reevaluate why you're taking each supplement, and eliminate those that aren't necessary. Contemplate how you might improve your diet with more wholesome foods and improve your health with better sleep and more exercise.

Chapter 10

Drugs for Heart Disease and Their Natural Alternatives

Heart disease is one of the leading causes of death in the United States, and heart disease drugs are among the top-selling prescription drugs. Heart disease drugs are also among the most dangerous prescription drugs you can take and are undoubtedly responsible for many thousands of deaths each year.

In spite of the dangers of heart drugs, American doctors continue to prescribe them routinely, without ever seriously addressing the issues of lifestyle and heart disease. Pick almost anyone in North America over the age of 50 off the street, and chances are he or she can tell you the major causes of heart disease: obesity, a high-fat diet, not enough exercise, stress, high cholesterol, and high blood pressure. Right? Well, partially.

There are many ways to measure risks for heart disease. Blood pressure numbers and cholesterol numbers are two ways to measure that risk, but they aren't necessarily the most accurate or most important indicators of heart disease. These indicators are used in Western medicine because there are specific drugs the doctor can prescribe to make the numbers go down. When the numbers go down, does this mean the heart disease is gone? Not at all. If you have existing heart disease or diabetes, or you smoke, drugs that push blood pressure and cholesterol numbers down can reduce your risk of having a heart attack. But they do little to address the underlying causes of your ill health and in fact will bring their very own harmful side effects into the mix and increase your risk of having other health problems.

We now know that other factors such as your homocysteine, C-reactive protein, and antioxidant levels are just as important as cholesterol and blood pressure, if not more so. However, the treatments for bringing down those numbers are available without a prescription and are very inexpensive.

The American Heart Association estimates that the cost of cardiovascular disease in 2006 was $403.1 billion, up from $298 billion in 2001. This includes the cost of physicians and nursing services, hospital and nursing home services, medications, and loss of productivity. The personal cost of heart disease is the biggest loss of all. Yet heart disease is one of the easiest diseases of all to prevent. Even if your parents and grandparents had heart disease, you can still prevent it in yourself.

If heart disease kills more people every year than anything else, why aren't these simple cures being shouted from the rooftops? Why isn't it the biggest topic of discussion on all the talk shows? First of all, it's too simple, too inexpensive, and not nearly dramatic enough for a talk show. Heart disease treatment in the United States, consisting mainly of surgery and drugs, is a multibillion-dollar industry. Why would those with a vested financial interest in heart disease treatment give it up for simple, natural, inexpensive remedies? That means that preventing and treating your heart disease is in your hands. It's your responsibility.

Simple cures seem to be the hardest thing to follow for many people, because they involve a change in lifestyle and daily habits. The only way to cure heart disease is to work on its causes. If you take the initiative to make positive changes in your diet, get some exercise, lose some weight, and take some supplements, you will begin to see improvement in your health very rapidly.

The single biggest factor contributing to heart disease in America is our poor diet. We eat too much unhealthy fat, too many processed foods, too many refined carbohydrates, and not enough fresh vegetables. In the 1950s, the Japanese diet was 16 percent fat, and they had almost no incidence of heart disease. Today their diet is 26 percent fat and includes many more Western foods and fast food, and heart disease is the second leading cause of death in Japan. Estimates are that Americans will spend in the neighborhood of $150 billion on fast food in 2008, up from $110 billion in 2001. The most popular vegetables are potatoes (in the form of French fries) and tomatoes (in the form of ketchup). Portion sizes continue to increase despite the widespread understanding that larger portions mean larger girths and higher risk of heart attack down the line. Although fast food chains have made some effort to offer some healthy meals, even these are overloaded with calories in the form of fat, refined carbohydrates, and sugar.

There is no question that people who eat less meat and more fish, fruits, and vegetables and drink more wine have significantly lower rates of death from heart disease. Those countries with the highest intake of antioxidants and bioflavonoids have the lowest death rates from heart disease. Furthermore, there is a strong correlation between diets high in polyunsaturated fatty acids (vegetable oils prone to oxidation and rancidity) and a high rate of death from heart disease and correspondingly less death from heart disease in those cultures that eat more monounsaturated fats such as olive oil. In fact, a study of 30 men with high cholesterol found that eating olive oil significantly reduced the tendency of their LDL cholesterol to oxidize. This is significant because oxidized LDL cholesterol creates inflammation, which causes plaque to accumulate in the arteries.

Most people who have been diagnosed with heart disease get on a medical treadmill that doesn't stop until the day they die. There are drugs for blood pressure and cholesterol control, all of which have their own uncomfortable side effects; there are the surgeries, including angioplasties and bypass operations; and there is the fear of the next heart attack, the next hospital stay, and, of course, of dying due to this disease.

In this chapter we will primarily cover drugs related to high blood pressure and high cholesterol because they are by far the most widely prescribed drugs in the United States. There are drugs prescribed for other specific symptoms of heart disease such as angina (chest pain caused when not enough blood gets to the heart muscles) and arrhythmias (irregular heartbeat), and they tend to be poorly studied, uniquely dangerous, and apt to cause deadly side effects. If your doctor prescribes a heart drug that's not listed here, be sure to carefully read the complete information sheet on it. If it's a new drug, be aware that many of the drug's side effects and interactions with other drugs are likely unknown and that you are, in effect, a guinea pig.

Should You Be Taking an Aspirin a Day?

If you read the headlines and listen to conventional physicians, you'll be convinced that aspirin is the miracle drug of the century. Not only does it banish pain and reduce inflammation and fever, it prevents heart disease. And now we're hearing that it prevents colon cancer. Yes, aspirin is a wonder drug. For short-term use there's nothing like a couple of aspirin to knock out a headache, to reduce the pain of a sprain, and even to quickly reduce heart disease risk while working on safer and more effective long-term solutions.

Used long-term, aspirin often does more harm than good. It causes gastric bleeding and ulcers, suppresses the immune system, and promotes macular degeneration, an irreversible eye disease that is the leading cause of blindness in the United States. A study published in the *British Medical Journal* found that the risk of gastrointestinal hemorrhage (bleeding) with aspirin doesn't change whether the dose is 50 mg or 1,500 mg. In other words, lowering your dose won't decrease the risk of this adverse effect. Taking buffered aspirin slightly helps counteract these side effects, but not significantly enough to make it safe to take long-term. And while aspirin decreases the risk of some types of strokes, it increases the risk of other types. Research has shown that taking ibuprofen (Motrin, Advil) with aspirin can negate the heart benefits of aspirin.

Aspirin essentially works by blocking the production of hormonelike substances called prostaglandins, which constantly regulate every cell in the body in many of their complex interactions. Some prostaglandins, when made in the body in excess, play a role in promoting heart disease, inflammation, and pain. The fact that aspirin very effectively blocks these prostaglandins would be good news, except that it blocks the formation of both "good" and "bad" prostaglandins, and in the process of suppressing the good prostaglandins, it also suppresses the immune system. (A little aside: Some of aspirin's benefits may also come from the use of magnesium in buffered aspirin, the form most often used in heart disease studies. A little magnesium every day could provide major benefits to the heart.)

While the bad prostaglandins can make your blood more likely to get sticky, clump together, and cause a stroke or heart attack, good prostaglandins lower blood pressure, inhibit blood aggregation and the production of cholesterol, and reduce inflammation reactions. Hmmmm. Sounds like "good" prostaglandins provide the same heart benefits that aspirin does—and they do. Much of heart disease has to do with the fact that bad prostaglandins are outweighing good prostaglandins.

Later in this chapter you'll find natural alternatives to aspirin that can reduce bad prostaglandins and increase good prostaglandins.

Natural Alternatives for Treating Heart Disease

In this section, you'll find general suggestions for preventing and treating heart disease, angina, and irregular heartbeat, and in the sections on high cholesterol and high blood pressure later in the chapter, you'll find specific suggestions for treating the underlying causes of these conditions.

Your number one, most important step in preventing and treating heart disease is to follow the Six Core Principles for Optimal Health. That is your foundation for all-around optimal health. Every single step in the plan is vitally important to a healthy heart.

Here are some further steps for taking care of your heart.

Use Alcohol in Moderation

Moderation is the ideal attitude to have when it comes to drinking alcohol. Studies show that a low alcohol intake, particularly of red wine, protects against heart disease when included as part of a healthy diet. However, even just a bit too much alcohol can bump up blood pressure and help create nutritional deficiencies that increase your risk of heart disease. This is even more true for women than for men.

Make Garlic a Staple of Your Diet

Garlic is the herb of legend and myth. It is mentioned in the Bible, in Homer's *Odyssey*, and in ancient Chinese texts, and it has been found in the tombs of ancient Egyptians. Now we have dozens of scientific studies to back up the folklore claims for garlic's prowess in keeping us healthy.

While garlic may or may not work to ward off vampires, it does a great job at neutralizing three risk factors for heart disease: high blood fats, high blood pressure, and abnormal blood clotting. After raw garlic, the most effective form of garlic appears to be aged extract of organic garlic with a high allicin content, but they all have some beneficial effects.

Keep Your Fibrinogen Low

You may not have heard a lot about fibrinogen as a risk for heart disease, but it is a key factor.

Fibrinogen is a protein substance found in blood that plays an important role in blood clotting. As with so many substances in the body, having enough fibrinogen is essential to good health, but too much can cause disease.

In nearly every study done on heart disease, high levels of fibrinogen in the blood were found to be directly related to coronary artery disease, probably by interfering with blood flow. Excess fibrinogen is also related to atrial fibrillation (rapid heartbeat), strokes, intermittent claudication (pain in the legs when walking), and high blood pressure. Reducing fibrinogen levels may be your single best protection against having a stroke. The good news is that most of the factors that raise or lower fibrinogen are the same ones that raise or lower other risk factors for heart disease.

What Makes Fibrinogen Levels Rise?

- Psychological and mental stress can increase fibrinogen levels.
- High blood sugar raises fibrinogen levels.
- Very high LDL cholesterol levels will raise fibrinogen levels.
- Excess natural estrogens and the synthetic estrogens found in birth control pills and conventional hormone replacement therapy (HRT) raise fibrinogen levels, which makes it ironic that the pharmaceutical industry was making claims that estrogen prevents heart disease—they are no longer allowed to make this claim. (You will read more about estrogens in Chapter 19 on HRT.)
- Smoking has a direct effect on raising fibrinogen levels.
- Obesity significantly raises fibrinogen levels.

What Lowers Fibrinogen Levels?

- Exercise is the single biggest factor in lowering fibrinogen levels.
- A glass of wine with dinner may slightly lower fibrinogen levels.
- Fish oil supplementation may lower fibrinogen levels.
- Eating plenty of garlic lowers fibrinogen.
- Olive oil lowers fibrinogen.
- Vitamin E lowers fibrinogen.
- Nattokinase may help lower fibrinogen.

Nattokinase and Heart Disease

Natto is a fermented soybean food that the Japanese have been eating for centuries. It's a cheese-like food with a distinct odor that is definitely an acquired cultural taste, but it may be one of the keys to the low risk of heart disease among the Japanese. In Japanese culture, various foods are often used as medicines, and natto has long been a popular Asian remedy for those suffering from heart disease.

Nattokinase is an enzyme that is extracted from natto, dried and used as a supplement. It was isolated in the early 1980s by Dr. Hiroyuki Sumi, a Japanese researcher working at the Medical School of the University of Chicago who was looking for a safer medicine that would reduce the blood clots associated with heart attacks and strokes. Subsequent test tube and rodent research has shown that nattokinase powerfully reduces blood clots by, in effect, dissolving fibrin and other substances that promote unhealthy blood clotting. The catch is that in spite of being on the market for many years, no formal, published research has been done with humans showing that nattokinase helps prevent heart attack and stroke. It's widely used among alternative health care professionals, but it would be nice to have the clinical trials to back up the observed benefits, because it's an inexpensive, natural, and safe supplement, unlike blood-thinning drugs such as Coumadin (warfarin).

If you're taking prescription blood thinners such as heparin or coumarin, talk to your doctor before taking nattokinase.

Keep Your Homocysteine Low

In the past few years, it has been very well scientifically documented that high levels of homocysteine, a by-product of metabolism of the amino acid methionine, is an important risk factor in heart disease and strokes associated with narrowed blood vessels. In fact, high homocysteine levels turn out to be a much more accurate marker of heart disease risk than cholesterol or blood pressure.

Researchers currently believe that excess homocysteine damages blood vessels, so it may turn out to be a primary cause of heart disease and not just an indicator. Homocysteine is an amino acid meant to exist only temporarily in the body. In a healthy body, it's quickly transformed into harmless substances. If you have a deficiency of certain B vitamins or a genetic predisposition that interferes with the metabolism of homocysteine, your blood levels will rise, and so will your risk of heart disease and stroke.

Excess homocysteine directly harms the cells that line the insides of the arteries, starting (and encouraging) the process that leads to heart attacks and strokes. In fact, when it's injected into the arteries of experimental animals, homocysteine causes the linings of those arteries to slough off. Eventually, lesions form that look very much like the clogs that form in the arteries of humans with heart disease. High homocysteine also causes the smooth muscle cells that line the artery walls to multiply, thickening them and making them less flexible. It interferes with the activity of blood components that prevent excessive blood clotting, and this sets the stage for clots that can plug up narrowed blood vessels, causing heart attacks, strokes, or thromboembolism (blood clot in the lungs). Excess homocysteine also prevents small arteries from dilating to allow more blood to flow through; it encourages the oxidation of LDL cholesterol, making this "bad" type of cholesterol even more dangerous to blood vessel health; and it generates free radicals. Antioxidants help significantly in reducing the amount of bad cholesterol in the blood, but if homocysteine levels remain high, the damage to arterial walls will continue.

According to a study done at Tufts University School of Medicine in Boston, if your homocysteine levels are just 20 percent above normal, your risk of cardiovascular disease is significantly increased. If your physician wants to measure your homocysteine levels, you should know that a normal homocysteine level is about 12 micromoles per liter (mmol/L), and cardiovascular risk increases at about 14 to 16 mmol/L.

The case for high homocysteine as a significant risk factor for heart disease has become incontrovertible. In fact, it's just as significant—if not more so—than cholesterol levels. One researcher states that homocysteine levels are up to 40 times better at indicating cardiovascular disease risk than cholesterol levels. (Of course, the drug companies can't make nearly as much money selling B vitamin supplements as they can selling statins, so we don't anticipate any major shift from the focus on cholesterol control anytime soon.)

Here are a few examples of the latest studies on the homocysteine–heart disease link:

- In one study, 131 subjects—each with one blocked coronary artery—were compared with about the same number of control subjects who were free of heart disease. With every 10 percent elevation in homocysteine levels came a 10 percent elevation in risk of developing severe coronary artery disease.

- A study of postmenopausal women found that elevations in homocysteine led to a higher incidence of coronary artery disease.
- In a study of people who developed deep vein blood clots, researchers found that subjects who developed them had much higher homocysteine levels than those who didn't.
- A study of 21,500 men between the ages of 35 and 64 found that those with the highest homocysteine (more than 15 mmol/L) were about three times more likely to die of heart disease.
- In another study, 587 men with confirmed heart disease had their homocysteine levels measured and were then followed for 4.6 years. Sixty-four of them died. Of those 64, 3.8 percent had homocysteine levels below 9 mmol/L; 8.6 percent had levels between 9 and 14.9; and 25 percent had levels of 15 or greater.
- In a study published in the *New England Journal of Medicine*, researchers evaluated the effects of homocysteine-lowering folic acid, B_{12}, and B_6 on artery narrowing in men who had required angioplasty to open up at least one clogged heart vessel. The men who took the supplements had lower homocysteine levels after six months, and their arteries were only half as likely to renarrow following their angioplasties.

One much-feared disease that is thought to be related to high homocysteine levels is Alzheimer's disease. This makes sense, because it's likely that the brain deterioration seen with this disease has something to do with the deterioration of blood vessels that feed brain tissues. In a study from Tufts University, researchers measured homocysteine levels in 1,092 subjects over a span of about a decade. Their average age was 76, and none of them had dementia. Eight years later, 111 of them had developed dementia, 83 of them from Alzheimer's disease. (In a few cases, dementia was caused by stroke or other vascular diseases that harm brain tissue.) When the researchers looked back at the homocysteine measurements they had taken, they found that those with homocysteine levels above 14 mmol/L were twice as likely to have developed Alzheimer's several years later than those with average levels. Those who had elevated levels come back from both tests were at the most risk. Milder elevations in homocysteine also caused risk to rise, but not as much. They concluded that if homocysteine were removed from the risk equation for Alzheimer's, 15 percent of cases would be prevented. As baby boomers age, this percentage would add up to tens of thousands of people.

Some drugs can cause high homocysteine levels, particularly those that interfere with folic acid, such as methotrexate, an immunosuppressive drug given to cancer, rheumatoid arthritis, and psoriasis patients; the anticonvulsant drugs phenytoin (Dilantin) and carbamazepine (Tegretol, Epitol); and the bile acid sequestrants for lowering cholesterol levels, cholestipol (Colestid) and cholestyramine (Questran). It's ironic that these cholesterol-lowering drugs, given to reduce heart disease, may actually cause it by raising homocysteine levels!

Other research has shown that homocysteine levels rise when daily folic acid intake is 200 mcg (micrograms) per day or less. This is a typical example of how inadequate the Recommended Daily Allowance (RDA) amounts are, because the current RDA for folate is 200 mcg.

Fortunately for nearly everyone, homocysteine can be easily and inexpensively lowered by taking some B vitamins. If you're taking a daily multivitamin that includes 400 mcg of folic acid, 50 mg of vitamin B_6, and 1,000 mcg of vitamin B_{12}, you should be covered. If your homocysteine levels are high, you should be getting an additional 200 mg daily of vitamin B_6 (pyridoxine) and 1 to 4 mg of folic acid daily until your homocysteine levels are back to normal.

Since a deficiency of vitamin B_{12} can also indirectly raise homocysteine levels, and since a high intake of folic acid can mask a vitamin B_{12} deficiency, make sure your intake of vitamin B_{12} is at least 1,000 mcg per day. Vitamin B_{12} is best taken sublingually (under the tongue) or as a nasal gel or spray. Low thyroid levels and excess alcohol can also raise homocysteine levels.

If your doctor asks you to get blood tests for heart disease, be sure to ask him or her to include homocysteine.

Keep Your C-Reactive Protein Low, Too

Inflammation is a necessary part of the immune system's response to infection or injury. It leads to the development of redness, heat, and swelling, and if it's properly controlled by the body, it breaks down damaged tissues and makes way for new, healthy tissue. In a body where prostaglandins are chronically out of balance, inflammation can easily run amok, harming healthy tissues.

Measuring the levels of a substance called C-reactive protein accurately indicates the amount of inflammatory activity going on deep within the body. Several studies involving tens of thousands of people have strongly linked high levels of C-reactive protein—a natural part of the

inflammatory response—with increased risk of dying of a heart attack. This connection makes good sense, because the formation of plaques in arteries involves inflammation, and high levels of inflammation have been found to make plaques prone to rupture or pinch off clots that can then clog arteries. It also makes sense because obesity, smoking, high blood pressure, and chronic periodontal disease all increase both cardiac risk and C-reactive protein levels. Some experts believe that the effects of statins, aspirin, and other nonsteroidal anti-inflammatory drugs (NSAIDs) on heart disease risk have more to do with their effects on inflammation than with their effects on cholesterol or blood clotting. The synthetic estrogens used in conventional HRT also increase C-reactive protein, which may explain why they don't help prevent heart disease. An article about C-reactive protein in the *New England Journal of Medicine* concluded, ". . . C-reactive protein level is a stronger predictor of cardiovascular events than the LDL cholesterol level."

Like other so-called cardiac "risk factors," high C-reactive protein is more an indicator of heart disease than a cause. To keep inflammation and C-reactive protein under control, balance your prostaglandins, shed excess pounds, and control high blood pressure (for more on how to do this, keep reading). Vitamin E and fish oil supplements can help lower C-reactive protein.

Get Plenty of Magnesium

Arnold is a fairly healthy guy in his mid-sixties who wound up in a hospital emergency room in the middle of the night, frightened and in pain, wondering if he was having a heart attack. It turned out he was suffering from a type of angina that causes spasms of the heart muscle. After giving him some drugs and monitoring him for a few hours, the doctors sent him home that night, telling him to make an appointment with his physician.

A few weeks later, Arnold's angina pain was returning, and his physician wanted to put him on a drug called a beta-blocker. Now Arnold takes pretty good care of himself (he does have a weakness for good ice cream), hates going to the physician, and really dislikes taking drugs. Finally he got the name of a physician using alternative health care approaches, who gave him some intravenous magnesium and prescribed a daily magnesium supplement. Not only did Arnold's angina pain totally disappear after the intravenous magnesium, but his energy level was higher than it had been in years. This was a happy guy!

The essential mineral that's the biggest key to prevention and treatment of heart disease is magnesium. Several recent studies have shown that if people who come into an emergency room with a heart attack are given intravenous magnesium right away, their chances of survival go way up, and if they continue to receive it, their survival rate continues to improve. It has been shown to help with angina and to improve the symptoms of congestive heart failure (CHF).

Magnesium works on several levels to keep the heart in good working order:

• **Prevents muscle spasms.** According to several Japanese studies published in the *American Journal of Cardiology*, the oxygen deficiency and spasms caused by magnesium deficiency narrows the coronary arteries, leading to angina. A great deal of angina pain could be relieved simply by bringing magnesium levels up to normal.

• **Keeps blood flowing smoothly.** Magnesium helps keep the blood from getting "sticky," a condition that can contribute to having a stroke.

• **Keeps cholesterol under control.** Another Japanese study found that patients with low HDL ("good") cholesterol had low magnesium levels and when they took magnesium supplements their HDL levels increased. In addition, animal studies have shown that when magnesium is deficient, the amount of oxidized LDL cholesterol increases, with a corresponding increase in arterial damage.

• **Maintains normal blood pressure.** At least 28 independent studies have shown that patients with hypertension (high blood pressure) have a magnesium deficiency. People who have long-term high blood pressure have magnesium levels that average at 15 percent below normal.

• **Keeps the heartbeat regular.** A magnesium deficiency can lead to irregular heartbeat (arrhythmia). If you're on the medication digitalis to treat heart disease, the medication can be toxic if you are deficient in potassium or magnesium.

It looks like magnesium is involved in just about every aspect of keeping a healthy heart, yet most Americans are deficient in this essential mineral. A large survey done by the U.S. Department of Agriculture found that only 25 percent of 37,785 individuals had magnesium intakes at or greater than the RDA, which is too low to begin with. Some 20 to 65 percent of critically ill hospitalized patients have a magnesium deficiency. A normal blood serum magnesium test will not give you an accurate indication of your magnesium levels. It's more accurate (and unfortunately more expensive) to measure intracellular magnesium levels.

Early symptoms of a magnesium deficiency can include muscle and nerve pain and an irregular heartbeat. A magnesium deficiency can also create potassium and calcium deficiency. Magnesium can be depleted by stress, excessive alcohol, sugar, diabetes, kidney disease, chronic diarrhea, not enough protein in the diet, too much protein in the diet, and thyroid disorders. Many researchers believe that alcoholics are at a much greater risk for heart disease because in excess, alcohol severely depletes magnesium.

Drugs That Deplete Magnesium

Aminoglycosides	Cisplatin
Corticosteroids	Cyclosporine
Diuretics	Foscarnet
Gentamicin	Pentamidine

Good food sources of magnesium include whole grains (especially oats, brown rice, millet, buckwheat, and wheat), legumes (lentils, split peas, and beans), bran, almonds and peanuts, and broccoli. Chocolate contains large amounts of magnesium, and a craving for chocolate may be an indicator of a magnesium deficiency.

Magnesium by itself can cause diarrhea, so unless you are constipated, be sure to take it in a multivitamin, in combination with calcium, or in the form of magnesium glycinate, gluconate, or citrate. You can take 300 to 400 mg of magnesium daily as a supplement.

Antioxidants, Antioxidants, Antioxidants

When a squirt of lemon juice helps food stay fresh, it is working as an antioxidant, protecting against the harmful effects of oxygen. Oxygen harmful? When an oxygen molecule loses an electron, it becomes an unstable molecule called a free radical, which tries to stabilize itself by grabbing another electron from a molecule of any body substance or tissue nearby, causing that molecule in turn to become unstable. Antioxidants are molecules that can donate an oxygen molecule to the free radical without becoming destabilized themselves.

This process of free radical creation is called oxidation, a normal and important part of your body's metabolism. It's when oxidation reactions overwhelm your body's ability to stabilize them that they do damage. Oxidation does damage when we're under a lot of stress, exposed to a heavy load of toxins, or don't have enough antioxidants in our diet.

Out-of-control oxidation is a causative factor in illness, including heart disease and strokes. Today's polluted world means our bodies have to cope with far higher levels of free radicals than ever before. Free radical culprits include smog, cigarette smoke, pesticides, and food additives. The average American doesn't eat nearly enough antioxidant-rich fresh fruits and vegetables to counteract these environmental toxins. Our bodies are in double oxidant jeopardy, which makes taking antioxidant supplements an important part of preventing heart disease.

Antioxidants come in many forms, from teas and herbal tinctures to foods and vitamins. Their marvelous power gives a shielding, protective effect against heart disease. Some work better than others to protect against heart disease.

Ginkgo biloba extract (GBE) is made from the tree of the same name. It is particularly rich in antioxidant substances that act synergistically. One of its properties leads to improvement in circulation to the heart. As might be expected, it also reduces oxidized LDL cholesterol levels and lowers LDL cholesterol generally. In addition, it raises "good" HDL cholesterol and lowers blood fat levels.

Ginkgo biloba can take from a few weeks to a month to produce its beneficial effects. GBE with at least 24 percent ginkgoflavonglycosides is the best form to take. Standardized, semipurified, and concentrated, GBE provides consistent levels of its most active compounds. Take the recommended dosage on the package.

Glutathione (GSH) is a tripeptide made from the amino acids cysteine, glycine, and glutamic acid. This humble little protein is found in the cells of nearly all living organisms on Earth, and its primary job is waste disposal. GSH has three main detox jobs in the body:

1. When there are free radicals lurking about, threatening to start an oxidation reaction, GSH catches them, neutralizes them, passes them on (often to another antioxidant such as vitamin E), and begins the cycle anew.
2. In the liver, GSH latches on to toxic substances and binds to them so the liver can excrete them without being damaged.
3. GSH prevents red blood cells from being damaged by neutralizing unstable forms of oxygen. We cannot survive without this miraculous antioxidant.

GSH's antioxidant work is the frontline defense for preventing oxidation of LDL cholesterol, which damages the arteries. It also protects the lymphatic system and the digestive system from an overload of unstable lipids (fats and oils). If glutathione levels drop anywhere in the body, the burden of toxic stress goes up.

GSH is one of the most abundant substances in the body, and as long as we have a good supply of its building block cysteine (the other building blocks, glycine and glutamic acid, are rarely in short supply) and its cofactor selenium, it will be hard at work doing its detoxifying chores. GSH levels drop

as we age and can be depleted by an overload of rancid oils (such as polyunsaturated and partially hydrogenated vegetable oils), overexposure to poisons such as pesticides, and pharmaceutical drugs that stress the liver, which is to say virtually all prescription drugs. Since glutathione often passes off its neutralized waste products to antioxidants such as vitamin C and vitamin E, a deficiency of these vitamins can impair its function.

Measuring GSH levels is expensive at this time, but if you have heart disease, are at a high risk for it, or have high LDL cholesterol levels, try raising your GSH levels. The best way to raise GSH levels is by taking a cysteine supplement, preferably in the more stable form of N-acetyl cysteine (NAC). Follow the directions on the container for dosages. Foods with high levels of cysteine include onions, garlic, yogurt, wheat germ, and red meat.

Green tea is a polyphenol, an aromatic, organic compound that acts as a potent antioxidant in the body. Like others in this family, it prevents the oxidation of LDL cholesterol, lowers cholesterol, raises "good" HDL levels, and lowers triglyceride levels. It also reduces blood coagulation and helps prevent the clumping of red blood cells, both good steps for the prevention of heart disease. Green tea extract is available in tablet form, without caffeine.

PCOs are procyanidolic oligomers, which are bioflavonoids found in grape seeds, lemon tree bark, peanuts, cranberries, and citrus peels. Known to improve circulation, PCOs strengthen blood vessel walls and prevent the clumping of blood-clotting substances, protecting against stroke. These properties come on top of PCOs' very strong antioxidant powers that preempt LDL oxidation.

To address high cholesterol with PCOs, 150 to 300 mg per day is recommended. Otherwise,

50 mg of PCOs daily makes a good supplement if you're over 50. Many studies have shown that PCO extract from grape seed is one of the most powerful antioxidants known. It also increases the performance of other antioxidants.

Vitamin D is an essential vitamin that is easily kept at healthy levels with regular exposure to sunshine. Unfortunately, thanks to intensive marketing by the sunblock industry, we have become sun-phobic in Western countries. Dozens of studies on vitamin D have been published in the past few years, and we now know that vitamin D is a must for good heart health and reducing the risk of stroke. In one study, men who were vitamin D deficient had a 63 percent higher risk of heart disease.

Sunshine is perfectly safe unless you get a sunburn. There is no solid evidence that normal sun exposure increases the risk of skin cancer and melanoma. The biggest risk factors for skin cancer and melanoma are having fair skin and getting sunburned. Thus the key is to enjoy the sun every day if possible, but to cover up and apply sunblock before you become burned.

For those who live in colder, cloudier, northern climates or who just can't get out in the sun enough, it's probably a good idea to take a vitamin D supplement. The RDA of 400 IU is clearly too low. It was put in place before Americans became sun-phobic. Vitamin D is a fat-soluble vitamin and as such can accumulate in the body and become toxic, so there has been justifiable concern about taking too much. Now that we have more research, it seems clear that we can safely take 2,000 IU daily in the D_3 cholecalciferol form to maintain our vitamin D levels. If your doctor wants to ratchet up your vitamin D levels quickly with large doses, be sure to test levels regularly. Check the "Resources and Rec-

ommended Reading" section in the back of the book for how to get a vitamin D test.

Vitamin E is your greatest ally and protector when it comes to vitamins and heart health; yet most people are deficient in vitamin E. In one study, the vitamin E intake of elderly, affluent Americans was less than three-quarters of the RDA.

Impressive results were shown in two major Harvard University studies of health professionals. A survey of over 39,000 male professionals showed that they enjoyed a 37 percent lower risk of coronary artery disease when they took 100 IU or more of vitamin E daily. The Nurses' Health Study of 87,000 women showed a 40 percent lower risk of heart disease for women on the same dose of vitamin E. More recent research has given us conflicting data about whether vitamin E helps prevent heart disease. However, nutrition studies show that without a doubt, eating foods high in vitamin E is protective.

A European population study looked at 100 apparently healthy men between ages 40 and 49 years old. Blood levels of vitamin E were found to be the most important risk factor for heart disease, even beyond smoking. There is evidence, too, that vitamin E can dissolve clots, helps the heart pump more efficiently, naturally makes arteries widen, and increases the oxygen available in the blood.

Vitamin E is a fat-soluble oil found in many foods, including unrefined vegetable oils, whole grains, butter, organ meats, eggs, a variety of nuts, sunflower seeds, fruit, soybeans, and dark green, leafy vegetables.

If you're going to take vitamin E supplements, we recommend that you take it in the form of mixed tocopherols and tocotrienols. These various forms of vitamin E occur together in food sources, and supplements that contain all of them are closer to what exists in nature. Studies from the University of Sweden in Uppsala and elsewhere have shown that when mixed, these various forms of vitamin E have much greater antioxidant power than d-alpha-tocopherol—generally known as natural vitamin E—alone. Do not use the synthetic form of vitamin E, called dl-alpha-tocopherol.

Although vitamin E is very safe even at high doses, 400 IU (dry form) daily should be an adequate dose for adults. The dry or succinate form is recommended for anyone sensitive to oils or with problems absorbing nutrients (if you're over the age of 65, you probably fall into the latter category). Vitamin E works well taken with its partners in the body, the nutrients vitamin C, beta-carotene and other flavonoids, and selenium.

Natural Remedies for a Stronger Heart

Natural remedies for strengthening the heart tend to help significantly with symptoms such as arrhythmia and angina, and can also make a big difference in people with CHF. Three of the most effective remedies are CoQ10, hawthorn berries, and carnitine.

Coenzyme Q10 (CoQ10)

CoQ10 has been shown to protect and strengthen the heart and lower blood pressure. CoQ10 is a vital enzyme, a catalyst to the production of energy in the mitochondria of our cells. Without it, our cells simply won't work. Its chemical name is ubiquinone or ubiquinol—it is ubiquitous, or everywhere, where there is life. Its levels in the human body are highest in the heart and liver. When we are ill or stressed, and as we age, our bodies are less able to produce CoQ10.

According to a study done by CoQ10 expert Karl Folkers, published in the *International Journal of Vitamin and Nutrition Research*, patients with a variety of cardiac disorders consistently demonstrate a blood deficiency of CoQ10. A double-blind Japanese study with 100 patients who had cardiac failure showed that only 30 mg per day of CoQ10 for two to four weeks produced a measurable improvement in symptoms. Many older people whose heart function has degenerated and who try CoQ10 report an almost immediate boost in their energy levels.

People who suffer from angina report that the pain disappears and they can exercise. In a double-blind placebo study using CoQ10 and other drugs traditionally used to treat angina, it was found that CoQ10 was far more effective in reducing or eliminating angina pain than any of the other medications. Other studies have shown that people on heart medications can greatly reduce their dosage of medicine if it is combined with CoQ10.

Statin drugs, which are being taken by millions of people to control high cholesterol, deplete the body's stores of CoQ10. In other words, by taking a drug that's supposed to reduce the risk of heart disease, these millions of people may actually be increasing their risk. If you have to take a statin drug, be sure to supplement with CoQ10.

This nutrient is also a valuable natural therapy for periodontal disease. Following the dosage instructions at the end of this section can have the fringe benefit of clearing up inflamed gums. Interestingly, people with chronic periodontal disease have significantly higher risk of heart disease. Some research indicates that this connection has to do with elevated inflammatory levels throughout the body, but it may also have to do with CoQ10 depletion.

In 2006 a new form of CoQ10 called ubiquinol became available. Ubiquinol is the more active and thus more bioavailable (more easily used) form of CoQ10, but it is very unstable and reverts back to ubiquinone when exposed to light and air. A Japanese company named Kaneka developed a method for stabilizing ubiquinol so it could be added to supplements. Within a year of making it available to the public, nearly every major vitamin company had incorporated some ubiquinol into its CoQ10 supplements. Although there are no formal or independently published clinical studies on ubiquinol yet, published research by Kaneka shows that ubiquinol raises CoQ10 levels in the blood eight to ten times more effectively than ubiquinone. An unpublished clinical trial in Texas with end-stage CHF patients who took ubiquinol for three months showed that it improved their cardiac function and may have extended life span.

Dosages for both forms of CoQ10 can range from 30 mg as a maintenance dose in a multivitamin to 400 mg daily of ubiquinone or 200 mg daily of ubiquinol for those with heart disease.

Hawthorn Berries (*Crataegus oxyacantha*)

Hawthorn berries have been used as a heart tonic for centuries and are widely used in Europe for angina and for lowering blood pressure. They are rich in bioflavonoids, which help strengthen the blood vessels. They are also a vasodilator, which increases the flow of blood and oxygen to the heart, lowers blood pressure, and strengthens the heart muscle. An analysis of studies on hawthorn showed that it offers significant relief from the symptoms of heart failure.

Hawthorn berries work gradually, and you may not notice a difference for a month or so. You can find hawthorn berry extract in capsule or tincture forms. Because the amounts vary widely, follow directions for use on the bottle. Some of the tinctures can be very powerful, so it is very important that you work with your doctor if you're already on heart medicine. However, in and of themselves, hawthorn berries are non-toxic and very safe.

Carnitine

This amino acid is another heart-strengthening nutrient that appears to be especially useful for treating angina and CHF. You can take 500 mg twice a day, preferably between meals.

Use L-Arginine with Caution

L-arginine is an amino acid that is the precursor of nitric oxide (NO), which plays a role in relaxing blood vessels and helps keep the lining of blood vessels healthy. There have been small studies with CHF and angina patients showing that L-arginine increased exercise tolerance and improved quality of life. However, a small government-sponsored study (National Institutes of Health) that compared L-arginine supplementation with a placebo in patients who recently had a heart attack found that more of those taking L-arginine died during the study. The numbers were very small but still statistically significant. L-arginine is, in general, a very safe supplement, but taking high doses of any one amino acid can have effects on many other systems of the body. Until more research has been done with high-dose amino acids, it would be wise to use them only under the care of an experienced health care professional.

Ban Pesticides from Your Life

Chronic exposure to pesticides is a known heart disease risk, but it is one that most people never think of when they have their lawn doused with chemicals, spray their garden, go after bugs in the house with a can of spray, or have their house fumigated. If you're pouring poisons down gopher or mole holes, or dousing your aphids with pesticides and your dog with flea dip, you're exposing yourself and your heart, not to mention your dog, to unacceptable levels of poisons.

These poisons may not kill you on the spot, but they will create free radical damage in your tissues and accumulate in the body. A study done of agricultural workers in the Ukraine showed that those frequently exposed to pesticides had a higher rate of heart disease as well as a higher rate of miscarriages and birth defects. There is also evidence that fetal exposure to pesticides can cause congenital heart disease.

Pesticides aren't the only toxins that can cause heart disease. Other toxins found in the workplace and in the garage include solvents, glues, and other binding materials, dyes, lacquers, paints, PCBs (polychlorinated biphenyls), metals, and vinylchloride. In many cases, workers only need to be exposed to fumes or dust from these materials to increase their risk of heart disease. For women, nail polish and

Reduce Your Exposure to Toxins

Here are some tips for reducing your exposure to pesticides and other environmental toxins:

• Control fleas on your pets and in your home with substances such as boric acid compounds (now found in most pet stores, or contact Fleabusters) and aromatic oils such as pennyroyal, rather than flea powders. (Women who are pregnant should not have direct contact with pennyroyal oil.)

• If you're a gardener, do it the organic way. There are plenty of books and magazines on the subject, and local classes are easy to find. You can create a beautiful lawn and garden without chemicals, and in the long run you'll have far fewer pest problems.

• Don't drink tap water if you have a city or county water supply. Get a good water filter, at least for the tap, that will remove heavy metals and pesticides.

• If you are exposed to pesticides, take a cool shower and drink plenty of clean water to help flush out the poisons.

• Wash, peel, or even scrub fruits and vegetables well, and eat organic produce whenever possible.

• If you think something at work is making you sick, pursue it. It could be mold or fungus in the heating or cooling system, fumes from wall paneling or carpets, or a coworker's liberally applied cologne or perfume. Virtually all perfumes and scented products, which we refer to as "fakegrances," are made from a nasty brew of chemicals, many of them toxic.

• Stop using fungicides, herbicides, and pesticides. Get out of the habit of blasting indoor and outdoor pests with a can of spray. Learn how to control pests naturally.

• Don't move in next door to an agricultural field or orchard unless you know it's organic and likely to stay that way.

nail polish remover are common and little-recognized sources of potentially damaging toxins.

Don't take it for granted that just because you buy a pesticide, herbicide, fungicide, cleaning solvent, paint, or other chemical from the hardware store it's safe. The industries that use these substances are largely unregulated. Thousands of these products on the shelves have *never* been tested for safety. In fact, you should assume they are harmful unless you find out otherwise, and avoid contact with skin and avoid breathing the fumes. Even such simple household chemicals as ammonia and chlorine can be harmful.

Try Not to Use Combination Drugs

Some drugs combine different types of heart drugs. It is not advisable to take the combination heart drugs; they have a terrible track record for dangerous side effects. It's difficult enough to combine and track the effects and side effects of heart drugs without putting them all in one pill. If they come in separate pills, you can take more or less of one (with your physician's supervision), and if you're experiencing side effects, it's easier to track down a cause. Remember, side effects are never your fault, and you should never feel you just have to suffer them. Furthermore, treating side effects with more drugs is a dangerous practice that conscientious doctors do not engage in.

A perfect example of this is Vytorin, a combination pill of the cholesterol-lowering drugs ezetimibe (Zetia) and simvastatin (Zocor), which lower cholesterol through different mechanisms. Recent research published in the *New England Journal of Medicine* revealed that although this drug combination does lower cholesterol, it doesn't reduce the risk of heart attack and stroke and may even speed up the buildup of plaque in the arteries. Other research shows that Vytorin may increase the risk of cancer. This information was not released by the drug company until two years after it was discovered, giving the manufacturers plenty of time to aggressively promote it on TV and rake in nearly $5 billion in sales of Vytorin in 2007 alone. This is a good example of a drug that was approved because it lowers cholesterol—without the long-term studies that would have shown whether it reduces the risk of heart disease.

Drugs for Arrhythmia, Angina, and CHF

Arrhythmia and angina (pain in the chest area) are symptoms of heart disease. They are together here because the drugs used to treat them are often the same.

Examples of Cardiac Glycosides (Digitalis Drugs)

Digoxin (Cardoxin, Digitek, Lanoxicaps, Lanoxin)

What Do They Do in the Body? The digitalis drugs are derived from the plants *Digitalis purpurea* and *Digitalis lanata*, otherwise known as foxglove. Although an exact description of their action on the heart is complicated and technical, in essence what they do is make the heartbeat strong and increase the heart's ability to pump blood.

What Are They Prescribed For? CHF and irregular heartbeat (arrhythmia).

What Are the Possible Side Effects? Although the digitalis drugs are used to treat irregular heartbeat, they can also cause it. Other adverse effects can include nausea, vomiting, loss of appetite, diarrhea, and stomach pain.

The primary danger of these drugs is too high a dose. The optimal dose and a toxic dose are not far apart with these drugs. Since the dosage can be inadvertently increased in many ways, overdosage is a very real concern. A long list of drugs can slow the clearance of digitalis drugs from the body or increase the effects of digitalis drugs. People taking this medication need to be very alert to what they are eating and drinking.

The early symptoms of an overdosage are nausea, vomiting, diarrhea, stomach pain, and loss of appetite. Other symptoms include headache, weakness, fatigue, sleepiness, confusion, restlessness, visual disturbances such as blurred vision, depression, skin rash, hives, irregular heartbeat, and gynecomastia. Your physician should be notified if you have any of these symptoms.

What Are the Interactions with Other Drugs? To be on the safe side, those who take the digitalis drugs should not take any prescription, over-the-counter, or herbal medicine without first checking for possible interactions.

What Are the Interactions with Food? Food in general slows the absorption rate of digitalis drugs but doesn't necessarily decrease levels. In other words, you'll get the same dose, but it will be delivered more slowly. However, a high-fiber meal can actually reduce the dose of a digitalis drug by carrying some of it through the intestines unabsorbed. High-carbohydrate meals may slow absorption more than balanced meals. High-fat meals may cause the body to reabsorb the drug, slightly increasing levels.

What Nutrients Do They Throw out of Balance or Interact With? The digitalis drugs increase the excretion of magnesium and potassium.

What Else to Take While Taking These Drugs. Be sure to take a good mineral supplement if you're taking digitalis drugs. Low potassium combined with high digitalis can be a deadly combination, causing irregular heartbeats, so it's

especially important to keep your potassium levels high by eating potassium-rich foods such as bananas, nuts, avocados, figs, prunes, tomatoes, and meat.

Along with diuretics, laxatives and licorice root can also deplete potassium.

Examples of Nitrates/Nitrites

Amyl nitrite

Isosorbide dinitrate (Isordil, Sorbitrate, Isosorbide, Dilatrate)

Isosorbide mononitrate (Monoket, ISMO, Imdur)

Nitroglycerin (Nitrostat, Nitrolingual, Nitrogard, Nitrong, Nitro-Bid, Nitrocine, Nitroglyn, Minitran, Nitrodisc, Deponit, Nitro-Dur, Nitrol)

There are no specific natural alternatives to these drugs. In other words, if you have such severe angina that not taking one of these drugs could put your life in jeopardy, it's important to keep taking it while you work to reduce your angina symptoms naturally. Since these drugs are most often taken only when an angina attack occurs, you'll naturally wean yourself off them as your angina is reduced. These drugs are somewhat outdated as heart attack and angina preventives; if you're taking daily doses whether or not you have an angina attack, ask your physician about switching to a safer drug.

What Do They Do in the Body? Reduce or relieve spasms in the heart muscle, thereby dilating blood vessels and lowering blood pressure.

What Are They Prescribed For? Angina attacks.

What Are the Possible Side Effects? Postural hypotension (feeling dizzy or faint when you stand from a sitting or lying position) can be a dangerous and possibly fatal side effect. These drugs can also damage organs. Other side effects include aggravation of some types of angina (chest pain) and some types of glaucoma, and they may cause severe headaches, blurred vision, and dry mouth.

Adverse reactions can include nausea, vomiting, diarrhea, heartburn, involuntary passing of urine and feces, impotence, urinary frequency, anxiety, restlessness, agitation, weakness, dizziness, fainting, rebound angina and hypertension, irregular heartbeat, insomnia, pounding heart, rash, flushing, twitching muscles, joint aches, bronchitis, sinus infection, sweating, and water retention.

CAUTION!

Think Twice About Taking These Drugs If . . .

- You have existing hypotension.
- You have kidney or liver disease.
- You have glaucoma.

What Are the Interactions with Other Drugs? Nitrates may reduce the effects of heparin, an antiocoagulant. Nitrates may interact dangerously with Viagra and other drugs for erectile dysfunction.

Alcohol, aspirin, and calcium channel blockers may increase the effects or prolong the action of nitrates.

Drugs for Preventing Strokes and Blood Clots

Examples of Blood Thinners

Coumarins: warfarin (Coumadin, Jantoven), anisindione (Miradon)
Heparins: enoxaparin (Lovenox), dalteparin (Fragmin)
Thienopyridine derivatives: clopidogrel (Plavix), ticlopidine (Ticlid)

What Do They Do in the Body? They are known as anticoagulants or blood thinners, and although their actions are complicated, in essence they thin the blood, reduce its stickiness, and reduce its tendency to clot.

What Are They Prescribed For? To reduce the risk of stroke or blood clots, for treatment after a stroke or heart attack; they are sometimes prescribed during or after surgery. Anticoagulants have been in the news because of overdoses of heparin given to premature infants prescribed anticoagulants to flush out IV catheters, and because a tainted batch of heparin from China was linked to multiple deaths and hundreds of allergic reactions.

What Are the Possible Side Effects? The major risk in taking the anticoagulants is that they will work too well and not allow the blood to clot when it needs to, causing a hemorrhage or uncontrolled bleeding. This can happen internally or externally. The anticoagulants are also affected by a wide range of other drugs, making dangerous drug interactions common. Easy bruising, nosebleeds, dark urine, and tarry or red stools may be the first signs of too high a dose or uncontrolled bleeding. People with bleeding ulcers can die if given anticoagulants.

A study published in the *New England Journal of Medicine* that compared patients taking aspirin and esomeprazole (Nexium, which blocks stomach acid) with those taking clopidogrel (Plavix) and esomeprazole found significantly more bleeding ulcers in the patients taking the clopidogrel.

CAUTION!

Think Twice About Taking These Drugs If . . .

- You have a bleeding ulcer.
- You have adrenal insufficiency.

- You have heavy bleeding during menstruation.
- You have liver or kidney problems.
- You have diarrhea.

Women and the elderly are more sensitive to these drugs.

What Are the Interactions with Other Drugs? If you are taking anticoagulants, do not take any new drug, even over-the-counter drugs, or supplements of any kind without checking first with your physician or pharmacist. Especially avoid NSAIDs (nonsteroidal anti-inflammatory drugs), which can cause gastrointestinal bleeding that can quickly spiral out of control under the influence of anticoagulants. Any product that contains salicylates should be used only with the supervision of your doctor, including aspirin, Pepto-Bismol, arthritis rubs that contain wintergreen oil (methyl salicylate), and wine. Specific supplements that may interact dangerously with anticoagulants include St. John's wort, gingko biloba, feverfew, fenugreek, chitosan, and nattokinase.

Vitamin K can also increase the effect of these drugs, and some doctors will warn patients to be careful about foods that contain vitamin K, especially dark, leafy greens such as kale, spinach, collards, and beet greens. This is backward! You should be encouraged to eat these foods, and the drug dose should be lowered.

The list of specific over-the-counter and prescription drugs that can interact dangerously with anticoagulants is pages long. The bottom line is that if you're taking an anticoagulant, make sure all health care professionals you're working with are reminded of this fact when they recommend you take any medicine, herb, vitamin, or other supplement.

What Are the Interactions with Food? Alcohol can increase the time it takes to clear anti-coagulants from the body, increasing the risk of bleeding. Over time, the opposite can happen: the drug may be cleared out faster than usual.

Cooking oils that contain silicone additives, such as sprays, may bind with these drugs and decrease their absorption. Eating a lot of foods very high in vitamin K could theoretically block the actions of these drugs. Foods high in vitamin K include dark, leafy green vegetables, lettuces, potatoes, fish and fish oils, fruits (especially citrus fruits), egg yolks, dairy products, and the cruciferous family of vegetables, including broccoli, cauliflower, cabbage, and brussels sprouts. Onions, garlic, and soy foods may increase the action of anticoagulants. If you eat lots of vegetables, don't stop just because you're taking this drug! Have your physician adjust the drug levels accordingly.

Don't drink tonic water if you are taking an anticoagulant. It contains an ingredient called quinine that can enhance the action of anticoagulants.

What Nutrients Do They Throw out of Balance or Interact With? Anticoagulants may attach to the metals in mineral supplements and not be absorbed. Take them separately from mineral supplements. Vitamin C interferes with the action of these drugs, reducing their effects. Vitamin E, which by itself "thins" the blood, may increase the effects of anticoagulants, although to date no studies have shown that it's harmful to combine vitamin E and anticoagulants.

Natural Alternatives to Drugs for Treating Strokes and Blood Clots

Your foundation for preventing strokes and blood clots is to follow the Six Core Principles for Optimal Health and the guidelines earlier in the chapter for a healthy heart. Especially important are getting plenty of exercise, drinking plenty of water, avoiding "bad" fats and oils, and keeping blood pressure moderate.

A stroke can be caused by either a blood vessel breaking or a blood clot blocking a blood vessel. Estrogens, including those used in birth control pills and for HRT, greatly increase the risk of some types of strokes. See Chapter 19 for natural approaches to HRT.

Garlic, onions, berries, and fish are foods that keep the blood and blood vessels healthy. The most important supplements for strong blood vessels are the bioflavonoids, including grapeseed extract, rutin, hesperidin, ginkgo biloba, green tea, and bilberry. Supplements important for healthy, "slippery" blood (follow dosage recommendations for daily vitamins in this book) include magnesium, vitamin B_6, folic acid, vitamin B_{12}, vitamin E, selenium, N-acetyl cysteine, lysine, and garlic.

If you have high levels of vitamin C, your risk of dying from a stroke may be half that of those with lower levels. This is according to a major study published in the *British Medical Journal* that tracked 730 elderly men and women for twenty years. Low levels of vitamin C were a strong predictor of death from stroke.

Some Drugs Delay Stroke Recovery

A stroke causes damage to the brain that can often be reversed with time and physical therapy. But it can be a long, slow, difficult road to healing, and those who are on that journey should be given every advantage. That's why you should know that some drugs can actually slow recovery after a stroke. The brain is particularly vulnerable after a stroke, and a recovering stroke patient shouldn't be given any drugs that aren't absolutely necessary.

According to a study done at North Carolina's Duke University that analyzed 96 stroke patients, 37 of them who were taking drugs such as benzodiazepines (Valium, Serax, Ativan, Xanax, etc.) took significantly longer to recover. In fact, even one dose of a drug such as the dopamine antagonist haloperidol (Haldol) can delay recovery by as much as two weeks. These human studies were a follow-up to animal studies that demonstrated the same result. Other drugs that appeared to delay recovery included prochlorperazine (another dopamine antagonist), antihypertension drugs such as clonidine and prazosin, and anticonvulsant drugs such as phenytoin and phenobarbital.

Having a stroke can be a very frightening and disorienting experience, but sedatives should not be used unless it's absolutely necessary. Before you resort to prescription drug sedatives, try some of the natural antianxiety remedies such as kava and St. John's wort.

Your first attempts at reassuring and calming a stroke victim should be the best sedatives of all: loving, supportive family and friends, gentle massage, humor, beautiful music, a good view out the window, good nutrition, and competent medical care and physical therapy.

Drugs to Lower High Blood Pressure

The dangers of high blood pressure (hypertension) have been extremely well publicized over the past decade. It's the dreaded silent killer, with no symptoms until you've got CHF, drop dead of a heart attack, or suffer a stroke. According to *Pharmacy Times*, drugs to treat high blood pressure made up two of the four most prescribed drugs of 2006, with the cholesterol-lowering drug Lipitor (atorvastatin calcium) at number one.

One could hardly call high blood pressure "silent" these days, because drug companies have spent millions if not billions over the past few decades to make sure everyone knows about it and to make it so scary that you'll take their hypertension drugs at the first sign of a higher-than-normal blood pressure reading. Anytime you walk into a physician's office, clinic, or hospital of any kind, the first thing they do is take your blood pressure.

While it's very true that chronically high blood pressure can be dangerous and should be treated aggressively, millions of North Americans with moderately high blood pressure are unnecessarily bullied by physicians into taking hypertension drugs without first making the diet and lifestyle changes that will lower almost all high blood pressure. This is a perfect example of how much quicker and easier it is to write a prescription for a drug that will make the numbers look better, without getting involved with the complexities of helping a person make lifestyle changes.

Hypertension drugs usually lower high blood pressure, but they have significant side effects and they treat the symptom, not the underlying cause. When you take them, the symptom of high blood pressure is suppressed and your numbers look good for your insurance company, but your disease continues to progress. It's important for you to be aware that unless you're one of the few people who have high blood pressure caused purely by genetics or an illness such as kidney disease, your high blood pressure is caused by diet and lifestyle choices.

If you're already on blood-pressure-lowering drugs, do not go off them suddenly. If you want to work on improving your lifestyle to reduce your blood pressure, work with an experienced health care professional to lower your blood pressure naturally while you wean yourself off the drugs.

Blood Pressure Facts

Your blood pressure rises above normal when too much fluid is being pumped through the blood vessels or the blood vessels constrict, putting greater pressure on your heart and blood vessels. It can also be caused when the arteries lose their elasticity. Consider the plumbing in a house: When water pressure is high, water comes out of the faucet with great force. When water pressure is low, it may only trickle out of the faucet.

Blood pressure readings show two numbers: the systolic pressure, which is the greatest amount of pressure exerted when the heart pumps or contracts, and the diastolic pressure, which is the lowest amount of pressure when the heart is in between beats, or relaxed. A "normal" blood pressure reading for a middle-aged adult is 130 (systolic) over 85 (diastolic), also shown as 130/85 mm Hg (millimeters of mercury, under pressure). A high diastolic blood pressure is more indicative of heart trouble in an older adult than a high systolic blood pressure.

Normal blood pressure increases as we age. As our blood vessels get saggier and baggier along with the rest of the body, we need increased blood pressure to circulate our blood effectively. Research shows that in the elderly it may be dangerous to bring the systolic blood pressure below 140 mm Hg. Most research shows that if you're over the age of 60, your systolic blood pressure may safely be as high as 160 mm Hg and your diastolic as high as 100 mm Hg.

Should you worry if your blood pressure varies some from these numbers? If you're overweight, stressed out, smoking, eating poorly, drinking too much alcohol or coffee, not exercising, or have heart disease, lung disease, or diabetes, then yes, because these are the risk factors for high blood pressure, and you need to get to work changing them—now. If you are following the Six Core Principles for Optimal Health and don't have any of the preceding risk factors or a family history of very high blood pressure, be aware that your blood pressure is high and consider treating it naturally to avoid the risks of hypertensive drugs. If you do need to use a hypertensive drug, ask your doctor to try a diuretic first, for reasons you can read about in detail later.

It's irresponsible for a physician to prescribe a blood pressure drug based on one reading. Your arteries are muscular and flexible, designed to change blood pressure constantly in response to the needs of your body. Blood pressure readings taken in a physician's office are usually higher than normal, and those taken in a drugstore are inaccurate as much as 60 percent of the time. If your physician feels your hypertension is severe enough to warrant taking drugs, you should be monitoring your blood pressure at home.

Your physician is in a very tough position when it comes to treating your high blood pressure. If your blood pressure numbers don't fit into the charts and your physician doesn't prescribe the drugs, he or she can be penalized by an insurance company and is vulnerable to malpractice suits.

How do we dare challenge blood-pressure-drug-prescribing habits? Numerous studies, including the famous Multiple Risk Factor Intervention Trial in the United States and the large Australian Medical Research Council Trial, have shown that people with mild to moderate high blood pressure who don't take prescription drugs to lower their blood pressure do better than those who do take drugs. At a recent American Heart Association meeting, it was reported that without treatment 1 percent of people with high blood pressure have a heart attack, but with treatment with a calcium channel blocker 1.6 percent have a heart attack. That's a 60 percent increase.

Unless you're under the age of 60 and your blood pressure is "severe" (e.g., above 180/110), there is little evidence that blood-pressure-lowering drugs (also called antihypertensives) actually reduce the risk of heart attack and stroke, or even the risk of dying. If you're in your seventies or older, multiple studies have shown that blood pressure drugs can do more harm than good. The exception to this is the Hypertension in the Very Elderly Trial (HYVET) study, published in the *New England Journal of Medicine* in 2008, which compared elderly patients taking either the diuretic indapamide alone or with an ACE (angiotensin-converting enzyme) inhibitor to patients taking a placebo. They found a significantly lower risk of fatal strokes, heart failure, and overall death rate in the treatment group. One reason this research may contradict similar studies is that it primarily used a diuretic, a type of hypertensive drug that has repeatedly been shown to be safer than others, such as beta-blockers and ACE inhibitors. Those who did take the ACE inhibitor in addition to the diuretic did so to reach a target blood pressure number of 150/80 mm Hg. One study showed that elderly patients on antihypertensive drugs whose systolic blood pressure dropped below 140 mm Hg had a significantly higher risk of dying. Another factor in this study is that patients were seen every three months and their medication adjusted at least that often if necessary. This rarely occurs in real life. One of the biggest dangers of antihypertensives in the elderly is that blood pressure drops too low; yet most doctor don't seem aware of this and tend to dismiss complaints of side effects as symptoms of aging.

Nearly all of the studies showing that antihypertensives do more harm than good were done with a placebo, meaning the group that did better did nothing to improve their blood pressure. Now imagine how bad the antihypertensives would look if they were measured against natural methods of lowering blood pressure, such as weight loss, exercise, diet, and stress reduction!

Drugs That Can Raise Your Blood Pressure

NSAIDs (aspirin, acetaminophen, ibuprofen)

Bronchodilators such as epinephrine, albuterol, and ephedrine

Corticosteroids (e.g., prednisone)

Bisphosphonates (e.g., Fosamax, Actonel, Boniva)

Nasal decongestants (e.g., phenylpropanolamine)

The migraine drug sumatriptan (Imitrex)

The benzodiazepine antianxiety drugs (e.g., Ativan, Xanax, Klonopin)

Many of the antidepressants, but especially venlafaxine (Effexor) and the MAOIs (Nardil, Parnate)

Types of Antihypertensives

There are four major types of drugs prescribed to lower blood pressure: diuretics, beta-blockers, ACE inhibitors, and calcium channel blockers. Diuretics lower blood pressure by reducing the amount of fluid in the body.

The rest of the drugs listed here lower blood pressure by suppressing body signals that it's time to raise blood pressure. This makes the numbers look good, but when you really need some blood pressure, it's not there, and that's the underlying cause of the deadly side effects of these drugs. For example, if you need to run or climb stairs, or you get a bad scare, your body will put out signals to raise blood pressure, but the drug will block those signals. The theory is that this will keep your blood pressure from going so high that it gives you a heart attack. But on the other side of the coin, there are good physiological reasons for your blood pressure to go up sometimes, and if your body can't meet those demands, it could kill you.

All of these drugs are used to control and suppress a wide variety of heart disease symptoms, but none have any healing properties. Diuretics are often prescribed to treat the water retention caused by liver and kidney disease, but since they can also aggravate kidney and liver disease, they can be counterproductive.

Which Are the Safest and Most Effective Blood-Pressure-Lowering Drugs?

Of the drugs that lower blood pressure, the newer and more expensive ACE-inhibitors and calcium channel blockers have never been proven to be safer or more effective than the simpler and time-tested diuretics. A government-funded study called the ALLHAT, or Antihypertensive and Lipid-Lowering Treatment to Prevent Heart Attack Trial, proved once and for all that for the vast majority of people with high blood pressure, a diuretic will work just fine. This was a large study with more than 33,000 participants that began in 1994 and ran for eight years. When all the data had been crunched, researchers found that those participants who took the calcium channel blockers had by far the *highest risk* of heart failure, and those taking the ACE-inhibitors the next highest risk, compared to those taking a diuretic. The diuretic was also more effective than either of the other drugs at lowering systolic blood pressure.

Drug companies had tried to justify prescribing ACE-inhibitors and calcium channel blockers by claiming they worked better for diabetics and prediabetics, but the ALLHAT study also disproved that claim. The diuretics work as well or better on all counts.

Diuretics

Diuretics, which are essentially designed to reduce fluid levels by making you urinate more, are one of the most common blood pressure medicines prescribed and, relatively speaking, the safest. One of the biggest problems with diuretics is the depletion of minerals. In addition to losing sodium, you lose most of the other minerals too, including potassium, magnesium, and calcium, which are essential to proper heart function, not to mention healthy bones. There's no sense in lowering your blood pressure to prevent heart disease if your method of lowering it is going to cause it anyway. Numerous studies have shown that people with high blood pressure tend to be deficient in magnesium, so the last thing they need is to lose more.

Diuretics also tend to deplete the B vitamins. If you're on a diuretic, be sure you're taking plenty of B vitamins and a good multimineral supplement. One of the most devastating side effects of diuretics for women is their tendency to promote the excretion of calcium in the urine, resulting in bone loss and osteoporosis.

Another side effect of diuretics is a higher susceptibility to heatstroke or heat stress, caused by the body's inability to cool off by sweating. This is particularly important for older people who live in a warm or hot climate. When it's hot and you're taking a diuretic, it's important to drink plenty of fluids.

Since diuretics tend to make you urinate more than usual, this can create an added discomfort for men with an enlarged prostate who often are already inconvenienced by having to urinate frequently. This side effect can also create more waking at night to urinate, which causes sleep loss, and in the elderly it increases the risk for a fall.

Although the side effects of the diuretics are not pleasant, they are minor compared to the potential side effects of the other antihypertensive drugs.

Examples of Thiazide Diuretics

Bendroflumethiazide (Naturetin)
Benzthiazide (Exna)
Chlorthalidone (Thalitone, Hygroton)
Chlorothiazide (Diuril, Hygroton)
Hydrochlorothiazide (Aquazide, Esidrix, HydroDIURIL, Microzide, Hydro-Par, Oretic, Ezide)
Hydroflumethiazide (Diucardin, Saluron)
Indapamide (Lozol, Lozide)
Methyclothiazide (Aquatensen, Enduron)
Metolazone (Zaroxolyn, Mykrox)
Polythiazide (Renese)
Quinethazone (Hydromox)
Trichlormethiazide (Metahydrin, Naqua, Diurese)

What Do They Do in the Body? Increase urination, reduce fluid and water retention.

What Are They Prescribed For? High blood pressure, edema (swelling, water retention, puffiness), and CHF.

What Are the Possible Side Effects? The most common and dangerous side effect of diuretics is excessive loss of minerals or an imbalance of minerals, called an electrolyte imbalance. Signs of a mineral imbalance can include dizziness, dry mouth, weakness, muscle pains or cramps, low blood pressure, rapid heartbeat, sleepiness, and confusion.

These drugs commonly cause dizziness, usually a signal that blood pressure is too low. Dizziness can lead to falls, dangerous driving, and mental fogginess—symptoms often attributed to aging, but which may be simply treated by reducing the dose of a blood pressure medication.

High uric acid levels can lead to gout, a painful inflammation usually in the big toe. Other possible side effects include kidney damage, hyperglycemia (may increase fasting blood glucose) or precipitation of underlying diabetes, raised LDL "bad" cholesterol and triglyceride levels, anemia, and sun sensitivity.

These drugs can also cause a wide variety of digestive problems, loss of appetite, vision problems, headaches, skin problems, restlessness, and impotence.

Even taking the preceding cautions into account, for most people diuretics are the safest prescription drugs for lowering blood pressure.

CAUTION!

Think Twice About Taking These Drugs If . . .

- You have lupus.
- You have kidney or liver problems.
- You have diabetes.
- You have urinary tract problems such as an enlarged prostate that interferes with urination. Diuretics can make you even more uncomfortable by increasing the number of times you have to urinate.

What Are the Interactions with Food? If you take too many electrolytes, such as in sports drinks, you may reduce the effectiveness of the drug.

It's good to eat plenty of high-potassium foods when taking diuretics that don't "spare" potassium. Some common high-potassium foods include bananas, citrus fruits, melons, almonds, green leafy vegetables, potatoes, carrots, avocados, and soybeans.

Licorice (not the candy made with anise, but the herb or root) can be an antidiuretic and reduce the actions of these drugs. It can also cause you to excrete higher-than-normal levels of potassium, the last thing you want on a diuretic that doesn't spare potassium.

Eating a lot of meat can increase uric acid even more, increasing the possibility of gout. If you are sensitive to monosodium glutamate (MSG), its negative effects can be exaggerated when you're taking diuretics.

Since the secondary purpose of taking diuretics is to reduce your levels of sodium, it's obviously wise to follow a low-sodium diet to reduce your need for the diuretics. One of the best ways to do this is to eliminate processed and packaged foods from your diet and concentrate on whole foods such as whole grains and fresh fruits and vegetables. When you do buy processed foods, read labels carefully. Many low-fat or sugar-free foods add lots of salt or MSG to improve taste.

What Nutrients Do They Deplete or Throw out of Balance? Minerals, especially sodium, potassium, calcium, and magnesium. Zinc is another important mineral that can be lost. Zinc is crucial to proper immune system functioning, wound healing, and thyroid function.

Diuretics can cause a depletion of vitamin A, which many Americans are already deficient in.

What Else to Take If You Take These Drugs. A good mineral formula that includes zinc, copper, boron, iodine, cobalt, manganese, molybdenum, vanadium, chromium, selenium, plenty of calcium and magnesium, and if you're a premenopausal woman, iron.

Be sure you're getting both beta-carotene and vitamin A in your multivitamin formula. Eat plenty of fresh fruits and vegetables.

Other Tips on These Drugs. They can skew the results of many blood and urine tests.

Examples of Loop Diuretics

Bumetanide (Bumex)
Ethacrynic acid (Edecrin)
Furosemide (Lasix)
Torsemide (Demadex)

What Do They Do in the Body? Increase urination, reduce fluid and water retention, largely by reducing sodium chloride (salt) uptake in your cells.

What Are They Prescribed For? High blood pressure, edema (swelling, water retention, puffiness).

What Are the Possible Side Effects? One of the most common and dangerous side effects of loop diuretics is dehydration caused by too much fluid loss. This can be deadly. An excessive loss of minerals or an imbalance of minerals, called an electrolyte imbalance, may result from taking these drugs. These diuretics are also more likely to cause hypotension, or blood pressure that is too low, which can also be dangerous, and such excessive potassium loss that it becomes life threatening. If your blood pressure is reduced too much, you may get dizzy when you stand up. In addition, high uric acid levels can lead to gout, a painful inflammation usually in the big toe.

Other possible side effects include kidney damage, reversible and irreversible hearing problems, diarrhea, hyperglycemia (diuretics can increase blood glucose) or precipitation of underlying diabetes, raised LDL "bad" cholesterol and triglyceride levels, and photosensitivity, a reaction to the sun. These drugs can also cause muscle pain and cramps, restlessness, a wide variety of digestive problems, vision problems, and skin problems.

CAUTION!

Think Twice About Taking These Drugs If . . .

- You have lupus.
- You have kidney or liver problems.
- You have diabetes.
- You have urinary tract problems such as an enlarged prostate that interferes with urination. Diuretics can make you even more uncomfortable by increasing the number of times you have to urinate.

What Are the Interactions with Food? The absorption of the drug may be reduced if you take it with food. Also, if you consume too many electrolytes, such as in sports drinks, you may reduce the effectiveness of the drug.

Signs of a Mineral Imbalance

Dizziness
Dry mouth
Low blood pressure
Muscle pains or cramps
Nausea and vomiting
Rapid heartbeat
Sleepiness and confusion
Weakness

It's good to eat plenty of high-potassium foods when taking diuretics that don't "spare" potassium. Some common high-potassium foods include bananas, citrus fruits, melons, almonds, green leafy vegetables, potatoes, carrots, avocados, and soybeans.

Licorice (not the candy made with anise, but the herb or root) can be an antidiuretic and reduce the actions of these drugs.

Eating a lot of meat can increase uric acid even more, increasing the possibility of gout.

If you are sensitive to MSG, its negative effects can be exaggerated when you're taking diuretics.

What Nutrients Do They Deplete or Throw out of Balance? Minerals, especially sodium, potassium, calcium, and magnesium. Zinc is another important mineral that can be lost. Zinc is crucial to proper immune system functioning, wound healing, and thyroid function.

Taken long-term, loop diuretics cause a depletion of the vitamin thiamine (B_1), which plays a key role in the functioning of the nervous system. A deficiency of thiamine can aggravate CHF or other heart problems. Chronic thiamine deficiency can also block enzymes involved in glucose metabolism, which may be why these drugs can cause hypoglycemia.

Diuretics can cause a depletion of vitamin A, which many Americans are already deficient in.

What Else to Take While Taking These Drugs. A good mineral formula that includes zinc, copper, boron, iodine, cobalt, manganese, molybdenum, vanadium, chromium, selenium, and if you're a premenopausal woman, iron. Eat plenty of fresh fruits and vegetables.

An extra B-complex vitamin supplement that includes at least 50 mg of thiamine. (It's best to take the B vitamins together.)

Be sure you're getting both beta-carotene and vitamin A in your multivitamin formula.

Other Tips on These Drugs. They can skew the results of many blood and urine tests. Take them with food, or they may upset your stomach.

Examples of Potassium-Sparing Diuretics

Amiloride (Midamor)
Spironolactone (Aldactone)
Triamterene (Dyrenium)
Combinations (Dyazide, Moduretic, Aldacta-
*   zide, Maxzide)*

The potassium-sparing diuretics are usually combined with one of the other diuretics to reduce excessive potassium depletion. However, the potassium-sparing diuretics in turn may cause excess potassium, called hyperkalemia, which can also be dangerous. Symptoms of too much potassium include muscular weakness, fatigue, numbness and tingling, and irregular heartbeat.

What Do They Do in the Body? Reduce fluid and water retention in such a way that the body retains potassium.

What Are They Prescribed For? In conjunction with loop and thiazide diuretics prescribed for high blood pressure and CHF, to reduce the loss of potassium, to treat aldosteronism (an excess of the adrenal hormone aldosterone, which causes the body to hold on to salt and excrete potassium), and to treat a variety of conditions involving potassium loss.

Spironolactone reduces the level of aldosterone, an androgen (male hormone), so it has been used to treat excess hair growth, acne, and other symptoms of excess androgens. Considering that this drug promotes tumor growth in rats and can cause unexplained uterine bleeding in women at high doses, it seems frivolous to use it other than short-term in life-threatening situations.

Triamterene is mainly used to treat edema, or water retention, especially when it is caused by aldosteronism.

What Are the Possible Side Effects? Excess potassium (hyperkalemia), dizziness, nausea, vomiting, and appetite loss. Liver and kidney problems may get worse. The peripheral neuropathy (numbness in the extremities) caused by diabetes may get worse.

Spironolactone affects sex hormones by reducing aldosterone levels. Aldosterone is an androgen, or male hormone. Taking spironolactone can cause a reduction in male hormones, and as a consequence, causes breast enlargement and other feminizing effects in men. It also promotes the growth of a variety of malignant tumors in rats. Spironolactone can cause lethargy, mental confusion, headaches, stomachaches, irregular menstruation, and thirst.

Triamterene may promote the formation of kidney stones and can raise blood sugar levels. It can also induce kidney failure.

CAUTION!

Think Twice About Taking These Drugs If . . .

- You have kidney or liver problems.
- You have diabetes.
- You have urinary tract problems such as an enlarged prostate that interferes with urination. Diuretics can make you even more uncomfortable by increasing the number of times you have to urinate.

What Are the Interactions with Food? If you consume too many electrolytes, such as in sports drinks, you may get too much potassium. Eating a lot of high-potassium foods in combination with taking the drugs can also raise potassium levels too high. Some common high-potassium foods include bananas, citrus fruits, melons, almonds, green leafy vegetables, potatoes, carrots, avocados, and soybeans.

Licorice (the root or herb used medicinally, or the candy with real licorice flavoring) can be an antidiuretic and may reduce the effect of these drugs. Licorice also contains a component called glycyrrhizin, which is similar to aldosterone, the very hormone that spironolactone is prescribed to reduce, so taking a lot of (real) licorice could negate those effects.

Eating a lot of meat can increase uric acid even more, increasing the possibility of gout.

Spironolactone levels may be increased by eating a lot of protein or fat at one sitting. Levels may be decreased by a high-fiber diet. If you're eating fiber-rich cereals or taking a fiber supplement such as psyllium, take it a few hours apart from taking this drug.

If you are sensitive to MSG, its negative effects may be exaggerated when you're taking diuretics.

What Nutrients Do They Deplete or Throw out of Balance? Minerals, especially sodium, potassium, calcium, magnesium, and zinc. Zinc is crucial to proper immune system functioning, wound healing, and thyroid function. Diuretics can cause a depletion of vitamin A, which many Americans are already deficient in.

What Else to Take While Taking These Drugs. A good mineral formula that includes zinc, copper, boron, iodine, cobalt, manganese, molybdenum, vanadium, chromium, selenium, and if you're a premenopausal woman, iron.

Be sure you're getting both beta-carotene and vitamin A in your multivitamin formula. Eat plenty of fresh fruits and vegetables.

Examples of Beta-Blockers

Beta-adrenergic-blocking agents: acebutolol (Sectral); atenolol (Tenormin); betaxolol

(Kerlone); bisoprolol fumarate (Zebeta); esmolol (Brevibloc) used for abnormal heartbeat; Levobunolol; metoprolol (Lopressor, Toprol XL); nadolol (Corgard); Oxyprenolol; Penbutolol sulfate (Levatol); pindolol (Betapindol, Calvisken, Decreten, Durapindol Visken); propranolol (Betachron E-R, Inderal, Inderal LA, Avlocardyl, Deralin, Dociton, Inderalici, InnoPran XL, Sumial); sotalol HCl (Betapace, Sotalex, Sotacor) used for irregular heartbeat; timolol maleate (Blocadren)

Alpha/beta-adrenergic blockers: arotinolol (Almarl), carvedilol (Coreg, Dilatrend, Eucardic, Carloc), celiprolol (Cardem, Celectol, Celipres, Celipro, Celol, Cordiax, Dilanorm, Selectol), labetalol (Normodyne, Trandate)

Beta-blockers, or beta-adrenergic-blocking drugs, are somewhat outdated, but some physicians still use them to treat high blood pressure. The downside of these drugs is that they can actually cause CHF, heart attacks, strokes, and asthma. Beta-blockers can cause serious arrhythmias (irregular heartbeats) and may worsen blood vessel problems that reduce circulation to the extremities, such as in diabetes. Asthmatics should never take a beta-blocker as it may trigger life-threatening airway spasms.

According to an article published in a 2007 issue of the *Journal of the American College of Cardiology* that reviewed 10 studies on using beta-blockers to control high blood pressure, diuretics and other blood pressure drugs work better to control blood pressure and have fewer side effects. The article points out that beta-blockers may be useful for treating patients who have had a heart attack or who have heart fail-

ure, but they shouldn't be routinely used to treat high blood pressure.

For years beta-blockers have been routinely given to patients who might be or are at risk of heart disease, before they have surgery. The practice is said to reduce the risk of heart attack and abnormal heart rhythms after surgery. The POISE (perioperative ischemic evaluation) study, a large, double-blind study out of Canada and published in the journal *The Lancet*, found that compared to a placebo, patients who were given beta-blockers before surgery were one-third more likely to die within a month, had doubled the risk of stroke, and were more likely to have clinically low blood pressure or low heart rate. The specific beta-blocker used in this study was metoprolol (Toprol).

Beta-blockers can cause serious new arrhythmias, dangerously low blood pressure, abnormally slow heart rates, CHF, heart attacks, gastrointestinal bleeding, liver and kidney damage, and reduced white blood cell count, and they interact dangerously with many other drugs.

What Do They Do in the Body? Beta-blockers reduce blood pressure by slowing the heart rate, reducing the force of contractions of the heart muscle, and relaxing the arteries.

What Are They Prescribed For? High blood pressure, especially in combination with a thiazide diuretic, and many other heart disease symptoms such as angina, irregular heartbeat, and recovery from some types of heart attacks, migraines, tremors, and anxiety.

What Are the Possible Side Effects? Dozens of "adverse effects" have been reported by people taking beta-blockers, which are listed on the drug information insert. If you have any type of new symptoms while on this drug, even if you have been on it for a long time, check with your physician and read the drug information insert. If you don't have the insert, either ask your pharmacist for one or look it up online. See the "Resources and Recommended Reading" section at the back of this book for online sources of drug information.

Dizziness and fatigue are two of the most common complaints of people on these drugs. That may mean they're taking too much. These side effects are considered "mild" by drug companies and physicians, but they can cause depression and reduce the activities you can participate in—yet another good reason to lower your blood pressure naturally!

A large, double-blind, multicenter randomized trial (the National Heart, Lung and Blood Institute's Cardiac Arrhythmia Suppression Trial) found that in certain types of heart attack patients, some beta-blockers caused a significantly higher death rate and risk of a second heart attack compared to patients who did nothing.

Beta-blockers can cause serious arrhythmias and may worsen blood vessel problems that reduce circulation to the extremities, such as in diabetes. They can also lead to cardiac failure by overdepressing the ability of the heart to contract.

Like all drugs that are prescribed to lower blood pressure, beta-blockers can easily send blood pressure too far in the other direction, causing hypotension, or low blood pressure. Symptoms of hypotension include dizziness when standing, sweating, and fatigue.

Other side effects can include muscle weakness, dizziness, hypo- and hyperglycemia, impotence, eye problems, worsening of lung problems, depression, joint pain, and rarely, anaphylaxis, a severe allergic reaction.

Kidney and liver damage may be made worse by beta-blockers and can cause unpredictable increases in drug levels.

Some beta-blockers can send your cholesterol levels in the opposite direction that you want them to go: increased LDL, VLDL, VH, and triglycerides, and decreased HDL.

Sudden withdrawal from beta-blockers can be dangerous.

The beta-blockers propranolol and atenolol reduce the nighttime production of melatonin, a brain hormone essential for good sleep. Melatonin deficiency has been implicated in breast cancer.

Beta-blockers can deplete CoQ10, which can cause fatigue and muscle pain.

CAUTION!

Think Twice About Taking These Drugs If . . .

- You have CHF or irregular heartbeat.
- You have asthma or other lung diseases such as chronic bronchitis and emphysema.

Most beta-blockers can suppress symptoms of diabetes and an overactive thyroid (hyperthyroidism). Since beta-blockers can cause or prolong hypoglycemia, use caution if you are diabetic.

What Are the Interactions with Food? Taking atenolol (Tenormin) and sotalol (Betapace) with food may reduce or slow their action. Taking labetalol (Normodyne, Trandate), metoprolol (Lopressor, Toprol), and propanolol (Inderal) with food may increase drug levels. Taking propanolol with a high-protein meal or with alcohol may increase drug levels even more.

Other Tips on These Drugs. They may interfere with glucose tolerance tests, insulin tests, glaucoma tests, and a variety of other blood and urine tests.

Examples of ACE inhibitors

Inhibitors of angiotensin-converting enzyme): benazepril (Lotensin), captopril (Capoten), enalapril (Vasotec, Renitec), fosinopril (Monopril), lisinopril (Lisodur, Lopril, Novatec, Prinivil, Zestril), moexipril (Univasc), perindopril (Coversyl, Aceon), quinapril (Accupril), ramipril (Altace, Tritace, Ramace, Ramiwin), trandolapril (Mavik), zofenopril

Angiotensin antagonists: losartan potassium (Cozaar), candesartan cilexetil (Atacand), eprosartan mesylate (Teveten), irbesartan (Avapro), telmisartan (Micardis), valsartan (Diovan)

What Do They Do in the Body? ACE inhibitors lower blood pressure by blocking the production of a series of chemicals, especially one called angiotensin, that the body releases to raise blood pressure. When blood pressure drops, the kidneys release a hormone called renin, which in turn stimulates the production of angiotensin, which has its own potent actions, including constricting the arteries to raise blood pressure. Angiotensin also stimulates the release of the adrenal hormone aldosterone, which gives cells signals to hold on to sodium and release potassium, thus allowing fluid buildup, another way of raising blood pressure.

Thus taking an ACE inhibitor has a very powerful effect on an important blood-pressure control mechanism, which is good news when your blood pressure needs lowering in the moment. But this can be bad news when it needs to rise, because the mechanism that allows it to do so is suppressed.

ACE inhibitors are a classic example of suppressing a symptom to treat a disease. The danger, of course, is that the disease progresses underneath, and a whole new set of symptoms and risks are created by the drug.

What Are They Prescribed For? High blood pressure, especially in combination with thiazide diuretics. Some of the ACE inhibitors are prescribed for CHF and for heart attack patients after a myocardial infarction, and sometimes for diabetic nephropathy (kidney disease).

What Are the Possible Side Effects? The most common side effect of ACE inhibitors is an annoying, persistent, nagging cough. While this isn't directly life threatening, it's a big energy drain and it's enough to create a loss of sleep. ACE inhibitors have probably gotten more people stuck on the drug treadmill than any other single drug. Why? They take an ACE inhibitor, get a cough, and then complain to their physician. Instead of taking them off the ACE inhibitor, the physician prescribes a cough suppressant, which causes insomnia, so the physician prescribes a sleeping pill, which is addictive, and so on.

The ACE inhibitor captopril (Capoten) can cause a large reduction of white blood cells (neutropenia), seriously compromising the immune system. This seems like an unacceptably severe side effect when there are so many alternatives. The risk of neutropenia is especially high for people with some kinds of kidney problems. There is some evidence that other ACE inhibitors could also cause neutropenia, although not as frequently. Captopril may also cause kidney damage.

ACE inhibitors can cause a serious allergy-type reaction (anaphylactic) that causes swelling, especially around the head and neck, which can be fatal when it obstructs airways.

Because ACE inhibitors block the release of the adrenal hormone aldosterone, which is an androgen, or male hormone, they have been known to cause symptoms of feminization in men such as breast enlargement. This same mechanism also blocks signals telling the body to release potassium, which can result in excessively high levels of potassium.

As with all drugs that lower blood pressure, there is always the risk that the blood pressure is lowered too much or that some other factor such as food, another drug, diarrhea, dehydration, exercise, or overheating will combine with the drug to lower blood pressure too far.

The ACE inhibitors ramipril (Altace) and fosinopril (Monopril) can aggravate existing liver disease. There have been cases where people taking ACE inhibitors suffered liver damage and liver failure (death), as well as kidney damage and kidney failure.

Other side effects of ACE inhibitors are dizziness (common with all drugs that lower blood pressure), headaches, irregular heartbeat, chest pain, diarrhea, nausea, fatigue, shortness of breath, rash, sexual dysfunction, vision disturbances, taste disturbances, and weakness.

There have been dozens of "adverse effects" reported by people taking ACE inhibitors, so don't rule out a symptom as a side effect of this drug just because it's not on this list. The latest to make the (unofficial) ACE inhibitor side effects list is sleep disturbances and nightmares, which apparently go away rapidly when the drug is stopped.

These types of drugs can cause injury and death to a developing fetus when taken in the second and third trimesters. Because of this, there doesn't seem to be any reason whatsoever for a woman of child-bearing age to take them.

CAUTION!

Think Twice About Taking These Drugs If . . .

Please think twice about taking an ACE inhibitor no matter what, especially captopril. They are especially risky for people with some types of kidney or liver disease, and the elderly, who tend to have decreased kidney function as a matter of aging. Don't go near this drug if there is any possibility of pregnancy.

What Are the Interactions with Food? Capsaicin, or cayenne, used as a spice and as an alternative medicine treatment for a variety of ailments, may make an ACE-inhibitor-caused cough worse. Capsaicin is also used topically to treat herpes zoster (shingles). Levels of captopril may be significantly reduced if it is taken with food, so take it an hour before or after eating. Other ACE inhibitors may be reduced less significantly. (Enalapril, benazepril, and lisinopril do not seem to be affected by food.)

Examples of Calcium Channel Blockers (Calcium Antagonists)

Amlodipine (Norvasc)
Barnidipine (HypoCa)
Diltiazem (Cardizem, Dilacor, Tiazac, Diltiazem HCl Extended Release)
Felodipine (Plendil)
Isradipine (DynaCirc, Prescal)
Nicardipine (Cardene)
Nifedipine (Adalat, Procardia)
Nimodipine (Nimotop)
Nisoldipine (Baymycard, Sular, Syscor)
Verapamil (Calan, Isoptin, Verelan, Covera)

What Do They Do in the Body? The movement of calcium in and out of some cells of the heart and arteries plays an important role in their contraction. Calcium channel blockers block the movement of calcium, lowering blood pressure by suppressing the contraction of artery muscles, dilating the arteries, and reducing arterial resistance to blood flow.

What Are They Prescribed For? Calcium channel blockers are prescribed for a variety of heart problems, including angina, arrhythmias (irregular heartbeat), rapid heartbeat, high blood pressure, and CHF. They are also prescribed for migraine headaches and Raynaud's disease. Those prescribed for high blood pressure include amlodipine, verapamil SR, diltiazem, nicardipine, nifedipine, isradipine, felodipine, and nisoldipine.

What Are the Possible Side Effects? Calcium channel blockers are among the most widely prescribed drugs in North America, and yet they are also among the most dangerous drugs you can take. Although they can be useful in normalizing an irregular heartbeat and spasms in the heart muscle, their long-term use for lowering blood pressure is very questionable.

There are at least two major studies showing that people who use calcium channel blockers to control high blood pressure have a higher risk of dying from heart disease and a higher overall risk of dying than people who use other antihypertensives.

In test rats they caused cancer, and the fast-acting forms of nifedipine have been shown in studies conducted by the National Heart, Lung and Blood Institute to increase the risk of a fatal heart attack.

Some of the more common "adverse reactions" include dizziness; swollen hands and feet (edema); chronic headaches; nausea; giddiness; nervousness; numbness and tingling; diarrhea; constipation; digestive problems such as stomach cramps, gas, and heartburn; dry mouth; gum disease; flushing; urinary tract problems; sexual problems; shortness of breath; muscle cramps and pains; and a cough.

The different types of calcium channel blockers can vary in their actions and side effects quite a bit, so if you must take one, be sure your physician is experienced in prescribing them and be sure to read the drug insert carefully for yourself. We're not aware of any evidence that using calcium channel blockers long-term will reduce the risk of heart attack or death.

CAUTION!

Think Twice About Taking These Drugs If . . .

You have kidney or liver disease. Calcium channel blockers are contraindicated with some types of heart disease, such as sick sinus syndrome. This differs with the type of calcium channel blocker. Talk to your physician, and read your drug information sheet. Dangerous side effects tend to occur more often in patients who are also on beta-blockers. This is a potentially dangerous combination.

What Are the Interactions with Food? Some calcium channel blockers are unaffected by food, some are decreased, and some are increased. Ask your pharmacist, and read your drug information insert. Taking felodipine and nifedipine with grapefruit juice can double drug levels, a potentially deadly interaction, and grapefruit juice can also affect the levels of other types of calcium channel blockers. In general, it's best not to take medicine with grapefruit juice unless your physician asks you to. Some calcium channel blockers may increase the amount of alcohol that gets into the blood when you have a drink or take medicine containing alcohol.

What Nutrients Do They Throw out of Balance or Interact With? Excess vitamin D may reduce the effectiveness of verapamil. Some calcium channel blockers, including nifedipine and verapamil, may bind with minerals in food or supplements, reducing the availability of the drug.

Other Tips on These Drugs. Calcium channel blockers can affect the results of blood and urine tests.

If you're taking a calcium channel blocker in the dihydropyridine class (i.e., felodipine [Plendil], nifedipine), watch out for dangerous interactions with erythromycin, an antibiotic, which can double felodipine levels. High felodipine levels can cause heart palpitations and low blood pressure.

Other Antihypertensive (Blood-Pressure-Lowering) Drugs

None of these drugs are considered primary or single treatments for high blood pressure. They are almost always used in combination with other drugs.

Examples of Antiadrenergic Agents, Centrally Acting

Methyldopa, methyldopate (Aldomet)

What Do They Do in the Body? Methyldopa and methyldopate lower blood pressure, probably by reducing levels of serotonin, dopamine, norepinephrine, and epinephrine and possibly by lowering renin, a substance released by the kidneys in response to low blood pressure.

What Are They Prescribed For? High blood pressure.

What Are the Possible Side Effects? Liver disease is a direct contraindication to taking methyldopa. This drug carries a high risk of damaging the liver and of causing blood disorders, including anemia, and can cause a syndrome of symptoms that resembles lupus. Other side effects include sedation or drowsiness (which may impair coordination and the ability to think clearly), fatigue, depression, fever, headache, dizziness, weakness, abnormally slow heartbeat, nausea, rash, breast enlargement in men and women, impotence, and decreased libido. As with all antihypertensive drugs, it carries the risk of abnormally low blood pressure.

CAUTION!

Think Twice About Taking These Drugs If . . .

Please think twice about taking these drugs, period. Many other newer drugs can do the same job without the high risk. Antiadrenergic agents have too many potent and negative effects on too many important bodily systems. If you have any type of liver disease, don't take them.

What Are the Interactions with Food? Methyldopa levels will be decreased if taken with food, especially protein. Eating too much salt while taking methyldopa could increase fluid retention and cause edema or water retention.

What Nutrients Do They Throw out of Balance or Interact With? Methyldopa decreases vitamin B_{12} levels and probably decreases folic acid levels as well.

What Else to Take While Taking These Drugs. Preferably, intravenous vitamin B_{12} and folic acid, but these drugs can cause sensitivity reactions so even that may be risky. At the very least, take sublingual vitamin B_{12} and folic acid supplements.

Be aware that the folic acid may hide evidence of anemia, a side effect of the drugs.

Other Tips on These Drugs. They affect many blood and urine tests.

Clonidine

Clonidine (Catapres)

What Does It Do in the Body? It has many effects on the body, including lowering blood pressure; reducing renin, aldosterone, and catecholamines (all important to normal bodily function); and stimulating growth hormone.

What Is It Prescribed For? Hypertension and many other miscellaneous conditions such as menopausal flushing (hot flashes) and diabetic diarrhea, reflecting its wide spectrum of effects on the body.

What Are the Possible Side Effects? The most dangerous aspect of this drug is that if you miss a dose or two, you could experience sudden and dangerously high blood pressure. Since everyone misses medication occasionally, this alone makes it not worth taking this drug. It has also caused degeneration of the retina in animals and has a long list of unpleasant side effects including dry mouth, dizziness, depression, sedation, constipation, fatigue, loss of appetite, nausea, rash, impotence, decreased libido, muscle weakness, dry eyes, and an odd mix of brain dysfunction symptoms such as hallucinations and nightmares.

CAUTION!

Think Twice About Taking This Drug If ...

Think twice about taking this drug, period. It's way too dangerous, and there are other better alternatives.

If you eat too much salt when you're taking clonidine, it can cause fluid retention.

Guanfacine

Guanfacine (Tenex)

What Does It Do in the Body? Lowers blood pressure and affects many other bodily systems, including the stimulation of growth hormone and the reduction of renin activity and catecholamine levels.

What Is It Prescribed For? High blood pressure, heroin withdrawal, and migraine headaches.

What Are the Possible Side Effects? Sedation, drowsiness, depression, fatigue, and if you forget to take a dose, it can cause nervousness, anxiety, and rebound high blood pressure. Other side effects are dry mouth, weakness, dizziness, constipation, impotence, vision and taste disturbances, palpitations, and rash.

CAUTION!

This is another drug that simply seems outdated and unnecessary most of the time.

Guanabenz

Guanabenz (Wytensin)

What Does It Do in the Body? Reduces blood pressure by acting on the brain centers that reduce blood pressure.

What Is It Prescribed For? High blood pressure.

What Are the Possible Side Effects? The most dangerous side effect of guanabenz is its tendency to rebound high blood pressure if you miss a dose or two. This makes it a potentially dangerous drug. It also can cause drowsiness, sedation, depression, fatigue, dry mouth, dizziness, weakness, and headache. It also interacts dangerously with many other drugs.

CAUTION!

Think Twice About Taking This Drug If . . .

Please think twice about taking this drug at all.

Antiadrenergic Agents, Peripherally Acting

Reserpine

What Does It Do in the Body? Lowers blood pressure by lowering levels of catecholamine and 5-hydroxytryptamine in many parts of the body, including the brain and adrenal glands.

What Is It Prescribed For? Schizophrenia, psychosis, and hypertension.

What Are the Possible Side Effects? Depression is the most common and most damaging side effect of reserpine. It shouldn't be used at all by people with any type of depression. It's also not a good drug for people with ulcers or kidney damage or disease, and it causes cancer in animals. Other side effects include dry mouth, dizziness, headache, irregular heartbeat, abnormally slow heartbeat, shortness of breath, a set of symptoms resembling Parkinson's, impotence, and rash.

CAUTION!

Think Twice About Taking This Drug If . . .

Please think twice about taking this drug, period. Major depression is too serious and insidious a side effect to take lightly. This drug is rarely used anymore because of its dangerous side effects.

Examples of Alpha-1 Blockers (Alpha-1-Adrenergic Blockers)

Doxazosin (Cardura, Carduran)
Prazosin (Minipress)
Terazosin (Hytrin)

What Do They Do in the Body? Lower blood pressure.

What Are They Prescribed For? Lowering blood pressure, benign prostatic hyperplasia, some types of CHF, and Raynaud's disease.

What Are the Possible Side Effects? Prazosin tends to cause sodium and water retention, something that is important to avoid when lowering blood pressure.

Like some of the other hypertensive drugs, prazosin, terazosin, and doxazosin can cause rebound hypertension if a few doses are missed and can cause dizziness and even fainting upon standing from a sitting or lying position.

These drugs should not be given to people who have liver damage.

Doxazosin caused reduced fertility in male rats, and testicular atrophy has occurred in dogs and cats given terazosin or prazosin.

Doxazosin can cause an abnormal reduction in white blood cell count.

People taking terazosin tend to gain weight.

These drugs affect cholesterol levels, but how they affect them seems to vary. Other side effects include dizziness, fatigue, weakness, drowsiness, headache, heart palpitations, nausea, shortness of breath, nasal congestion, and vision disturbances.

CAUTION!

Think Twice About Taking These Drugs If . . .

- You have liver disease or damage.
- Your immune system is compromised or suppressed.
- You are obese.
- Your cholesterol is high.

Vasodilators

Hydralazine (Apresoline)

What Does It Do in the Body? Lowers blood pressure by interfering with the ability of calcium to move in and out of cells and effect the contraction of some parts of the heart and artery muscles. At the same time, it increases heart rate and output. It also increases renin levels, which stimulates the production of angiotensin, which is exactly what other hypertensive drugs block.

What Is It Prescribed For? High blood pressure.

What Are the Possible Side Effects? Hydralazine can cause a set of symptoms that resembles lupus, which may not necessarily all go away when the drug is stopped. This happened in 5 to 10 percent of patients, which is a high number.

It can cause nerve pain in the hands and feet, blood abnormalities, and angina, and has been implicated in myocardial infarctions, a type of heart attack.

Side effects include headache, loss of appetite, digestive problems, angina, vision problems, numbness and tingling, dizziness, tremors, depression, anxiety, rash, nasal congestion, flushing, water retention, muscle cramps, shortness of breath, difficulty urinating, and of course, abnormally low blood pressure (hypotension).

CAUTION!

Think Twice About Taking This Drug If . . .

You have coronary artery disease, have had a stroke or are at risk for one, have lung disease, have blood abnormalities, or have lupus. This drug should not be at the top of anyone's list for treating high blood pressure, for obvious reasons.

What Are the Interactions with Food? Taking with food will increase drug absorption. Eating a lot of salty foods will increase water retention.

What Nutrients Does It Throw out of Balance or Interact With? Hydralazine depletes vitamin B_6. Foods containing a relative of hydralazine called tartrazine, a yellow dye, will also deplete vitamin B_6. Symptoms of B_6 deficiency are numerous and include depression, memory loss, pain in the fingers and feet, carpal tunnel syndrome, and menstrual symptoms, to name a few.

What Else to Take While Taking This Drug. Take 50 mg of vitamin B_6 daily in addition to your daily multivitamin.

Minoxidil (Loniten)

What Does It Do in the Body? Lowers blood pressure, grows hair.

What Is It Prescribed For? High blood pressure, male pattern baldness.

What Are the Possible Side Effects? This is such a dangerous drug that it is recommended only as a last ditch effort if no other hypertensive drugs have worked. It can cause a serious condition called pericardial effusion, and it can make angina worse. In animals it caused all kinds of gross abnormalities of the heart, as well as lesions and infertility.

It can cause fluid and mineral imbalances that are the opposite of what would benefit someone with high blood pressure, as well as an abnormally strong heartbeat and kidney impairment.

CAUTION!

Think Twice About Taking This Drug If . . .

- You have kidney problems.
- You have angina or have had a heart attack.
- Please think twice about taking this drug, period. It's way too dangerous, and there are many better alternatives.

What Are the Interactions with Other Drugs? This is a bad drug to combine with guanethidine, because it can make the already considerable orthostatic hypotension risks of guanethidine even worse.

Natural Alternatives to High Blood Pressure Drugs

High blood pressure is caused by arteries in distress and is one of the easiest symptoms of poor health to treat with simple, natural remedies.

Since medicines that lower blood pressure do have side effects—many of them risky and unpleasant—it's important to always begin by treating high blood pressure with nondrug methods. If you're taking medicine for high blood pressure, your physician should be monitoring you regularly and should have a goal of getting you off the medication. Having said that, almost all physicians consider their patients to be on antihypertensives for life once they begin taking them. This is lazy medicine and is not in the best interests of the patient.

When you're taking drugs to lower blood pressure, it's important not to take herbs that directly lower blood pressure, such as hawthorn, without checking with your doctor and monitoring your blood pressure so you can make the necessary reductions in medication. The following blood-pressure-lowering program works effectively to lower blood pressure, so if you are also taking a hypertension drug, you will need to measure your blood pressure daily at home to be sure it doesn't drop too low. Everyone taking an antihypertensive should have a blood pressure monitor at home and use it daily. This will help monitor changes in blood pressure as well as increase awareness of what raises or lowers blood pressure.

If you suddenly find you have high blood pressure, be sure to check with your doctor to rule out heavy metal poisoning (i.e., lead, mercury, cadmium) and kidney disease.

Weight Loss and Exercise

If you are overweight, the first and most important step in lowering blood pressure, even if it is genetic, is to lose weight. People with high blood pressure weigh an average of 29 pounds more than people with normal blood pressure. For every 2 pounds of weight you drop, your blood pressure will drop at least 1 point in both the systolic and diastolic readings.

The natural partner of weight loss is exercise, which also improves circulation. If you exercise, you are 34 percent less likely to develop hypertension than if you're a couch potato. Just a brisk half-hour walk three or four times a week can lower blood pressure from 3 to 15 points in three months. Exercise will also help reduce stress, an important component in hypertension.

The Six Core Principles for Optimal Health are your foundation for treating hypertension naturally. When you're treating hypertension, it's especially important to keep your antioxidant levels high, eat plenty of fiber-filled vegetables and whole grains, and drink plenty of water.

Keep Sodium, Potassium, Magnesium, and Sugar in Balance

For about 30 percent of the population, reducing salt in the diet will help lower blood pressure naturally. Keep your salt intake moderate regardless, at 2,000 to 3,000 mg per day. Studies have shown that an extremely low-sodium diet causes more problems than it solves, so don't overdo it. Excessively low sodium, also called hyponatremia, is most common among elderly women and is poorly recognized by doctors. Hyponatremia can be caused by many drugs, but especially the diuretics, SSRI antidepressants, and antipsychotic and antiepileptic drugs. Hyponatremia can be hard to recognize because, especially in the elderly, the symptoms can be attributed to so many other factors, but they can include nausea, loss of appetite, fatigue, lethargy, muscle cramps, headache, confusion, and when severe, delirium, seizures, coma, and respiratory arrest. Remember, only 30 percent of the population have high blood pressure that's helped by a low-sodium diet—the rest of us simply need to be moderate in our salt intake. If you avoid processed foods, it's highly unlikely that you'll get too much salt in your diet.

Reducing your salt intake won't be effective unless your potassium intake is also high, and yet people who take diuretic drugs to treat hypertension often become potassium-deficient. Signs of potassium deficiency include muscle cramps, weakness, and an irregular heartbeat. Since potassium supplements may cause problems of their own, including diarrhea and nausea, eating a potassium-rich diet is the best way to maintain healthy potassium levels. Most fresh fruits and vegetables contain potassium. Those highest in potassium are bananas, apples, avocados, lima beans, oranges, potatoes, tomatoes, peaches, cantaloupes, and apricots. Fish and meats also contain potassium.

Sufficient magnesium is essential for healthy blood pressure. It plays a key role, with sodium and potassium, in maintaining fluid balance in the cells and regulating how much water the cells hold. When your cells are holding onto water, your blood pressure can go up. Just taking a magnesium supplement can significantly reduce blood pressure. Magnesium deficiency can cause a variety of heart problems, including irregular heartbeat, and it contributes to diabetes.

Recent research shows that beet juice can help reduce blood pressure. An article published in the journal *Hypertension* found that three hours after intake of 2 cups of beet juice, blood pressure was lowered by an average of 10 points, which is about what you will achieve with most blood-pressure-lowering drugs. Researchers concluded that natural nitrates in the beet juice converted to nitrites, which increased nitric oxide levels, which relaxed blood vessels and lowered blood pressure. Pomegranate juice, dark grape juice, and dark chocolate may have similar effects. When you purchase commercial fruit juices, be sure that they are minimally sweetened and do not contain corn sweeteners, which can cause unstable blood sugar and excessive weight gain.

Cutting way back on sugar and refined carbohydrates such as white flour may be as important as cutting down on the salt. The insulin and adrenaline released when your blood sugar spikes cause the body to retain sodium and hold water, which raises blood pressure.

Coffee also stimulates the release of adrenal hormones and can cause a rise in blood pressure.

The Best Cure-All

One of the best ways to reduce blood pressure, which you may find hard to believe because it's so simple, is to drink plenty of clean water.

Stress Hormones Raise Blood Pressure

If you do all of the preceding and your blood pressure is still high, take a good look at the stress in your life and take steps to manage it better or reduce it. The adrenal hormones released when you're under stress automatically raise blood pressure; so if you're chronically stressed, you may have chronic hypertension.

A Natural Blood-Pressure-Lowering Program

Maintain a healthy weight.

Get some moderate exercise at least 30 minutes every day or 45 minutes three to four times a week.

Eat a low-fat, moderate-sodium, low-sugar diet emphasizing whole, fresh foods, especially vegetables, grains, and plenty of fiber.

Avoid refined, packaged, and processed foods.

Limit alcohol consumption to two drinks per day or less.

Avoid coffee.

Stop smoking.

Avoid drugs that raise blood pressure.

Drink plenty of water.

Daily Vitamins (add to the basic vitamin plan in Chapter 9)

Vitamin C, 1,000 to 2,000 mg (reduce the dose if it causes diarrhea)

Vitamin E, 400 IU daily (800 IU total)

Magnesium, 500 to 800 mg

Calcium, up to 500 mg

Zinc, 10 mg daily

Carnitine, up to 1,000 mg, three to four times daily between meals

CoQ10, 30 to 90 mg daily

Herbs

You can take these herbs alone or in a formula that combines them. They come as tablets, as capsules, or in a liquid tincture. Check with your pharmacist about any herb-drug interactions that might be a concern if you're taking one or more prescription or nonprescription medications.

Cayenne

Dandelion (acts as a diuretic)

Dong quai

Garlic (eat fresh or take the odorless pills three times a day)

Gingko biloba (improves blood flow to the extremities)

Ginseng

Hawthorn (strengthens the heart)

Foods

Fresh fruits and vegetables

Fresh celery (four stalks a day has been known to significantly reduce blood pressure—try drinking a carrot and celery juice mix daily)

Cold-water, deep-sea fish (cod, mackerel, sardines, salmon, herring)

Olive oil (instead of vegetable oils or butter)

Onions

Reducing stress may mean cutting down on your commitments, getting more sleep, or making more time for recreation. Managing stress better may mean learning how to meditate; learning relaxation exercises; taking yoga, tai chi, or qi gong classes; or talking to a friend or therapist. Most of us know exactly what our life stressors are. It's a matter of making your health and well-being important enough to make the needed changes.

Cholesterol-Lowering Drugs and Their Natural Alternatives

Cholesterol is a fatlike material that is found in the brain, nerves, blood, bile, and liver. Although it has been a victim of negative press, it is an essential component in the production of the steroid hormones and in nerve function as well as other essential body processes. When it is present in the blood in excess and in one of its destructive oxidated forms (e.g., LDL), it is one of many contributors to hardening of the arteries, or arteriosclerosis, better known as heart disease.

If you do a study of heart disease patients and cholesterol, you will find that cholesterol levels are higher in those with heart disease, and you will find cholesterol-laden fatty deposits blocking the arteries of many people with heart disease. But to then assume that simply lowering cholesterol levels will make heart disease go away is a huge fallacy. High cholesterol does not cause heart disease; it is a symptom of heart disease! When you get a high cholesterol reading on a blood test, that can be an early warning signal that you need to take better care of yourself, but it's certainly not a reason to take cholesterol-lowering drugs before you've given diet, exercise, and supplements a good try.

Heart disease isn't the only disease that causes high levels of blood cholesterol. Diabetes, hypothyroidism, kidney disease, and liver disease can also significantly raise cholesterol levels. Your doctor should first rule out these diseases as a cause of high cholesterol before prescribing you a cholesterol-lowering drug.

Debunking the Cholesterol Myths

In 2001, a federally sponsored report published in the *Journal of the American Medical Association* strongly urged that the 13 million Americans taking statin drugs should be joined by 23 million more. According to this report, taking such a step would offer Americans effective protection against ever having a heart attack. With this strong a push from mainstream medicine in favor of pharmaceutical cholesterol control, it's hard to keep a clear head on the real facts about cholesterol. Unfortunately this bastion of "evidence-based medicine" has no evidence to back up this claim. We'd like to set the record straight for you.

Since the publication of the famous Seven Countries Study in the 1970s, the notion that a diet high in animal fat and cholesterol amplifies the risk of suffering a fatal heart attack has been virtual gospel in mainstream medicine. Reports from the early years of the ongoing Multiple Risk Factor Intervention Trial (MRFIT), involving over 360,000 men, cemented the notion that a diagnosis of high blood cholesterol greatly increases heart attack risk. Scores of smaller studies appeared to further support the diet-heart hypothesis that a high-cholesterol diet causes high blood cholesterol and that high blood cholesterol causes heart disease.

As a result, mainstream medicine has adopted cholesterol-lowering therapies as its first-line defense against heart attack. Millions of people swallow drugs each day to keep their cholesterol low, and drug companies continue to campaign aggressively to get more people to take these medications. Millions have reduced or eliminated sources of animal fat from their diets to reduce their cholesterol consumption, thinking that replacing those foods with vegetable oils, grain-based foods, and low-fat versions of other foods will protect them against heart attack—still the number one cause of death in the United States.

The first problem with this approach is that the diet-heart hypothesis is a myth. Nearly all of the studies frequently cited as supportive of the diet-heart hypothesis are, in fact, methodologically or statistically weak. The second problem is that the focus on cholesterol control has caused much of the medical research community to quit seeking out other avenues for heart disease prevention and to pay only lip service to the lifestyle modifications that truly work to prevent heart attacks.

Uffe Ravnskov, M.D., Ph.D., is a Swedish physician and researcher who has eloquently debunked the cholesterol hypothesis in his book *The Cholesterol Myths* (New Trends Publishing, 2000). Dr. Ravnskov points out that according to the graphs created by Dr. Ancel Keys and the other authors of the Seven Countries Study, the correlation between risk of fatal heart attack and fat consumption seems inarguable. The lower the fat consumption, the less people died from heart attacks, and vice versa. Each country appears to fall perfectly in place on the curve. He also points out that a total of 22 countries were evaluated for this study, and only 7 were included in the final work. If all 22 had been included, the points on the graph would have looked more like a scatterplot than a straight, strong, upwardly curving line.

Dr. Ravnskov also discusses the MRFIT trial, which found that those with the highest blood cholesterol levels (over 265 mg/dL) had an incredible 433 percent greater risk of fatal heart attack than those with the lowest (under 170 mg/dL). A closer look at this study reveals that the researchers' choice to express risk in this manner exaggerates the actual difference between the groups. While 1.3 percent of the subjects with the highest cholesterol levels died from heart attack during the six years of the study, 0.3 percent of the subjects with the lowest levels also died from heart attack. While 1.3 is 433 percent greater than 0.3, the fact is 98.7 percent of the highest cholesterol group did not die of heart attack, and 99.7 percent of the lowest cholesterol group also did not die of heart attack. When you look at it this way, there is only a 1 percent difference between the two groups!

The evidence that contradicts the diet-heart hypothesis is more solid than the evidence that supports it. In the Framingham, Massachusetts, population—a group of thousands of people who are the subjects of ongoing research on several chronic diseases—the cholesterol levels of people who had heart attacks were almost as likely to be low as high. Other studies imply that high cholesterol is protective against heart disease mortality in elderly men and women and that very low cholesterol can be dangerous in women. Cattle-herding Masai in Kenya—who live on diets that consist almost entirely of flesh foods—have some of the lowest blood cholesterol levels and rates of death from heart disease on the planet. A majority of individuals who suffer heart attacks have blood cholesterol levels that fall within the range of normal, while many with high cholesterol never suffer a heart attack.

How Low Is Too Low?

There is absolutely no evidence anywhere that normal cholesterol floating around in the blood does any harm. In fact, cholesterol is the building block for all your steroid hormones, which includes all the sex hormones and the cortisones.

Even slightly low levels of cholesterol are associated with depression, suicide, and lung cancer in older women. A study in Great Britain found that low levels of cholesterol can cause schizophrenia. A controversial article published in the *Journal of the American College of Cardiology* in 2007 suggests that people who take statins and have very low cholesterol levels have a higher risk of cancer, finding ". . . a highly significant inverse relationship between achieved LDL-C levels and rates of newly diagnosed cancer." In other words, the lower the number, the higher the risk of cancer. Or to put it another way, there may be some benefit to normalizing cholesterol levels, but taking cholesterol below normal may be risky. What *will* harm you is oxidized cholesterol, but we'll talk about that in a minute.

Does Eating High-Cholesterol Foods Raise Cholesterol Levels?

How about the myth that eating high-cholesterol foods raises cholesterol levels? This is true for only about 30 percent of the population. For most people, eating high-cholesterol foods does not raise cholesterol. The body manufactures about 75 percent of its own cholesterol from the breakdown products of foods we eat, primarily sugars and carbohydrates. The rest we get directly from what we eat, meaning foods that contain cholesterol. If we eat more cholesterol, the body makes less or it is broken down by the liver and excreted. People who eat extremely excessive amounts of cholesterol-containing foods so that the body is unable to keep up with the elimination process or people whose livers are not functioning properly may have high cholesterol due to their eating habits, but this is an exception, not the rule. OK, if you're having bacon for breakfast, a hamburger for lunch, and steak for dinner, your cholesterol might go up!

If you want to find out if you are one of the 30 percent for whom eating cholesterol does raise blood levels, try this. Have your HDL and LDL cholesterol levels measured; then cut way down on high-cholesterol foods for three months. After the three months, go back and have your cholesterol levels measured again. If your cholesterol count is influenced by your cholesterol intake, your LDL (bad) cholesterol level should have dropped and your HDL levels should be the same or higher.

If Cholesterol Doesn't Cause Heart Disease, What Does?

Heart disease has multiple causes that most Americans are familiar with by now. The most familiar is diet. But why is diet so important? Why do people who eat lots of vegetables and less red meat have healthier hearts? Primarily because people who eat that way also tend to eat less sugar and refined carbohydrates, foods that powerfully promote the oxidation, inflammation, and nutritional deficiencies that are the foundation for most heart disease.

If you want to dramatically reduce your risk of heart disease, and every other chronic disease that's rampant in Westernized countries such as diabetes and arthritis, then dramatically reduce your consumption of sugar and refined carbohydrates. The easiest way to accomplish that is to avoid processed foods.

Vegetables are powerful weapons against heart disease. They are high in antioxidants and hundreds of phytochemicals (plant chemicals) that are natural artery "Roto-Rooters" that disarm harmful oxidized cholesterol and keep it from clogging arteries. Vegetables are also high in fiber, which helps sweep toxins out of your digestive system.

Another potent risk factor for heart disease is low glutathione levels, which interfere with the body's ability to clear out harmful types of cholesterol and toxins that damage arteries.

Some villains in the heart disease drama directly harm artery walls. One of these villains is high homocysteine levels, often caused by a deficiency of B vitamins. Another such villain is rancid oil, such as unsaturated vegetable oils teeming with unstable molecules.

The partially hydrogenated vegetable oils are equally if not more toxic to the heart, and although they've almost been eliminated from supermarket shelves, they're still widely found in fried fast food.

Low magnesium levels do damage by weakening the heart muscles and interfering with nerve impulses and heartbeat.

And we all know by now that depression, high levels of chronic unresolved stress, and lack of exercise are potent risk factors for heart disease.

Why Does Cholesterol Accumulate in the Arteries?

Drug company advertising for cholesterol-lowering drugs gives the impression that excessive cholesterol in the blood simply deposits itself on the artery walls and that lowering cholesterol levels with drugs stops that process. It would be nice if it was that simple, but once again the magic pill theory falls short.

High cholesterol is a symptom of an underlying nutritional deficiency or toxicity (such as those previously mentioned) that damages the arteries. Cholesterol takes many forms, and some forms act as a component in the repair glue that the body calls on to repair damaged artery walls. If the cholesterol called in to do repair work is oxidized, the artery continues to get the message that it's damaged, and more cholesterol gets piled on. In a kind of double whammy, the same nutritional deficiencies and toxins that allow cholesterol to become oxidized also impair the ability of the liver and other organs to do their cleanup work to eliminate harmful fatty acids in the blood. The inflammatory process that kicks in to try to repair artery damage only accelerates the expansion of the artery wall, contributing to the chain reaction of cholesterol accumulation and causing further cholesterol oxidation. One of the ways cholesterol becomes oxidized is when you don't have high enough levels of antioxidants in your body to neutralize the harmful cholesterol.

Myth of the Cholesterol Count

Another cholesterol myth perpetuated by the drug companies is that everyone with a total cholesterol count over 200 mg/dL should be concerned. This claim is not backed up by research. Our individual biochemistry allows for a wide range of cholesterol levels. Your relative levels of HDL and LDL cholesterol are more important than your total cholesterol. A very high level of LDL "bad" cholesterol probably indicates that your body is not efficiently removing cholesterol from your blood, but that inefficiency, and the heart disease that may accompany it, is most likely caused by poor nutrition, a sedentary lifestyle, and stress.

What is more important is that your HDL "good" cholesterol levels stay high and your LDL "bad" cholesterol levels stay low, relative to each other. However, keep your focus on high levels of HDL. A recent study in China found that people with low counts of LDL and low counts of HDL still have high coronary risk. We'll give specific suggestions later in the chapter for raising HDL levels.

The best way to evaluate your cholesterol status using the measurements given in most blood chemistry panels is to measure the ratio of your total cholesterol to your HDL count. For example, if you are a man and your total cholesterol count is 250 and your HDL is 85, you divide 250 by 85 and your ratio will be 2.9. When you calculate your ratio, compare it to these numbers: the average ratio for women is 4.4; for men, it is 5.0. If your ratio number is low, that's a fair indicator that your cholesterol balance is healthy.

Here's a general rule for total cholesterol levels: if your total cholesterol levels are under 200, consider this a green light. Don't worry, be happy! If your cholesterol levels are over 200, be aware that this might be an indication of some damage to your arteries. If you're leading a healthy lifestyle, don't be overly concerned, but be watchful. Consider this a yellow light. If your cholesterol levels are over 300, your body is trying to tell you something: "Help! You're plugging up my arteries!" Consider this a red light. You need to seriously evaluate your diet and lifestyle.

No matter what category you fall into, please do not try to totally eliminate cholesterol from your diet. It is the fundamental building block of all your sex hormones and the adrenal hormones, and it plays an important part in the excretion of fats. Cholesterol is also found in high amounts in the brain and nervous system, where hormones play a critical part in balancing all bodily systems. We all need some cholesterol in our diet. If your cholesterol levels are high, your answer probably lies in overall diet and lifestyle changes.

There's More to Heart Health than Lower Numbers

While a cholesterol-lowering drug will usually do a very good job of lowering your cholesterol, there's scant, if any, evidence that it will help you live longer or reduce your risk of a heart attack unless you are extremely ill or have just suffered from a heart attack. There are no studies showing that women benefit from cholesterol-lowering drugs. Nor are there any studies showing that these drugs reduce heart attacks or death in men from ages 65 to 75. Since heart disease takes decades to develop, it's highly unlikely that cholesterol-lowering drugs will help anyone over the age of 75. That leaves men from ages 35 to 55, but even here the evidence of benefit is slim, and the possible side effects are sobering.

Believe it or not, there is complete consensus (or should we say lip service) among drug companies, physicians, and organizations such as the American Heart Association that the first step in lowering cholesterol should be a "vigorous" attempt to improve diet and increase exercise. Sadly, few physicians are following this advice, and drug company advertising and marketing certainly doesn't reflect it. But it's well-known that cholesterol-lowering drugs can cause severe side effects and that long-term follow-up studies are sadly lacking. The studies that do exist juggle numbers and play with statistics to the point where the information becomes meaningless.

Every information sheet on the most commonly prescribed cholesterol-lowering drugs will tell you that they cause cancer in rodents when taken long-term in relatively normal doses. It's also well-known that they can cause severe emotional imbalances in men, along with a wide array of life-threatening side effects. A study done at the Henry Ford Medical Center in Detroit showed that men taking cholesterol-lowering drugs had a higher risk of suffering from depression, crying spells, anxiety, worry, and suicidal thoughts. Yet physicians routinely prescribe these drugs indefinitely for their older patients.

The wisest course of action is to avoid these drugs unless you are in imminent danger of a heart attack due to clogged arteries. If that's the case, it's important to do everything possible to reverse your heart disease using the cholesterol-lowering plan outlined here and to get off the drugs as soon as possible. These drugs can have ominous side effects, especially when used on a long-term basis. The *New England Journal of Medicine* published research showing that genetics likely plays a role in the muscle pain, weakness, and nerve damage that can be a side effect of statins.

Cholesterol-Lowering Drugs

Examples of Bile Acid Sequestrants

Cholestyramine (Questran, Prevalite)
Colesevelam (Welchol)
Colestipol HCl (Colestid)

The bile acid sequestrants, also known as "bile-blockers," such as cholestyramine (Questran) and colestipol HCl (Colestid) are resins, often taken in powder form, that block the production of bile. Cholesterol is the building block of bile, a substance normally released via the liver to break down fats in the intestines and enhance their absorption. After bile breaks down fats, it is reabsorbed back into the liver. The bile-blockers bind to bile in the intestines so it can't be reabsorbed and is instead excreted in the feces. This forces the liver to take up more cholesterol from the blood to produce more bile, in effect lowering cholesterol levels (and making your liver work a lot harder).

Seems like a neat solution, but the bile-blockers also bind to the fat-soluble vitamins such as A, D, E, and K, so that instead of absorbing these vitamins you excrete them. (Sound familiar? Olestra, the fake fat, does the same thing.) Ironically, a shortage of vitamin E can be a direct cause of heart disease, which is what the drugs are meant to prevent in the first place.

There is some evidence that along with blocking cholesterol absorption these drugs are blocking the absorption of the important EFA (essential fatty acids) oils that are essential to good health. Bile-blocking resins also lower folate (folic acid) levels, which raises homocysteine levels, another potent risk factor for heart disease.

Here's a medical maze for you. Physicians prescribing bile-blockers will read on the drug information sheet that anticoagulant, blood-thinning drugs such as warfarin (Coumadin) can become less effective when prescribed along with a bile-blocker. Yet long-term use of a bile-blocker can cause a deficiency of vitamin K, which will increase the tendency to bleed, making the drugs more effective. In other words, what will happen when you combine these two types of drugs is truly unpredictable—and that is very dangerous.

What Do They Do in the Body? Lower cholesterol by blocking the reabsorption of bile.

What Are They Prescribed For? Lowering cholesterol levels.

What Are the Possible Side Effects? Constipation occurs in up to 50 percent of all patients who use these drugs! Constipation can be severe, especially if you already have a problem with constipation or hemorrhoids.

Chronic use of these resins can lead to excessive bleeding or poor clotting from a vitamin K deficiency. Vitamin D deficiency can also be a problem, resulting in rashes and irritations on the skin, tongue, and anus, as well as poor bone formation. Vitamin D deficiency also increases the risk for heart disease and many types of cancer.

In addition, osteoporosis, liver dysfunction, and disturbances of the acid-base balance of the body are side effects of these drugs.

They can also raise triglyceride levels. High triglyceride levels increase the risk of heart disease.

Most alarming, however, is the research that reports cancer as a possible side effect. Several studies stated that some rats who were given bile acid sequestrants grew cancerous intestinal tumors.

CAUTION!

Think Twice About Taking These Drugs If . . .

- You have constipation, especially if you are over 60 years of age.
- You have blood clotting problems, osteoporosis, or severe vitamin deficiencies.
- You have a gallbladder obstruction (bile duct obstruction).
- You have phenylketonuria, a genetic disease; hypothyroidism; diabetes; kidney and blood vessel disorders; dysproteinemia; obstructive liver disease; or ischemic heart disease.

What Are the Interactions with Other Drugs? Because bile acid sequestrants may delay or reduce the absorption of other drugs you take with them, it's best to take other medication at least one hour before or four to six hours after taking bile acid sequestrants.

What Are the Interactions with Food? These drugs decrease the absorption of nutrients you get from your foods such as sugars, fats, vitamins, and minerals.

What Nutrients Do They Deplete or Throw out of Balance? Calcium, carotene, electrolytes, folic acid, iron, and the fat-soluble vitamins, A, B_{12}, D, E, and K.

What Else to Take While Taking These Drugs. Take supplements of vitamins A, B_{12}, D, E, and K as well as folic acid, iron, electrolytes, beta-carotene, and calcium.

To reduce constipation, drink plenty of water and eat foods high in fiber such as whole grains, vegetables, and fruit.

Other Tips on These Drugs. Because of the absorbing mechanism of these drugs, take other medications or supplements at least one hour before or four to six hours after a bile acid sequestrant.

Examples of Statins (HMG-CoA Reductase Inhibitors)

Atorvastatin (Lipitor)
Fluvastatin (Lescol)
Lovastatin (Mevacor, Altocor, Altoprev)
Mevastatin
Pravastatin (Pravachol)
Rosuvastatin (Crestor)
Simvastatin (Zocor)

These drugs are known as the cholesterol-blockers or statins, and if you live in the United States and watch TV, you've seen endless expensive ads for these drugs. The statins may be the most heavily and aggressively marketed drugs in history. The drug companies are working overtime to manipulate you, us, and everyone else from Congress to the American Medical Association (AMA) to the American Heart Association to the individual doctor to get us all on statin drugs. Every few years they manage to get "normal" cholesterol level numbers reduced so that today, virtually everyone over the age of 50 would need to take statins based on their cholesterol numbers. And it's working! In 2006 Lipitor (atorvastatin calcium) was the top-selling drug in the United States. There is *zero* (that's right— zip, zilch) evidence that statins reduce the risk of heart disease or death for women, and yet women spend billions of dollar a year on them.

Statin drugs directly block an enzyme (HMG-CoA reductase) needed to make cholesterol in the liver. These drugs originate from an ancient Chinese medicine called red yeast rice, which is rice fermented with red wine and the yeast *Monascus purpureus*. Lovastatin is actually the name of a compound found in red yeast rice. The rest of the statins are essentially lovastatin "tweaked" to create more potent and patentable drugs, which also have more side effects.

The biggest danger and most common side effect of taking statin drugs is liver damage. It's frightening to imagine what's happening to a liver subjected to, say, a dose of Mevacor (lovastatin), a couple of martinis, and a Tylenol (acetaminophen), all of which compromise liver function. This type of triple whammy could be enough to cause serious problems in someone already ill or weak, yet few physicians would think to mention this to their patients. American medicine has a tendency to pay no attention to the liver until it is very damaged.

Remember, cholesterol is the basic building block for the cortisones, testosterone, estrogen, progesterone, and DHEA. Is it any wonder that people taking cholesterol-blocking statins suffer from steroid-hormone-related complaints, such as men growing breasts and being impotent, women becoming bald, and both suffering from insomnia and fatigue? Cholesterol is essential for proper brain function. Is it any wonder that men with very low cholesterol are depressed and suicidal, and that memory problems are a complaint of those on this drug?

But perhaps even more serious than the preceding side effects is the fact that the same mechanism that blocks cholesterol production also blocks the production of CoQ10, a substance essential to a healthy heart and muscles. Your physician may tell you that you'll never have a shortage of CoQ10, but this is not borne out by the facts. The truth is that heart disease patients are consistently found to have low levels of CoQ10. About 1 out of every 200 people who use the statins has side effects of muscle pain and weakness, which can be a sign of even more serious problems, leading to kidney failure and even death. All indications are that the cause of these symptoms is a deficiency of CoQ10. So once again, we have a cholesterol-lowering drug supposedly given to reverse heart disease but causing a deficiency of a substance crucial to a strong and healthy heart.

Keeping cholesterol in a healthy range is a good idea, and taking a statin drug short-term may be a wise choice, but the concept that these drugs are harmless and can be taken for life is misguided and dangerous. As you'll discover later in this chapter, you can also choose to take a red yeast rice supplement, which is the natural form of the statin drugs and has been shown to safely and effectively lower cholesterol. But keep in mind that it, too, is a statin and also has the potential to cause the same kinds of problems.

What Do They Do in the Body? These drugs directly block an enzyme needed to make cholesterol in the body.

What Are They Prescribed For? Lowering cholesterol levels.

What Are the Possible Side Effects? The most common side effects of the statins are stomach ulcers, liver damage, and a dangerous disease called rhabdomyolysis that actually destroys muscle tissue. Baycol (cerivastatin), a statin that was recalled in 2000, caused at least 31 fatal cases of this disease. The risk of rhabdomyolysis increases as the statin dose increases and in those with diabetes and kidney disease. In fact, rhabdomyolysis can cause kidney damage.

The watchdog group Public Citizen has petitioned the Food and Drug Administration (FDA) to ban rosuvastatin (Crestor) because of concerns of rhabdomyolysis and kidney toxicity. According to Public Citizen, some of the major U.S. health insurers have refused to reimburse for Crestor because of safety concerns.

Other side effects of the statins include back pain, insomnia, heartburn, greater susceptibility to upper sinus infections, alteration of taste, dizziness, memory loss, numbness in the extremities, tremors, loss of libido, impotence, enlarged thyroid, and skin conditions such as bumps and rashes. They also tend to increase the formation of cataracts, and they cause cancer and birth defects in rodents and dogs. Some patients have experienced steroid-hormone-related complaints such as impotence, insomnia, and fatigue.

Be aware! Many of these symptoms are attributed to aging rather than to the statin side effects, resulting in a poor quality of life for potentially millions of people. These side effects are also likely to get you on the drug treadmill, as your doctor prescribes sleeping pills for insomnia, acid blockers for heartburn, antibiotics for sinus infections, and erectile dysfunction drugs for impotence. No wonder the statins are such a cash cow for the drug companies!

CAUTION!

Think Twice About Taking These Drugs If . . .

- You have a stomach ulcer.
- You have the following conditions: infection, a suppressed immune system,

hypertension, trauma, uncontrollable seizures, or endocrine or electrolyte disorders. These drugs can cause kidney failure in patients with severe cases of these conditions.
- You have liver disease, poor liver function, kidney disease, or poor kidney function, or you drink substantial amounts of alcohol. They can damage your liver and kidneys significantly.
- You are scheduled soon for surgery. Ask your physician how you can safely discontinue using these drugs.
- You have any disease that contributes to increased blood cholesterol such as hypothyroidism, diabetes, kidney and blood vessel disorders, liver disease, or dysproteinemia.

What Are the Interactions with Food? Take lovastatin and fluvastatin with meals. Pravastatin and simvastatin are taken without regard to food.

What Nutrients Do They Deplete or Throw out of Balance? CoQ10.

What Else to Take While Taking This Drug. CoQ10 (ubiquinone or ubiquinol), 30 to 200 mg daily. To support your liver, you can take the herb silymarin (milk thistle), the supplement alpha-lipoic acid, and NAC (N-acetyl cysteine).

Other Tips on These Drugs. Because of the real threat of muscle destruction, contact your physician immediately if you notice muscle pain, tenderness, or weakness, particularly if a fever accompanies these symptoms.

In addition, your physician should monitor your liver and kidney functions regularly when you are taking these drugs (few physicians actually do this).

Ezetimibe (Zetia)

What Does It Do in the Body? Reduces cholesterol levels by reducing the intestinal absorption of cholesterol.

What Is It Prescribed For? Lowering cholesterol levels.

What Are the Possible Side Effects? Liver damage, abdominal pain, diarrhea, muscle pain, back pain, joint pain, chest pain, cough, hoarseness, sinusitis, fatigue, dizziness, headache, viral infection, depression, mood changes, and memory impairment.

CAUTION!

Think Twice About Taking This Drug If . . .

Please think twice about taking this drug, period, whether alone or combined with another drug (e.g., Vytorin). This is a relatively new drug, it's a potent drug, and there's no evidence that it benefits patients with heart disease. Furthermore, there is evidence that Vytorin (Zetia and Zocor) may increase the risk of cancer.

Dextrothyroxine sodium (Choloxin)

What Does It Do in the Body? Reduces cholesterol levels by stimulating the liver to excrete it faster.

What Is It Prescribed For? Lowering cholesterol levels.

What Are the Possible Side Effects? This drug stresses the heart tremendously. It can cause heart attacks and increase the size of the heart.

This drug can also cause nausea, vomiting, constipation, diarrhea, gallstones, jaundice, hair loss, rashes, itching, menstrual irregularities, water retention, muscle pain, tremors, nervousness, and dizziness.

CAUTION!

Think Twice About Taking This Drug If . . .

- You are scheduled for surgery in the next two weeks. Avoid it.
- You have liver or kidney disease.
- You have asthma.
- You have a heart condition.
- You are severely overweight.

Please think twice about taking this drug, period. It's too hard on the heart, the liver, and the kidneys, and there are too many other, relatively safer alternatives available. In also interacts dangerously with many other drugs.

Clofibrate (Atromid-S)

What Does It Do in the Body? Lowers triglycerides and very low-density lipoprotein (VLDL) cholesterol levels. It does not predictably lower LDL levels.

What Is It Prescribed For? Lowering high triglyceride levels.

What Are the Possible Side Effects? This drug can cause anemia, liver and kidney dysfunction, gallbladder problems, peptic ulcers, abnormal heartbeat, and flulike symptoms.

Liver cancer is also a possible side effect of this drug. It produced tumors in the livers of rodents and humans in published research. A World Health Organization (WHO) study found that clofibrate may increase the risk of cancer, liver disease, and pancreatitis.

CAUTION!

Think Twice About Taking This Drug If . . .

- You have a peptic ulcer.
- You have liver or kidney disease.
- You have a gallbladder obstruction.

- You haven't tried diet and exercise changes first. There are too many serious side effects, and it is a poorly studied drug.

What Nutrients Does It Deplete or Throw out of Balance? Minerals, carotenes, fats, iron, sugars, and vitamins A, B$_{12}$, D, E, and K.

What Else to Take with This Drug. Supplements that replenish the preceding vitamins, minerals, and nutrients.

Gemfibrozil (Lopid)

What Does It Do in the Body? Its major effect is to lower triglycerides and VLDL (very low-density lipoprotein), but it may also lower LDL levels, and it may raise HDL levels.

What Is It Prescribed For? Reducing triglycerides.

What Are the Possible Side Effects? As is true with most of the other cholesterol-lowering drugs, this drug is essentially toxic and therefore stresses your liver and kidneys. As a result, liver dysfunction, hyperglycemia, and kidney failure are possible side effects of this drug. It may also increase the risk of cancer.

Other side effects include hypokalemia (excessively low sodium), muscle pain, eczema, fatigue, drowsiness, vertigo, convulsions, appendicitis, gallbladder disease, abdominal pain, upset stomach, taste perversion, water retention, lupuslike syndrome, jaundice, pancreatitis, anemia, impotence, vitamin deficiencies, and irregular heartbeat.

Liver cancer and cataracts occurred in rats tested with this drug.

CAUTION!

Think Twice About Taking This Drug If . . .

- You have an underactive thyroid or diabetes.

- You have liver, kidney or gallbladder disease.
- You have poor liver or kidney function.

What Are the Interactions with Food? Absorption of nutrients from food is reduced.

What Nutrients Does It Deplete or Throw out of Balance? Vitamins A, B$_{12}$, D, E, K, calcium, iron, magnesium, and potassium.

What Else to Take While Taking This Drug. Vitamins A, B$_{12}$, D, E, and K; calcium; iron; magnesium; and potassium.

Other Tips on This Drug. Be especially cautious when driving or doing any activity that requires alertness, coordination, or physical dexterity. This drug can make it difficult to focus and concentrate.

Fenofibrate (TriCor)

What Does It Do in the Body? Increases the body's breakdown of triglycerides in the bloodstream by inhibiting specific enzymes. It also alters cholesterol particles in the bloodstream, causing them to be broken down and excreted more rapidly.

What Is It Prescribed For? Reducing total cholesterol, LDL cholesterol, and triglycerides. It also slightly increases HDL.

What Are the Possible Side Effects? Diarrhea, nausea, constipation, abnormal liver function tests, respiratory disorders, runny nose, back pain, headache, gallstones, pancreatic inflammation, kidney failure, and rhabdomyolysis (the same dangerous muscle disorder that can strike people who use statin drugs). Studies on animals found that dosages within the limits used on humans caused cancer.

Eight Steps You Can Take to Lower Your Cholesterol Naturally

1. Eat more fiber. Studies show that fiber has a direct and dramatic cholesterol-lowering effect. You can get plenty of fiber by eating fresh, whole, unprocessed foods and a plant-based diet. Pectin, a soluble form of fiber found in apples, blueberries, and grapefruit, particularly helps reduce cholesterol. If you want to add more fiber, take 1 teaspoon a day of psyllium with 8 ounces of water or juice. Psyllium is the active ingredient in Metamucil, but the latter also has sugar, preservatives, and food colorings. Stick to the plain psyllium found in your health food store—it's cheaper, too. Whole oat cereal manufacturers are FDA-approved to claim that their product reduces cholesterol levels. True, and so do the other sources of fiber.

2. Make olive oil and fish oil your predominant dietary fats. They both can actually lower LDL cholesterol. However, don't entirely neglect the other fats: keep your nutrition in balance.

3. Add garlic to your diet. Garlic is a powerful cholesterol-lowering substance. It also lowers blood pressure and makes the blood less sticky. Add it liberally to your diet.

4. Have a glass of red wine with dinner, or take a bioflavonoid supplement such as grapeseed extract or green tea daily. Both are known to have a cholesterol-lowering effect. However, too much alcohol (more than two drinks per day) will raise cholesterol levels.

5. Take niacin, in the form of inositol hexanicotinate.

6. Take your cholesterol-busting supplements.

7. Eat your cholesterol-busting foods.

8. Exercise, which will directly raise HDL cholesterol. It's a must for healthy arteries.

CAUTION!

Think Twice About Taking This Drug If . . .

You have any type of kidney or liver impairment.

Natural Alternatives to Cholesterol-Lowering Drugs

It is so easy for nearly everyone to significantly lower LDL cholesterol and raise HDL levels with diet, exercise, and supplements that it seems extreme for physicians to prescribe cholesterol-lowering drugs before other, simpler measures have been taken and failed. The exception to this would be if you are in imminent danger of having a heart attack and need to take extreme measures.

Niacin Is a Potent Cholesterol Buster

Taking niacin (vitamin B_3) is one of the safest and most effective ways to lower LDL or "bad" cholesterol and raise HDL or "good" cholesterol. It also effectively lowers triglycerides. It's at least as effective as the cholesterol-lowering drugs and much less expensive. However, there are some downsides to niacin.

Niacin is a vasodilator, meaning it expands the blood vessels, bringing more blood into the upper part of the body. In large doses, it can cause a "niacin flush" around the head, neck, and shoulders. The skin becomes flushed and red, and this is accompanied by a burning or tingling sensation, which most people find uncomfortable and annoying. While a niacin flush is harmless, in high doses niacin can cause stomach cramps, diarrhea, and nausea, and high doses taken for an extended period of time may adversely affect the liver. People with ischemic heart disease should be cautious with niacin. For these people, niacin can cause abnormal heartbeats.

The key to taking niacin successfully to lower cholesterol levels is to start with a small amount, 50 mg twice a day, and gradually work up to 400 mg three times a day over a period of two to three months. It's also important to take a "no-flush" niacin formula that delivers all of the benefits of niacin without the unpleasant side effects. These formulas are made with inositol hexanicotinate. If your doctor prescribes nicotinic acid, tell him or her about inositol hexanicotinate. It's the same thing in a safer form. If you stick to a healthy lifestyle, you shouldn't have to take the niacin for more than a year at the most. Please remember to taper it off gradually.

If your physician has you on cholesterol-lowering drugs, don't stop taking them without supervision.

Estrogen Lowers Cholesterol: Fact or Fiction?

That hormone replacement therapy (HRT) protects against heart disease was an accepted "fact" in conventional medicine until the Women's Health Initiative and European research finally showed this "fact" to be fiction. Now women are being told not to take HRT to prevent heart attack. HRT with estrogens and progestins (synthetic progesterone) actually increases the risk of heart attack and stroke, and its effects on bone health are minimal. Natural hormones, however,

may be a safe option for some women. Natural estrogens, when used wisely, can help maintain healthy blood vessels. You'll read more about this in Chapter 19. If you're over the age of 50 and contemplating HRT, we'd like to recommend that you read one of the books that Virginia Hopkins coauthored with Dr. John R. Lee, *What Your Doctor May Not Tell You About Menopause*, or if you're between the ages of 35 and 50, *What Your Doctor May Not Tell You About Premenopause*.

Do Fish Oil Supplements Really Lower Cholesterol?

Fish oil is excellent not only for reducing overall cholesterol, but also for increasing your HDL or "good" cholesterol. The best source of fish oil is fish eaten during your daily meals. There has been a lot of speculation that taking a fish oil supplement can give you the same benefits as eating fish, but the data published from several studies indicate that it just isn't true. In fact, taking a supplement of fish oils may make your cholesterol worse! It's possible that fish oil supplements are rancid by the time they get to our refrigerators. Some studies done with fish oil preserved with vitamin E are encouraging, but your best bet is to eat fish (and not deep fried!) at least twice a week.

Cholesterol-Busting Supplements

If your cholesterol is over 300, you'll want to consider taking the following vitamins and minerals in addition to those suggested in the Six Core Principles for Optimal Health. Most of these essential nutrients are antioxidants that help lower your LDL or "bad" cholesterol levels:

• **Vitamin C.** 1,000 mg three times daily. If this high a dose gives you diarrhea, reduce the dose until it goes away.

- **Magnesium.** 300 mg daily.

- **Calcium.** 200 mg daily.

- **Vitamin E (mixed tocopherols).** 400 IU twice a day (total 800 IU daily). In one study, ingesting this amount daily caused a 26 percent reduction in LDL or "bad" cholesterol production.

- **Psyllium (fiber).** 1 to 2 teaspoons a day. Be sure to drink plenty of water.

- **N-acetyl cysteine (NAC).** 500 mg three times a day. This will help raise your glutathione levels, which will support your liver so it can more efficiently excrete cholesterol.

- **Green tea.** The active beneficial ingredients in green tea are called polyphenols, substances that act as antioxidants, neutralize harmful fats and oils, strengthen the liver, and lower LDL cholesterol, while increasing HDL levels. You can either drink green tea or take it in a concentrated form as a supplement.

- **PCOs or proanthocyanidins.** PCOs (e.g., grapeseed extract) work specifically to stop "bad" cholesterol from forming and sticking to artery walls.

- **Cayenne.** This spice lowers cholesterol. Take a daily supplement of cayenne in capsules, or use it liberally on your food.

- **Curry.** Another spice that lowers cholesterol.

- **Guggul.** Taking guggul is a new but old way to lower cholesterol. Ayurvedic medicine is an ancient form of healing from India that relies largely on dividing people into body and personality types and then prescribing a variety of treatments that include plant medicines. Lately we've been learning more about the large number of safe, effective medicines Ayurveda has in its pharmacy, and scientific research is following. One of the best known Ayurvedic medicines is called guggul, a plant traditionally used mainly to treat arthritis and obesity. Studies have shown that guggul significantly reduces cholesterol levels without side effects. One study used an active component of guggul called guggulipid, which participants took for 12 weeks. In 80 percent of the patients, serum cholesterol was lowered by an average of 24 percent and serum triglycerides were lowered by an average of 23 percent, which is comparable to the prescription drugs. Of these, 60 percent showed an increase in their HDL (good) cholesterol. When guggulipid was compared to the drug clofibrate (Atromid-S), it came out about the same, without the side effects.

- **Red yeast rice.** This is actually an ancient Chinese medicine and condiment made from specially fermented rice and red wine. The reaction between the rice, wine, and yeasts used for fermentation yields natural statin substances. Red yeast rice has been used safely to strengthen circulation and help digestion in Chinese medicine for hundreds of years. In two studies presented at the American Heart Association's conference in 1999, red yeast rice—sold under the brand name Cholestin—was found to lower blood cholesterol levels. In another study, published in the *American Journal of Clinical Nutrition*, red yeast rice was found to lower total cholesterol, LDL, and triglycerides (another type of blood fat that has been linked with heart disease).

When the company that makes Cholestin put their product through rigorous scientific testing to prove its efficacy and safety, do you think the FDA, an organization that constantly harasses supplement makers because of a so-called lack of such research, applauded or supported their efforts? Of course, they didn't. Instead, they tried to call Cholestin a drug and ban supple-

Top Cholesterol-Busting Foods

Alfalfa sprouts

Berries, especially blueberries and raspberries

Brewer's yeast

Carrots (raw)

Eggplant

Fenugreek (an herb)

Fish, especially salmon, mackerel, herring,
    sardines, cod, tuna, and trout

Garlic

Grapefruit

Legumes

Oat bran

Olive oil

Onions

Prunes

Soy products such as miso, tempeh, and tofu

Whole grains, including rice, barley, millet,
    oats, wheat, and rye

Yogurt

ment manufacturers from selling it at all. Afraid of competition against expensive, bestselling cholesterol drugs, the FDA told federal judges that allowing Cholestin to be sold would reduce the incentive of the pharmaceutical industry to develop new medicines—reasoning that seems outrageous to anyone who believes that the FDA is supposed to be watching out for consumers, not big drug companies. Fortunately, the judges ruled in favor of the supplement makers, and red yeast rice is now a safe, effective, inexpensive, and widely available alternative to statin drugs for which no prescription is needed.

• **Policosanol.** Supplements containing this substance have been found to work well to balance cholesterol counts. Biochemically speaking, policosanol is made up of a series of what's known as fatty alcohols. If you want to know what these fatty alcohols naturally look and feel like, scrape a little bit of the waxy film off the leaves of a tree or the peel of a citrus fruit. Commercially sold policosanol supplements are usually made from either sugarcane or beeswax. Citrus peels, wheat germ, and caviar are other rich sources of policosanol.

Policosanol has been shown to lower LDL cholesterol levels by up to 20 percent, and it raises HDL by an average of 10 percent—without the side effects caused by statins. As a matter of fact, in a study of nearly 28,000 people who used policosanol for two to four years, less than half of 1 percent of the subjects experienced notable adverse effects from their daily dose.

In one study, published in the journal *Gynecological Endocrinology*, researchers enlisted 244 menopausal women for whom six weeks on a conventional cholesterol-lowering diet did no good. The women were given either a placebo pill or 5 mg of policosanol each day for 12 weeks. The women given policosanol were then given 10 mg for 12 more weeks. By the end of the study, the policosanol users had some amazing changes in their cholesterol levels: their LDL fell by 25.2 percent, their total cholesterol fell by 16.7 percent, and their ratio of total cholesterol to HDL fell by 27.2 percent. This is big news because the statins do not raise good HDL cholesterol and may even slightly lower it.

What Boosts Good (HDL) Levels

Carnitine, an amino acid

Fish

Guggul

Yams

Policosanol

Another study—this one from the *International Journal of Clinical Pharmacology*—compared the effects of policosanol to those of pravastatin, a commonly used statin drug, in elderly patients with high cholesterol and high risk of heart attack. These patients took 10 mg of policosanol or pravastatin for eight weeks. Those who took policosanol lowered their LDL by an average of 19.3 percent, their total cholesterol by an average of 13.9 percent, and their ratio of total cholesterol to HDL by 24.4 percent. Pravastatin reduced LDL by 15.6 percent and the total-cholesterol-to-HDL ratio by 15.9 percent, but didn't raise levels of artery-cleaning HDL. In this study, policosanol also stood out for its ability to inhibit the tendency of blood to clot together and clog blood vessels.

Policosanol causes none of the adverse effects statins can cause. It appears to work by slowing the production of cholesterol in the liver while increasing the liver's ability to reabsorb LDL. The most frequently cited side effect? Weight loss—not exactly an undesirable side effect for most people at risk of developing heart disease. Unlike statins, policosanol causes no decrease in libido, and there's a hint of evidence from an animal study that it may actually increase libido slightly! Policosanol also inhibits the oxidation of LDL cholesterol, the free radical attack that makes LDL so much more dangerous to blood vessel health.

In animal studies, it decreased the uncontrolled inflammation and cell growth known to lead to artery disease. Policosanol also helps thin the blood, decreasing the chances of a clot forming to plug up an artery and cause a heart attack or stroke.

Levels of a specific type of proinflammatory biochemical called thromboxane can rise too high as a direct result of a poor, refined-food diet and can cause artery walls to clamp down tight, decreasing blood and oxygen flow to the heart and elsewhere. Some studies have shown a decrease in levels of this type of thromboxane with policosanol.

Lowering Triglycerides Naturally

Triglycerides are a type of fat that circulates in the blood. There is good evidence that elevated triglycerides are at least as big a risk factor for heart disease as high LDL cholesterol. If your triglycerides are high, there's a pretty good chance you're eating way too many refined carbohydrates—think sugar, cookies, candies, pastries—and not getting enough exercise. Excess alcohol will also raise triglycerides. Supplementing with niacin (in the form of inositol hexanicotinate) can help lower triglycerides, as can guggulipid (see earlier section on cholesterol-busting supplements) and fish oil supplements. For most people, cutting out the refined carbs and getting some exercise will lower triglycerides.

Chapter 11

Drugs for the Digestive Tract and Their Natural Alternatives

A healthy digestive tract is an essential cog in the wheel of a healthy body. If you're serious about living a long, healthy, vibrant life, your digestive system needs to be able to break down and assimilate your food efficiently and effectively. The millions upon millions of cells that make up your body wouldn't know what to do with a whole piece of fruit. They can use only the simplest breakdown products of food to fuel their activities, and they can use the vitamins and minerals locked away in that juicy apple only once they are released in their simplest forms.

Digestion begins in the mouth. As soon as you take a bite of food, enzymes and mucins in your saliva begin to break it down and lubricate it for a trip down the esophagus. Meanwhile, down in the stomach, the taste, smell, or even the thought of food stimulates the secretion of hydrochloric acid and the enzyme pepsin, which digests protein. Enzymes from the gallbladder and pancreas are also stimulated by the smell and taste of food.

Chewing is another potent trigger of acid and enzyme secretion. Your mother was absolutely right when she reminded you to chew your food thoroughly. The longer you chew, the more time the rest of your digestive tract has to prepare for its role in the process. Smaller particles of well-chewed food are, for practical purposes, predigested. This helps ensure optimal breakdown and absorption of what you eat.

Stomach Acid, Heartburn, and Ulcers

In the stomach, muscular contractions thoroughly mix food with hydrochloric acid. Stomach acid—powerful enough to strip paint—is a vital part of good digestion. A thick mucous layer protects the stomach walls from harm as the acid kills bacteria and parasites and frees up minerals (such as magnesium and potassium) and the B vitamins folate and B_{12} so that they can be absorbed in the small intestine.

If sufficient stomach acid isn't produced, digestion suffers. The passage of food out of the stomach into the small intestine is delayed, which can lead to heartburn as the stomach pushes food mixed with acid back into the esophagus. Burning is caused by acid coming in contact with the lining of the esophagus, which isn't protected by a mucous layer like the stomach is. Heavy, fatty meals; large meals; eating on the run or while under stress; lying down just after a meal; or eating just after heavy exercise also set the stage for heartburn.

Contrary to what the huge drug companies that make antacids and H2 blocker drugs such as Tagamet and Zantac say, excessive acid production is almost never the reason for heartburn or ulcers. It is estimated that more than half of all bleeding ulcers are caused by taking NSAID drugs such as aspirin and ibuprofen. In many cases, the antacids and H2 blockers given to alleviate the symptoms of stomach pain mask the symptoms until the problem is life threatening.

Antacids and H2 blockers alleviate symptoms for a short while by buffering acid and decreasing acid secretion, but they can actually aggravate the underlying problem: too little acid in the stomach. With chronic use of these medications, digestion is compromised and decreased absorption of some vitamins and minerals can result. Once the food finally makes its way into the intestines, it isn't broken down enough for it to be properly absorbed.

Research shows that long-term use of both H2 (e.g., Tagamet) and proton pump inhibitors (e.g., Nexium) can increase the risk of community-acquired pneumonia and other infections, probably because the reduced stomach acid fails to kill the bacteria that can cause infections.

Other factors contribute to low secretion of stomach acid. Drinking icy cold liquids with meals can suppress it, and stomach acid levels decline with age. A large percentage of people over 50 make too little stomach acid for thorough digestion of food.

A few years ago, if you asked your physician what causes ulcers, he or she would promptly reply that too much stomach acid was to blame. Now we know that a spiral-shaped bacteria called *Helicobacter pylori* (*H. pylori* for short) is the primary culprit. It suppresses acid production and creates holes in the stomach's protective mucous layer, allowing acid to seep through and burn holes in the delicate tissue underneath.

An *H. pylori* infection can also cause symptoms of indigestion and heartburn.

The Small Intestine and Its Enzymes

Food leaving the stomach is squirted in small amounts into the duodenum, which is the first part of the small intestine. The pancreas and small intestine secrete the enzymes amylase (to digest starches), protease (to digest proteins), and lipase (to digest fats) when they detect food in the duodenum. These enzymes break food down into parts your body can use, including carbohydrates, amino acids, free fatty acids, vitamins, and minerals. The pancreas also makes bicarbonate that buffers acid so that the food won't burn holes in the small intestine. Bile that has been made in the liver and stored in the gallbladder to emulsify fats is released into the duodenum as food passes through.

Enzymes play a major role in all of the body's functions. Digestive enzymes are only one variety of these important catalysts of biological reactions and are named for the substance they break down. For example, the enzyme that breaks down sucrose (table sugar) is called sucrase; cellulose (plant starch) is broken down by cellulase. The absence or shortage of a single digestive enzyme can have serious consequences. Abdominal cramping and diarrhea after drinking milk are the symptoms of a deficiency of lactase, the enzyme responsible for the digestion of the sugars in milk (lactose).

Digestive enzymes are built from amino acids and vitamin or mineral cofactors, or coenzymes. Zinc and magnesium are two of the most common digestive enzyme cofactors. The B vitamins thiamine, riboflavin, pantothenic acid, and biotin, as well as the minerals molybdenum, manganese, copper, iron, and selenium,

play the role of coenzymes as well. Each time the enzyme does its job, it uses up its coenzyme, which then needs to be replaced. Eating foods rich in vitamins and minerals will ensure that your digestive enzymes will be able to quickly reactivate. Raw foods contain their own enzymes that help your digestive tract do its job.

The surface of the small intestine is designed to absorb the nutrients your body has worked so hard to extract from your food and turn them over to the bloodstream and liver for processing. Your small intestine is 22 feet long, with an inside surface lined with tiny fingerlike protuberances called villi (think of a microscopic shag carpet). These protrusions greatly increase the available surface area for absorption of nutrients to a whopping 2,000 square feet—a little bigger than half a football field.

Leaky Gut Syndrome, Food Allergies, and Digestive Disorders

Your small intestine is vulnerable to harm due to poor diet, certain drugs, or disease. If the villi are damaged, food isn't well absorbed and what is known as "leaky gut syndrome" can result. In a healthy intestine, nutrients are "tagged" by specialized immune cells so that the body will recognize them as safe. Without these tags, needed nutrients are treated as foreign invaders and your immune system creates antibodies to destroy them. In a damaged gut, your tagging mechanism is not up to par and food allergy—an immune response that can microscopically damage the intestinal wall—results. The symptoms of food allergy can be as diverse as fatigue, a chronic rash, headaches, and arthritis.

Food allergy is created in a damaged gut when microscopic holes in the intestinal lining allow undigested food molecules to escape into the bloodstream. The immune system can't recognize these molecules, so it sends out its battalions in an effort to destroy them. An immune system that's working overtime will definitely keep you from feeling your best, as anyone with allergies knows from experience. Food allergies have been implicated in a wide variety of digestive problems including constipation, diarrhea, Crohn's disease, and irritable bowel syndrome (IBS).

If you think you might have leaky gut syndrome, you can ask a health professional to give you what's called the lactulose/mannitol absorption test. Levels of lactulose, a large molecule that shouldn't be passed into the bloodstream, are measured. Elevated levels are a good indication that your gut is leaky.

Even as conventional physicians deny the existence of delayed food allergies, they can't cure many of the chronic digestive diseases such as Crohn's disease, IBS, arthritis, and autoimmune diseases. Meanwhile, health care professionals such as naturopathic doctors who are treating these diseases as symptoms of food allergies are having success.

The causes and effects of food allergies are hard to separate. If your secretions of digestive juices aren't adequate, more undigested food particles pass into the small intestine and then potentially into the bloodstream through the damaged gut lining. Some damage may be done to the intestines by foods you have become allergic to. Some people are more susceptible to food allergy than others; if you weren't breast-fed and were introduced to difficult-to-digest foods such as grains or cow's milk too soon, you probably have some leaky gut and food allergy problems. When a child's delicate digestive system isn't ready to assimilate a food, it's quickly labeled as potentially harmful by the immune system. Immediate reactions such as diarrhea or vom-

iting can result, or there may be inflammatory responses such as asthma and eczema.

For adults, some of the causes of food allergy can be chronic stress, drugs that knock the secretion of digestive juices out of balance, poor diet, or overindulgence in alcohol. Any number of environmental toxins, including pesticides, food additives, intestinal parasites, and heavy metals, can bring on delayed food allergy in adults.

The Large Intestine and Probiotics

Once your meal has passed through the twists and turns of the small intestine, the nutrients available for absorption have been drawn into the bloodstream. In the lower part of the small intestine, where it meets the large intestine, the vitamins A, B_{12}, D, and E are absorbed. A sphincter called the ileocecal valve controls the flow of waste into the large intestine. If your digestion isn't good, there is probably some undigested food remaining as well, which can cause gas and bloating as colon bacteria break it down by fermenting it. IBS is what physicians often diagnose in people with this complaint and a wide variety of other gastrointestinal complaints, including constipation, diarrhea, and abdominal cramping. As waste moves through the colon, water and minerals are pulled from it back into the body. A solid mass of feces is formed and is eventually excreted through the rectum and anus during a bowel movement.

The bacteria that reside in your colon are indispensable for good digestive health. Generically known as probiotics, these friendly bacteria are also found in the urinary tract, the mouth, and the vagina. In the intestines, probiotics have a variety of jobs. They do battle with foreign bacteria that might otherwise cause infection; they manufacture some vitamins, such as vitamin K;

and they keep the growth of a fungal yeast called *Candida albicans* under control. All told, we play host to 100 trillion friendly bacteria belonging to at least 400 different species.

Prescription drugs such as antibiotics and steroids, undue stress, and nutritional imbalances all contribute to the demise of good bacteria. When their numbers are low, bad bacteria and *Candida albicans* become overgrown. Yeast overgrowth in particular can cause many unpleasant symptoms. If you suffer from bloating, gas, unusual fatigue, diarrhea, constipation, skin problems, headaches, mental fogginess, joint pains, or environmental allergies, yeast overgrowth could be a culprit. This problem is especially common during and following treatment with antibiotics, so you should always follow a course of antibiotics with two weeks or more of probiotic supplementation.

You can buy capsules or a refrigerated liquid containing acidophilus, bifidus, and other friendly strains of bacteria in your local health food store. Fructooligosaccharides (FOS), a kind of sugar found plentifully in bananas that enhances the growth of probiotics, are another ingredient you should look for in a probiotic supplement.

How to Prevent Colon Cancer

Living a lifestyle that maintains a healthy colon will protect you against colon cancer, a disease that strikes about 160,000 people each year and kills more than 57,000 people each year. It is estimated that 68 percent of colon cancers could be prevented, and the evidence is piling up. A genetic predisposition in some people can't be discounted, but no matter what your genes are programmed for, you can reduce your risk by doing a few simple things to prevent constipa-

tion and to keep the bowel from being exposed to toxins day in and day out.

Your first step toward good colon health is to eat more fiber and avoid constipation. Fiber is an effective sponge that absorbs cancer-causing toxins and sweeps them out of the body in the feces. Hard, difficult-to-pass stools sit in the colon for too long. Toxins that should have been passed out of the body unabsorbed are more likely to seep back into the bloodstream or to cause damage to the colon itself.

The trace mineral selenium is your top colon health supplement. People who live in areas where the soil is high in selenium have dramatically lower rates of colon cancer.

The other biggest known risk factors for colon cancer are vitamin D deficiency, folic acid deficiency, and high alcohol consumption (which interferes with folic acid synthesis). In fact, a folic acid deficiency is associated with many types of cancer, and supplementing it has repeatedly been shown to reverse cervical dysplasia, a precancerous growth in the cervix. A small but pioneering study done some 10 years ago showed that supplementation with folic acid significantly decreased precancerous lung cells in smokers.

Folic acid is a B vitamin found in fresh, leafy, dark green vegetables such as spinach and kale, turnips, endive, asparagus, wheat bran, yeasts, and liver. It plays an important role in the synthesis of RNA and DNA, and thus in the process of cell division and growth. Chromosomes are more likely to have breaks if the cell is deficient in folic acid, creating the cell changes associated with cancers.

People who take aspirin regularly have been found to have lower rates of colon cancer, but aspirin may be acting as a stand-in for folic acid. Aspirin and folic acid compete for some of the same receptor sites in cells. If you're concerned about preventing colon cancer, be sure to take a daily folic acid supplement and save the aspirin for occasional use only.

If you're taking the recommended dosages of daily vitamins (see Chapter 9), you're getting all the folic acid you need. If you have had colon cancer or are at a high risk for colon cancer, you can take an additional 400 mcg of folic acid daily as a preventive measure, as well as 1,000 mcg daily of sublingual or intranasal vitamin B_{12}, which works hand-in-hand with folic acid. You can find both vitamins at your health food store.

Prescription and Over-the-Counter Drugs for the Digestive System

Examples of H2 Blockers

Cimetidine (Tagamet)
Famotidine (Pepcid)
Nizatidine (Axid)
Ranitidine (Zantac)

What Do They Do in the Body? H2 blockers block acid production in the stomach. They make up a class of drugs that block the stomach's response to acid stimulators such as food, caffeine, insulin, and histamine. The H2 blockers, once sold as antiulcer drugs, are now being marketed as antiheartburn agents sold over the counter. They are different enough so that even though they are in the same class of drugs, we'll cover each drug and its effects separately.

You know from the first few pages of this chapter that ulcers aren't caused by excessive stomach acid production but by bacteria. Most adults actually produce too little stomach acid. When ulcers are already established, it may help in the healing process to further reduce acid

production, but in the long run, this strategy can be counterproductive and doesn't deal with the root of the problem, which is probably *H. pylori* infection. Some of these drugs are used as part of an *H. pylori* eradication regime.

H2 blockers can cause mineral imbalances in the body. Calcium, phosphorus, and magnesium levels are affected. Vitamin B_{12} isn't absorbed well by people using H2 blockers. If you have an allergy to one of the H2 blockers, you shouldn't use any of them. If you are using H2 blockers over-the-counter, don't use the maximum dose for more than two weeks at a time without consulting with your physician. If you have symptoms such as difficulty swallowing or persistent abdominal pain, you should think twice about using H2 blockers sold over the counter.

Any acid-blocking medication interacts with the food you eat. Inadequate acid production in the stomach means that your ability to digest what you eat is impaired, and your body may not be able to absorb nutrients properly. The valve that must open to allow food to pass from the stomach into the small intestine is triggered by the acidity of the stomach's contents, and heartburn can result if acid levels are low and food sits too long in the stomach.

If you are using an acid-reducing medication for more than a week, be sure to use an intranasal or sublingual vitamin B_{12} supplement in addition to your multivitamin.

All of the H2 blockers interact with a long list of other drugs, usually blocking or reducing their effects. If you are taking other drugs, please check their drug information sheets carefully for interactions with heartburn drugs.

Ranitidine (Zantac)

What Is It Used For? Treatment of duodenal or gastric ulcer, gastroesophageal reflux disease (heartburn), erosive esophagitis, heartburn, *H. pylori* eradication, treatment of Zollinger-Ellison syndrome (a condition that causes oversecretion of stomach acid), prevention of damage of the gastrointestinal lining that can result from long-term use of nonsteroidal anti-inflammatory drugs (NSAIDs), prevention of stress ulcers, and control of upper gastrointestinal bleeding.

What Are the Possible Side Effects? Zantac adversely affects the liver's ability to detoxify other drugs you may be taking. That could mean that other drugs will have magnified effects on your body. Other possible side effects include severe headache, sleepiness or fatigue, diarrhea, stomach pain, and itching. Very rarely there may be a decrease in the number of blood cells, vertigo, blurred vision, and blood pressure and liver function changes.

CAUTION!

Think Twice About Taking This Drug If . . .

- You have any of a group of disorders known as porphyria.
- You have kidney or liver problems.
- You are under 16 years of age.

Famotidine (Pepcid, Pepcid AC)

What Is It Used For? Duodenal and stomach ulcer, heartburn, acid indigestion, sour stomach, and Zollinger-Ellison syndrome (a condition that causes oversecretion of stomach acid).

What Are the Possible Side Effects? Headache, sleepiness, fatigue, dizziness, confusion, diarrhea, growth of breasts in males (gynecomastia), kidney or liver impairment, impotence, loss of appetite, dry mouth, musculoskeletal pain, numbness, acne, dry or peeling skin, flushing, ringing in the ears, changes in sense of taste, fever, heart palpitations, and itching.

CAUTION!

Think Twice About Taking This Drug If . . .

You have kidney or liver problems.

What Are the Interactions with Food? Food increases the absorption of famotidine.

Nizatidine (Axid)

What Is It Used For? Duodenal and stomach ulcer, heartburn, acid indigestion, sour stomach, erosive esophagitis, gastroesophageal reflux disease, and prevention of upper gastrointestinal bleeding.

What Are the Possible Side Effects? Sleepiness, fatigue, dizziness, diarrhea, constipation, sweating, heart rhythm irregularities, a rise in uric acid levels in the bloodstream, changes in blood cell counts, and fever.

What Are the Interactions with Other Drugs? Nizatidine increases blood levels of salicylates (aspirin). It can make alcohol's effects on you more pronounced. If you are using antacids, they can make nizatidine less effective.

Cimetidine (Tagamet, Tagamet HB)

What Does It Do in the Body? Cimetidine blocks acid production in the stomach.

What Is It Used For? Duodenal and stomach ulcer, heartburn, acid indigestion, sour stomach, erosive esophagitis, gastroesophageal reflux disease, Zollinger-Ellison syndrome, and prevention of upper gastrointestinal bleeding. It has also been used to treat hyperparathyroidism, chronic viral warts in children, stress ulcers, herpes virus infections, excessive body hair growth in women, and dyspepsia (general symptoms of stomach upset, heartburn, nausea, and lack of appetite).

What Are the Possible Side Effects? Headache, sleepiness, fatigue, dizziness, confusion, hallucinations, diarrhea, breast development in males (gynecomastia), and impotence. Rarely, side effects can include inflammation of the pancreas, effects on the liver, changes in blood cell counts or immune function, skin problems, cardiac arrhythmias or arrest, joint pain, and hypersensitivity reactions.

In people with arthritis, cimetidine may aggravate joint symptoms; stopping the drug reverses this effect. Severely ill people, especially those with compromised liver or kidney function, may experience mental confusion, agitation, psychosis, anxiety, or disorientation when given this drug (which is reversible when the drug is discontinued).

There is some evidence that cimetidine may impair male fertility.

CAUTION!

Think Twice About Taking This Drug If . . .

You have impaired kidney or liver function. People with liver or kidney disease can't clear the drug from their systems as rapidly as others, and so blood concentrations may be too high. This is a common concern for elderly people.

What Are the Interactions with Food? Tyramine-rich foods such as aged cheese, processed meats, avocados, bananas, sauerkraut, most soy products, and some wines and beers can cause severe headache and temporarily raise your blood pressure when eaten while using cimetidine. Food delays the absorption of cimetidine.

Examples of Proton Pump Inhibitors

Omeprazole (Prilosec)
Lansoprazole (Prevacid)
Pantoprazole (Protonix)
Rabeprazole (Aciphex)
Esomeprazole (Nexium)

They suppress stomach acid production by inhibiting the cellular mechanism that pumps acid into the stomach.

What Do They Do in the Body? Suppress stomach acid production. They are much more powerful than the H2 blockers in this respect.

What Are They Used For? Gastric or duodenal ulcer, gastroesophageal reflux disease (heartburn), to maintain healing of erosive esophagitis, with antibiotics for eradication of *H. pylori*, treatment of Zollinger-Ellison syndrome (a condition that causes oversecretion of stomach acid). Omeprazole is the only drug in this class that has been subjected to long-term trials; all of the other drugs should not be used for more than four to eight weeks at a time.

What Are the Possible Side Effects? Increased risk of hip fracture, headache, dizziness, fatigue, weakness, diarrhea, abdominal pain, nausea, vomiting, constipation, upper respiratory infection, rash, cough, back pain, and constipation.

Combination therapy with the antibiotic clarithromycin and omeprazole may cause your sense of taste to change or may result in tongue discoloration, runny nose, inflammation of the pharynx, or flulike symptoms.

Long-term treatment with omeprazole has been linked to a serious condition called atrophic gastritis, where the stomach becomes inflamed and parts of it die.

Dozens of other cardiovascular, nervous system, gastrointestinal, urinary, metabolic, musculoskeletal, and respiratory symptoms have been reported but are rare. Severe rash (Stevens-Johnson syndrome) and changes in blood cell counts, liver function, hearing, and taste are other rarely observed side effects.

Animal tests have found that omeprazole, rabeprazole, and pantoprazole cause cell changes that could lead to cancer. Human studies have shown similar results with regard to rabeprazole and pantoprazole.

CAUTION!

Think Twice About Taking These Drugs If . . .

- You are elderly.
- You have osteoporosis or are at risk for osteoporosis.

Because of their profound, long-lasting inhibition of stomach acid secretion, proton pump inhibitors can interfere with drugs that require a specific pH for absorption. The effects of the antifungal drug ketoconazole, the antibiotic ampicillin, iron salts, and the heart drug digoxin can be decreased if given with these drugs.

What Are the Interactions with Food? If taken after meals, the drugs' effects are minimized. Take proton pump inhibitors on an empty stomach.

What Else to Take If You Take These Drugs. A sublingual vitamin B_{12} supplement. These drugs can interfere with B_{12} absorption.

Miscellaneous Drugs for Heartburn and Other Stomach Disorders

Sucralfate (Carafate)

What Does It Do in the Body? It creates a sticky gel in your stomach or small intestine that binds to ulcers, protecting them from further burning and ulceration by stomach acid.

What Is It Used For? Treatment of stomach and duodenal ulcers.

What Are the Possible Side Effects? Constipation, dry mouth, diarrhea, nausea, stomachache, gas, indigestion, headache, insomnia, sleepiness, dizziness, and back pain.

CAUTION!

- If you develop a rash or swelling, or have trouble breathing, you may be allergic to sucralfate.
- Those with kidney problems should not take this drug with aluminum-containing antacids. Sucralfate contains aluminum, and the two combined could bring too much of the mineral into the body at once for weakened kidneys to handle.
- This drug should be used with caution if you have kidney failure or need dialysis.
- Because of its high aluminum content, there doesn't seem to be any good reason to use this drug.

What Are the Interactions with Food? Take this drug on an empty stomach, at least one hour before meals.

Examples of Antacids

Aluminum carbonate gel (Basaljel)
Aluminum hydroxide gel (Amphojel, Alu-Tab, Alu-Cap, Dialume)
Calcium carbonate (Amitone, Mallamint, Dicarbosil, Equilet, Tums, Chooz, Maalox Antacid caplets, Mylanta)
Magaldrate (Riopan, Iosopan)
Magnesium hydroxide (Milk of Magnesia)
Magnesium oxide (Mag-Ox 400, Maox 420, Uro-Mag)
Sodium bicarbonate (Bell/ans)
Sodium citrate (Citra pH)

Antacids are some of the biggest-selling over-the-counter drugs in pharmacies. But not only do these drugs *not* treat the underlying problem, they may actually make the symptoms worse.

Although antacids such as Mylanta, Rolaids, and Tums can temporarily suppress the symptoms of heartburn, in the long run they'll likely do you more harm than good. You may even become dependent upon them. These over-the-counter medications help neutralize the acid in your stomach for up to an hour. That's fine for the moment, but your stomach may respond an hour later by producing even more acid to make up for what was neutralized, causing you to reach for more antacids. They also contain aluminum, silicone, sugar, and a long list of dyes and preservatives. Your stomach acid is one of your frontline defenses against harmful bacteria. Suppress it, and the rest of your systems have to work overtime to protect you.

What Do They Do in the Body? Antacids neutralize stomach acid. By increasing the pH of the stomach and duodenum (the first part of the small intestine), they also inhibit the action of the enzyme pepsin, which breaks down proteins. Antacids also increase the tone of the sphincter between the esophagus and the stomach, which decreases the likelihood of gastroesophageal reflux (heartburn).

What Are They Used For? Relief of upset stomach, heartburn, acid indigestion, and sour stomach. Aluminum- and magnesium-based antacids are also used to prevent stress ulcer bleeding, and antacids are often used in the treatment of ulcers.

What Are the Possible Side Effects? Magnesium-containing antacids can cause diarrhea.

Aluminum-containing antacids can cause constipation, intestinal blockage, or dangerously high body levels of aluminum. There is no conceivable reason to use aluminum-containing antacids.

Antacids may cause rebound acid production, where acid levels rise above normal once the antacid wears off.

Use of high doses of calcium carbonate and sodium bicarbonate at the same time can lead to milk-alkali syndrome. Symptoms are headache, nausea, irritability, weakness, electrolyte imbalances, and kidney damage.

Long-term use of aluminum-containing antacids can lead to phosphate depletion (hypophosphatemia) if intake of this mineral isn't adequate. Hypophosphatemia can lead to loss of appetite, exhaustion, weakness, and bone problems.

Antacids can deplete calcium levels. Using antacids such as Tums as a source of calcium is not useful, since at best it will replace what the antacid is blocking.

CAUTION!

Think Twice About Taking These Drugs If . . .

- You have hypertension, congestive heart failure, or kidney failure, or you are on a low-sodium diet. Most antacids are very high in sodium, so look for a low-sodium version.
- You are undergoing dialysis. Avoid aluminum-containing antacids. (We recommend avoiding aluminum-containing antacids, period.)
- You have had recent gastrointestinal hemorrhage. Use aluminum hydroxide with care.

How Do Antacids Interact with Nutrients? Aluminum- and magnesium-containing antacids can bind with phosphate and deplete the body of calcium, resulting in weakening of bones. Phosphate depletion can cause muscle weakness.

Vitamins A, B₁ (thiamine), and D are not well absorbed or are destroyed if antacids are in your system. In general, antacids block the action of stomach acid, reducing the absorption of nutrients.

Examples of Antidiarrhea Drugs

Difenoxin with atropine sulfate
Diphenoxylate with atropine sulfate
Loperamide
Bismuth subsalicylate

Diarrhea is your body's way of getting rid of harmful substances. When you have diarrhea, food containing bacteria or viruses can be flushed out of the body quickly. You may also have diarrhea when you eat certain foods that don't agree with you. If diarrhea goes on for more than five days, you may have a medical problem that needs attention. Severe diarrhea in infants, children, or the elderly should get medical attention within three days, since they can rapidly become dangerously dehydrated.

Difenoxin with atropine sulfate (Motofen)

What Does It Do in the Body? Slows the contractions of the intestines so that their contents move through more slowly.

What Is It Used For? Treatment of diarrhea.

What Are the Possible Side Effects? Nausea, vomiting, dry mouth, upset stomach, constipation, dizziness, light-headedness, drowsiness, headache, burning eyes, and blurred vision.

In some people, especially children, atropine (an ingredient of this drug) may cause skin and mucous membrane dryness, flushing, low body temperature, fast heartbeat, and difficulty urinating.

CAUTION!

Think Twice About Taking This Drug If . . .

- Your diarrhea could be caused by bacteria such as *E. coli*, salmonella, or shigella.
- You have been taking broad-spectrum antibiotics.
- You have colitis.
- You have jaundice.
- You have narrow-angle glaucoma or adhesions between the iris and lens of the eye.
- You have a heart condition such as rapid heartbeat or angina, gastrointestinal obstructive disease, urinary problems, or myasthenia gravis.
- You have liver or kidney disease. Use difenoxin with caution.

Diphenoxylate with atropine sulfate (Logen, Lomotil, Lonox, Lomanate)

What Does It Do in the Body? It has a constipating effect, making feces more solid.

What Is It Used For? Treatment of diarrhea.

What Are the Possible Side Effects? If you are hypersensitive to diphenoxylate, you may experience rash, swelling in the gums and elsewhere, or a life-threatening allergic reaction called anaphylaxis.

Other potential side effects include dizziness, drowsiness, sedation, headache, general feeling of not being well, lethargy, euphoria, depression, confusion, numbness of the extremities, loss of appetite, vomiting, abdominal discomfort, problems with the natural movements of the intestines, and inflammation of the pancreas.

CAUTION!

Think Twice About Taking This Drug If . . .

- Your diarrhea could be caused by bacteria such as *E. coli*, salmonella, or shigella.
- You have been taking broad-spectrum antibiotics.
- You have colitis.
- You have liver or kidney disease. Use diphenoxylate with caution.

Loperamide (Diar-Aid, Imodium A-D, Kaopectate, Maalox, Neo-Diaral, Pepto Diarrhea Control)

What Does It Do in the Body? Decreases the movement of the intestines and slows water and electrolyte transfer into the bowel.

What Is It Used For? Treatment of diarrhea.

What Are the Possible Side Effects? Usually minor, they include abdominal pain, distention, or discomfort; constipation; dry mouth; nausea; vomiting; tiredness; dizziness; and skin rash.

CAUTION!

Think Twice About Taking This Drug If . . .

- You have a disease that would be worsened by constipation.
- You have bloody diarrhea or a fever above 101° F.
- Your diarrhea could be caused by bacteria such as *E. coli*, salmonella, or shigella.
- You have been taking broad-spectrum antibiotics.
- You have acute ulcerative colitis.

Loperamide can cause your colon to become very distended and unable to do its job properly.

Use with caution if you have kidney problems.

Bismuth subsalicylate (Bismatrol, Pepto-Bismol)

What Does It Do in the Body? It suppresses secretions into the intestines, decreases inflammation, and has some antimicrobial effects.

What Is It Used For? Treatment of diarrhea, nausea, indigestion, and abdominal cramps. It is also used with antibiotics to treat *H. pylori* infection.

What Are the Possible Side Effects? Severe constipation can occur in debilitated people and infants. Feces may temporarily be gray or black.

CAUTION!

Think Twice About Taking This Drug If . . .

- Diarrhea is accompanied by high fever or continues for more than two days.
- Constipation is not relieved with laxatives.
- There is rectal bleeding, muscle cramps, weakness, or dizziness. Call your health professional.
- You are on a salt-restricted diet. Look for low-sodium versions of these antidiarrheal drugs.
- You have congestive heart failure or kidney disease. Dangerous electrolyte imbalances can occur.
- Check with your doctor before taking this drug if you are taking blood thinners.

Drugs for Constipation

Drugs for constipation fall into several categories, all with different mechanisms of action for bringing about a bowel movement. Some are taken orally, while others can be used as suppositories or enemas. Any of these laxatives can result in dependency if used for too long. Your digestive system essentially "forgets" how to have a bowel movement without them.Constipation drugs include saline laxatives, irritants/stimulants, bulk-producing laxatives, lubricants, and surfactants.

Examples of Saline Laxatives

Epsom salts
Milk of magnesia
Magnesium citrate
Sodium phosphates (Fleet Phospho-Soda)

What Do They Do in the Body? Draw water and electrolytes into the intestines to make feces softer.

What Are the Possible Side Effects? These drugs may alter the body's fluid and electrolyte balance.

What Else to Do When Taking These Drugs. Drink plenty of water, and use a mineral supplement containing magnesium and potassium.

Examples of Irritants/Stimulants

Cascara sagrada
Senna (Ex-Lax, Senolax, Senokot, Senexon)
Bisacodyl (Bisco-Lax, Evac-U-Gen, Dulcolax, Dulcagen, Fleet bisacoydl, Modane, Feen-a-mint)
Castor oil

What Do They Do in the Body? Stimulate the intestinal walls to move feces through the intestinal tract. They also alter water and electrolyte secretion into the gut. Evacuation is rapid and complete, so these drugs are often used before surgery or in very severe cases of constipation.

What Are the Possible Side Effects? Too-frequent use results in loss of electrolytes (especially potassium) and dehydration; the colon may become unable to contract on its own. Cascara sagrada and senna can discolor feces.

Examples of Bulk-Producing Laxatives

Methylcellulose (Citrucel, Unifiber)
Psyllium (Fiberall, Genfiber, Hydrocil, Konsyl, Maalox Daily Fiber, Metamucil, Mylanta Natural Fiber, Reguloid, Serutan, Syllact, Modane Bulk, V-Lax)
Polycarbophil (FiberCon, Equalactin, Mitrolan, FiberNorm, Fiber-Lax)
Malt soup extract (Maltsupex)

What Do They Do in the Body? These drugs are basically fiber, which holds water in feces to make them softer and easier to evacuate, and gives them bulk.

What Are They Used For? Psyllium is useful in IBS, spastic colon, and hemorrhoids. LDL cholesterol can be lowered up to 20 percent with psyllium.

Polycarbophil also is used to treat IBS and diverticulosis.

What Are the Possible Side Effects? Bulk-forming agents are the safest method to use for relief of constipation. Excessive bowel activity (diarrhea, nausea, vomiting), anal irritation, bloating, flatulence, abdominal cramping, weakness, dizziness, fainting, sweating, and palpitations happen rarely.

Esophageal, stomach, small intestinal, and rectal obstruction have been reported with bulk laxatives. Be sure to take them with plenty of water.

Examples of Lubricants

Castor oil (Fleet Flavored Castor Oil, Purge, Neoloid)
Mineral oil (Milkinol)

What Do They Do in the Body? These oils don't allow water from the feces to be absorbed back into the body through the walls of the colon, and thus prevent the bowel contents from drying out.

What Are the Possible Side Effects? Large doses of mineral oil can cause leakage from the anus, anal itching, irritation, hemorrhoids, and general anal discomfort.

What Are the Interactions with Food? Lubricants may decrease the absorption of fat-soluble vitamins such as A, D, and E.

Examples of Surfactants

Docusate (Dialose, Regutol, Colace, Disonate, DOK, DOS Softgel, Regulax, Dioeze, Correctol, Sulfalax Calcium, Diocto-K)

What Do They Do in the Body? Surfactants help mix fats with the contents of the colon, which makes stools softer and bowel movements easier.

What Are They Used For? Treatment of diarrhea or in conditions such as anal fissure or hemorrhoids where passing firm stool is painful.

Miscellaneous Laxatives

Glycerin suppositories draw extra water into the colon and cause slight irritation of the colon walls, stimulating contractions.

Lactulose (Chronulac, Constilac, Duphalac) brings more water and electrolytes into the colon. Diabetics shouldn't use lactulose. It can cause flatulence, belching, abdominal cramping, nausea, and vomiting.

Natural Alternatives for Treating Diarrhea

Although it's uncomfortable and inconvenient to have diarrhea, your best bet is to let nature take its course. Allow your body to cleanse itself unless the diarrhea is severe or lasts for more than a day or two. Drink plenty of water while you have diarrhea. You can try a sports drink that contains replacement electrolytes as long as it's not too high in sugar. Stay away from caffeine, soft drinks, and sugary foods. As soon as you feel well enough, eat foods such as rice, cereal, bananas, and potatoes, which are rich in carbohydrates and gentle on your stomach.

If you have chronic diarrhea, try to figure out whether foods or drugs are causing it. Heartburn drugs such as H2 blockers (Tagamet, Zantac) and proton pump inhibitors (Nexium, Prilosec) can cause diarrhea. Lactose intolerance, an allergy to milk sugars, can cause diarrhea when dairy products are eaten.

Use probiotics or yogurt to help get your body back into balance after a bout of diarrhea. A mineral supplement containing magnesium and potassium will restore your body's depleted electrolyte stores.

Natural Alternatives to Ulcer Drugs

The bacteria *H. pylori* is found in 90 percent of duodenal ulcer and 70 percent of stomach ulcer patients. This bacteria increases your risk of insufficient acid secretion (atrophic gastritis), ulcer, and stomach cancer. Your doctor can give you a test in his or her office to find out if this bug is at the root of your problem. If it is, you'll be put on a course of antibiotics and a bismuth preparation (you know it as Pepto-Bismol) for a week. This is one instance in which conventional medicines may be your best bet. Quick eradication of *H. pylori* is important for healing of ulcers. There are some herbal remedies you can try first, however, if you want to avoid antibiotics.

Licorice extract (deglycyrrhizinated licorice, or DGL) is a wonderful herbal healing aid for ulcers. It increases the production of protective mucus in the stomach. Use 300 mg four to six times a day. Unripe banana also has antiulcer effects, as do the herbs slippery elm (*Ulmus fulva*; take 200 mg four to six times a day), marshmallow root (*Althaea officinalis*; take 200 mg four to six times a day), and the juice of raw cabbage. You can buy extract of unripe plantain banana (*Musa paradisiaca*); take 150 mg four to six times a day.

If you have any type of ulcer, be sure to eliminate gastrointestinal irritants such as tobacco, NSAIDs, coffee, and alcohol.

Once your ulcer has healed, try taking steps to enhance your body's secretion of digestive acids and enzymes to prevent a recurrence.

Natural Alternatives for Treating Heartburn and Insufficient Acid Secretion

If you have chronic heartburn, you probably know exactly what triggers it. If you don't, here are the most common culprits: overeating, or too much fat or fried food; processed meats with nitrates or nitrites in them; too much sugar, alcohol, chocolate, drugs, or stress; clothes that fit tightly around the waist; obesity; and pregnancy. Obesity, tight clothes, and pregnancy put excess pressure on the esophageal muscle. Pregnancy also stimulates the release of hormones that relax the muscles so they will stretch to accommodate the growing baby—the esophagus muscles relax along with all the other ones.

Eating a balanced diet of unprocessed, organic whole foods is your foundation for a healthy stomach. Eat a green salad or raw vegetables at least once a day. Sprouted legumes and seeds are excellent sources of enzymes. Chew your food thoroughly.

Drinking cold or hot liquids with meals decreases stomach acid production. To help

Drugs That Can Cause Heartburn

Many prescription and over-the-counter drugs can cause or aggravate heartburn. Drugs that specifically relax the esophageal sphincter muscle, allowing stomach acid to reflux up, include anticholinergics (such as drugs to treat Parkinson's), calcium channel blockers (heart disease drugs), nicotine, and beta-blockers (to lower blood pressure and prevent spasms in the heart muscle).

Here is a list of other common offenders:

Antacids (can cause acid rebound and
    dependency)
Antibiotics
Antidepressants (fluoxetine, buspirone)
Asthma drugs (aminophylline, theophylline)
Chemotherapy drugs
Corticosteroids (prednisone)
Drugs that affect the heart and blood vessels,
    including drugs for lowering cholesterol and
    blood pressure, diuretics, and beta-blockers
Painkillers and narcotics (aspirin, acetamino-
    phen, ibuprofen, naproxen, codeine, piroxicam,
    indomethacin)
Synthetic estrogens and progestins (Premarin,
    Provera)
Tranquilizers and barbiturates
Ulcer drugs (sulfasalazine, sucralfate,
    misoprostol)

increase stomach acid, you can drink a glass of water at room temperature a half-hour before eating. If that doesn't help, you can add a tablespoon of apple cider vinegar. If neither of those solutions work, try taking a betaine hydrochloride (HCl) supplement with your meal. Follow the directions on the bottle, starting with the smallest dose and increasing it if needed. Do not take HCl supplements when you have an ulcer. Since stomach acid production declines as we age, HCl supplementation can be a good antiaging strategy.

Natural heartburn therapies include deglycyrrhizinated licorice extract, or DGL. Try one or two 380-mg tablets chewed and swallowed on an empty stomach, three to four times a day. A glass of water at room temperature, raw cabbage or potato juice, or herbal teas such as fenugreek, slippery elm, comfrey, licorice, and meadowsweet (lukewarm, no lemon) can bring quick relief. Fresh papaya or banana can help as well.

If you do need to lower your stomach acidity, you can use a form of organic sulfur called methylsulfonylmethane (MSM) in supplement form, 1,000 mg daily. Don't eat a lot of fat, either, as fat slows the emptying of the stomach. Use alcohol and chocolate in moderation. Eat several small meals a day so you don't overeat at any one meal. Don't eat on the run or right before exercising. Don't lie down after eating. Reduce stress with exercise and meditation.

Natural Alternatives for Constipation

Bulk laxatives such as psyllium are your best bet for safe, quick relief. Once you're moving again, it's up to you to change your habits to prevent a recurrence. Here are some guidelines to follow to avoid constipation:

Ten Good Reasons to Throw Away Your Antacids

1. They can cause rebound acid.
2. They block action of aspirin.
3. They block action of antibiotics.
4. They block action of quinidine.
5. They decrease iron and calcium absorption.
6. Metoclopramide (Reglan, Maxolon) increases absorption of alcohol.
7. An overly alkaline environment causes imbalances of intestinal flora, stresses kidneys, and causes urinary tract infections.
8. Aluminum may be connected to Alzheimer's disease and slows digestion.
9. They may cause diarrhea or constipation.
10. They have high sodium content.

• One of the simplest and most effective things you can do to banish constipation is to drink more water. If you aren't getting enough water, your stools will be hard and dry, and straining to pass them can result in hemorrhoids or anal tears and bleeding.

• Eat more fiber. Fresh vegetables are full of fiber, as are fruit, legumes, and whole grains. These foods should make up a generous portion of your diet. Use extra bran or nibble on prunes if you don't feel your bowels are moving regularly and easily. (If you have IBS, bran might not be the best solution for you, as it tends to worsen bloating and gas for people with this problem.)

• If you're having trouble getting enough fiber in your diet, use psyllium in the morning before breakfast. Use 1 to 3 teaspoons in at least 8 ounces of water or juice. Drink it immediately after you stir in the psyllium.

• Go when the urge strikes you. If you habitually hold back bowel movements, constipation can result.

• Get some exercise. Moving your whole body keeps things moving in the digestive tract.

• Check your medicine cabinet for drugs that cause constipation. Diuretics, painkillers, tranquilizers, antidepressants, antihistamines, narcotics, and decongestants are potential culprits. The overuse of over-the-counter laxatives can cause dependency, as the colon is cleaned out so completely with one use that it may take a couple of days for another bowel movement to happen naturally. If you don't realize this, you might take another dose too soon, thinking that you are constipated again. Damage to the lining of the large intestine and loss of the bowel's ability to do the work of moving the bowel contents often result from overuse of laxatives.

• Sitting for hours on planes or in cars, changes in quality of water and food, and change from your ordinary routine can make you "irregular." When you travel, pack natural remedies such as prunes, psyllium, or bran.

• Herbal remedies that contain cascara sagrada or senna stimulate contractions in the large intestine and rectum, moving the contents of the bowel. Don't use them more than once in a while, because you can quickly develop a dependency on them.

• Supplementation of magnesium at 600 to 900 mg a day helps relieve constipation by drawing water into the contents of the large intestine and by relaxing irritated, constricted intestinal walls. Many vegetables are good sources of magnesium, and herbs such as gotu kola, skullcap,

horsetail, alfalfa, nettle, hawthorn berry, and wild oat seed are also rich in this essential mineral.

• If you're on a very low-fat diet, you may want to try adding a tablespoon of olive or avocado oil a day. A little extra oil may be what's needed to make transit through the bowel smooth and easy.

• Probiotic supplements containing acidophilus should help with constipation and gas. Use a refrigerated supplement from your health food store.

• Green foods such as spirulina, chlorella, wheatgrass juice, or even liquid chlorophyll added to water can help get bowels moving. Here's an added benefit: chlorophyll, which is found abundantly in all green foods (it's what makes them green), has a deodorizing effect in the large intestine.

• If you're constipated and really uncomfortable and don't feel like swallowing anything, try an Epsom salts bath. You can buy Epsom salts (magnesium salts) in your local market or drugstore. Dump an entire box into a bath, sit in it for 20 minutes, and within a couple of hours you'll have a bowel movement.

Beat IBS and Treat Food Allergies Naturally

Identification and treatment of food allergies is the most important step you can take to cure yourself of IBS. How do you know whether you have food allergies? There is some controversy about this subject, but let's keep it simple. Think of negative reactions to foods as either immediate or delayed. If you respond to a food by sneezing, itching, wheezing, breaking out in hives, or by experiencing watering and itchy eyes, a runny nose, or even a life-threatening reaction called anaphylaxis (this involves sudden swelling of the throat that can close off the airway), you have an immediate allergy to that food. Most of the immediate allergic reactions to foods happen in children and are outgrown. Strawberries, seafood, beans, and milk products are the most common culprits.

Delayed allergies are much more difficult to pinpoint. Because symptoms may not occur until days after the food is eaten, the exact cause is not always obvious. Symptoms can include headache, other allergies such as hay fever, stiff and achy joints, indigestion, and fatigue. If allowed to progress, food allergy can lead to impaired digestion and general symptoms of malnutrition, including dry skin, dull hair, and increased susceptibility to illness. Most problems caused by food allergies aren't quite serious enough to stop people from getting through their days, but they have little energy and don't look healthy.

Digestive disturbances, rashes, minor aches and pains, and vague health problems that can't be attributed to anything specific are common complaints of those with delayed food allergies. These unfortunate individuals may simply decide that it's an inevitable part of growing older. Don't let yourself fall into this way of thinking! The difference between feeling like you're sick all the time and feeling great might be one or two of the foods in your diet.

Start to keep a record of the foods you eat. Look for the most common triggers of delayed food allergies: wheat, corn, dairy products, soy, citrus fruit, nightshade vegetables (tomatoes, potatoes, eggplant, red and green peppers, cayenne pepper), peanuts (usually due to aflatoxin, a fungus found in most peanuts), eggs, beef, and coffee. Ironically, foods that you feel you "must"

have every day are most often the culprits. The release of the offending foods into your bloodstream causes the body to release adrenal hormones that give you a temporary surge of energy.

IBS is often a result of allergy to dairy products. People with celiac sprue, which is an allergy to gluten, are allergic to wheat, rye, barley, oats, and all other gluten-containing grains. Food additives and colorings such as BHT, BHA, MSG, benzoates, nitrates, sulfites, and red and yellow food dyes cause delayed allergic reactions in many people, especially children.

Watch out for antibiotics and NSAIDs (e.g., aspirin and ibuprofen), which are very hard on the stomach. Just a few ibuprofen a month can cause a chronically upset stomach.

Artichoke leaf (*Cynara scolymus* L., Asteraceae)—not Jerusalem artichoke, but the kind of artichoke that's delicious steamed and eaten with melted butter—has been used since antiquity as a medicine for gastrointestinal problems, including gas, intestinal spasms, and vomiting. A study in the journal *Phytotherapy Research* found that an artichoke leaf extract (ALE) significantly reduced symptoms of constipation-predominant IBS. This German study looked at 279 German patients with at least three of five IBS symptoms. All of them took an extract called Hepar-SL forte, which contains 320 mg of dry extract of artichoke leaf, with meals. After six weeks, they reported improvements ranging from a 65 to 77 percent decrease in symptoms. Eighty-six of the patients reported that ALE was more effective than previous treatments they'd tried.

Peppermint oil has also been used for gastrointestinal complaints throughout history. In studies conducted in Germany, more modern formulations including peppermint oil and caraway oil in an enterically coated capsule (one designed to break down only once it has passed into the stomach) have shown promise as IBS therapies. Don't take peppermint oil that is not enterically coated, because it can cause damage to the esophagus. Strongly brewed peppermint tea might be helpful if you can't find peppermint extract.

Medical testing for delayed food allergy is a tricky business. The existing tests vary in reliability and can be very expensive. Fortunately, self-diagnosis can be done with what is known as an elimination diet.

How to Do an Elimination Diet

You can do an elimination diet with the support of a health care professional if you don't feel able to tackle it on your own. A terrific resource on food allergy and elimination diets is *Optimal Wellness*, a book by Ralph Golan, M.D. (Ballantine Books, 1995). Precede the two-week period with 10 days of eating your normal diet, keeping careful track of *everything* you eat and drink and of any symptoms. Then make a list of the foods you eat every day and a list of the foods you ate more than five times during your record keeping. After you finish your 10-day period of eating your regular diet, eliminate all of the foods on your "everyday foods" list and "more than five times in 10 days" list, as well as any other suspected allergens, for two weeks. Continue to record everything you eat and how you're feeling. Be very careful to eliminate all potential sources of allergenic foods. Vitamins often contain fillers and fibers that may be allergens. Common food allergens such as wheat, corn, dairy products, and eggs are hidden in many processed foods. Be careful not to get into a pattern of eating some other food frequently during this time, or you may set yourself up for sensitivity to yet another food.

Vary what you eat throughout the day and from day to day.

At the end of the two weeks, reintroduce foods one at a time. No more than one food should be reintroduced every 24 hours. Your response to foods you have allergies to will be pronounced. Continue to record all symptoms you experience. If you are allergic to a food you have avoided for two weeks, you may experience rapid or uneven heart rhythms, sudden sleepiness, stomach cramps, bloating, gas, diarrhea, constipation, headache, chills, sweats, flushing, and achiness.

If you notice that you are feeling very good on the limited diet, this is an important piece of feedback that you're on the right track. Your intestinal wall is shed and regenerated completely every three days, so healing of a leaky gut happens quickly.

While you're on an elimination diet, you can take some supplements to aid in healing your intestines. Glutamine is an amino acid essential for healthy gut mucosa; take 500 mg three times a day. Essential fatty acids, found in borage and evening primrose oils, help prevent inflammatory reactions in the gut and throughout the body. The B vitamin pantothenic acid (B_5) is an important building block of the intestinal walls. Use 500 mg twice a day.

During an elimination diet, be sure to drink plenty of clean water every day, and take supplements to help heal your small intestine.

If you've suffered for many years from chronic, low-grade health problems caused by food allergy and leaky gut, you may be dealing with other problems such as nasal allergy, sinus infection, arthritis, autoimmune disease, or candida overgrowth.

Once you've pinpointed problem foods, omit them from your diet for two months. Try reintroducing them again, one at a time, at that point. If you still have a reaction, wait six months and try again. You should eventually be able to reintroduce food allergens into your diet and enjoy them occasionally, but chances are that if you start eating them every day again, you'll become sensitive to them again.

Children generally outgrow food allergies, but it can be frustrating for the family to deal with a child's sensitivity to common foods such as wheat or dairy products. The improvement in health, however, should be well worth a few months of deprivation.

Chapter 12 — Cold, Cough, Asthma, and Allergy Drugs and Their Natural Alternatives

These days we are aware that stress, a weakened immune system, and poor nutrition can all tip the scales in favor of coming down with a cold or flu. Pay attention to your body's signals. It will tell you, in no uncertain terms, when it is fighting off a cold or flu. You already know the signals. Your sinuses may be painful when you wake up in the morning. You may feel especially tired and achy after work or develop a sore throat, headache, achy muscles, sneezing, or chills. If you apply the natural remedies described in the latter part of this chapter as soon as you get these signals, your immune system will have a fighting chance to knock out that bug before it gets the best of you.

If a full-blown cold or flu can't be averted, you can find many ways to suppress cold and flu symptoms at any drugstore. But suppressing symptoms with drugs may turn out to be counterproductive, for reasons you'll discover more about in this chapter. Those symptoms are, in fact, important aspects of your body's immune defenses against these diseases. In the case of a viral infection—which is what colds and flu are—your body's natural mechanisms for beating the illness need support, not suppression.

Physicians adamantly push flu shots at everyone these days, but little good evidence has found them to be an effective form of prevention. A close look at the studies on flu shots—as well as their track record in actually reducing flu infections or death from flu—shows that a flu jab isn't as good an insurance policy against flu as many believe.

Is It a Cold, Flu, or Allergy?

Allergies and asthma affect rising numbers of people worldwide, probably due to a combination of factors: increasing air pollution, consumption of highly processed foods tainted with artificial additives, and a more or less constant barrage of medications from infancy on that alter the natural function of the immune system, causing it to become overreactive. While allergies are rarely more than a nuisance, asthma—a form of allergic reaction—can and does kill, and is a serious public health problem.

The symptoms of common-cold-induced nasal congestion may be very similar to the congestion caused by allergies. The underlying causes of both have to do with a malfunctioning immune system. How do you know whether you're allergic or infected?

Cold viruses are always in our environment, and whether you "catch" a cold is a function of how healthy you are and how well your immune system is working. Cold symptoms are caused when a cold virus attacks and kills cells, which then release substances that cause inflammation, mucus production, and infection, and possibly a slight fever. Most colds will resolve within five to seven days. If you take care of yourself by getting plenty of rest and warm fluids and eating wholesome food, a cold can resolve itself within three days.

Symptoms of influenza or flu virus tend to be more severe, including a higher fever, aches, chills, and nausea.

Neither a cold nor flu can be effectively treated with an antibiotic. Antibiotics kill bacteria, and colds and flus are caused by viruses. While a cold or flu can cause a bacterial infection, you are best off allowing your own body to fight it and heal it unless a doctor determines that you are at risk for pneumonia or some other serious infectious disease.

Allergy symptoms, on the other hand, result when the immune system overreacts to an irritant such as dust mites, pollen, perfumes, air pollutants, pet dander, or food. When the immune system mistakes these harmless invaders for deadly enemies, it sends out the histamines to attack, which in turn cause inflammation.

Inflammation caused by allergy can occur almost anywhere in the body. The most common sites are the mucous membranes of the nose, eyes, ears, and throat. However, inflammation in the joints (arthritis), the brain (headaches, confusion, fatigue), lungs (asthma, cough), gastrointestinal system (cramps, indigestion, diarrhea), and skin (hives, rash) can also be caused by allergies.

What we're most often concerned about in the spring is known as allergic rhinitis, or hay fever, which usually consists of a runny, itchy nose and watery eyes. About 20 percent of the population of the United States suffers from hay fever, and the incidence is rising. Thirty years ago, estimates were that under 100,000 people suffered from hay fever. Today that number has risen to more than 40 million. Allergies are also on the rise because children's immune systems are under attack from vaccinations, antibiotics, and the constant use of medicines such as Tylenol (acetaminophen) that harm the liver, our most important organ of detoxification. A growing body of research demonstrates that children who are medicated frequently with antibiotics and fever-reducing drugs are more likely to end up with allergies and asthma. After starting out with a compromised immune system, most children are then fed foods devoid of nutrition but loaded with additives, dyes, preservatives, pesticides, and hormones. They are also exposed to the toxic effects of "fake" fragrances (fakegrances) found in everything from laundry soap and fabric softeners to so-called air fresheners and perfumes. Children with an unrecognized sensitivity to dairy products, wheat, or sugar, for example, who have also had their immune systems and intestinal systems compromised by constant antibiotics, are primed for a lifetime of allergies and other environmental sensitivities. Adults are in the same boat, but to a less sensitive degree.

Spring is a big season for hay fever because that's when trees pollinate. In the late spring and summer, grasses pollinate. In the fall, weeds are the culprits. Nonseasonal indoor causes of allergies include food, dust mites, cigarette smoke, aerosol sprays, room deodorizers, insecticides, cleaning products, fresh paint or varnish, mold, fungi, and pets.

How can you tell if your runny nose is being caused by hay fever? According to W. Stephen Pray, a pharmacist, professor, and allergy expert from the Southwestern Oklahoma State University College of Pharmacy, some of the differences between a cold and an allergy are:

- A runny nose caused by allergies is usually clear, while a cold causes a yellow discharge within a few days, indicating infection. Chronic, long-term allergies can eventually cause a sinus infection, but in general, discharge from the nose will be clear.
- The nose is itchy with hay fever, usually not with a cold.
- Sneezes come in groups during a hay fever attack, sometimes as many as 10 to 20 sneezes one right after another. Sneezes caused by a cold generally come on one at a time.
- Watery, itchy eyes tend to be a sign of hay fever rather than a cold.

The ears are often involved in an allergy, causing hearing problems, popping, and sometimes ringing in the ears. More than 80 percent of people who suffer from frequent ear infections have allergies as well. Older children and adults who get a cold don't often get an ear infection with it.

A classic sign of chronic allergies and particularly food allergies has been dubbed the "allergic shiner," a semicircular area below the eyes that is dark or bluish in color. Long-term blocked nasal passages interfere with the ability of blood to flow away from below the eyes, resulting in an accumulation of blood in that area and a darkening under the skin that makes it look bruised.

Chronic allergies can cause many side effects, especially in children, that may go unrecognized. Some of these side effects include fatigue, headaches, irritability, a poor sense of smell and taste, hearing problems, fatigue in the morning, and snoring. Chronic eye, ear, nose, and throat infections can take hold because of the constant irritation and inflammation caused by allergies. In children, permanent facial changes can be a result of chronic allergies.

It's helpful (if not pleasant!) when our bodies fight off a real invader such as a virus with an immune reaction, which we call a cold or flu. This immune response eventually rids the body of the invader. But when we react to allergens, there may be no end in sight, and this can interfere with our enjoyment of life.

Childhood Exposures Decrease Allergy and Asthma Risk

During the past decade, researchers have found that exposure to dust and dirt during early childhood, especially in the first year of life, may be protective against allergy. Such exposure is thought to "activate" aspects of immunity that keep allergy and asthma at bay.

In a study from the Institute of Social and Preventive Medicine in Basel, Switzerland, researchers evaluated 812 children living in rural parts of Austria, Germany, and Switzerland. They compared children who lived on farms—where they are constantly exposed to animal dander and bacteria from animal waste—to children who did not live on farms. Samples of dust from the children's mattresses were analyzed for endotoxin (substances known to cause allergic irritation in sensitive people) content, and blood samples were analyzed for markers of allergic inflammation. Far more endotoxins were found in the farm children's bedding, but higher endotoxin levels correlated with decreased blood markers of allergic inflammation. The likelihood of asthma, hay fever, and atopy (allergic skin irritations) was approximately 50 percent lower in farm children, and their immune systems did not respond dramatically to the endotoxins. In other words, their immune systems were better at discerning what was actually a threat.

Children don't need a spic-and-span environment, and their attraction to dirt and grime may be Mother Nature finding a way to expose them to endotoxins that help their immune systems

develop properly. Unfortunately, if a child has already developed allergies, exposing him or her to potential allergens may do more harm than good. Later in the chapter, we'll explain how to keep an allergic or asthmatic person's environment as clear of allergens as possible.

When bacteria cause an infection, it appears that allowing children's bodies to fight it off without antibiotics may protect against future allergies and asthma. When researchers from British Columbia combined the results of seven studies involving about 12,000 children, they found that when a child receives a course of antibiotics before his or her first birthday, that child is twice as likely to end up developing asthma than a child who receives no antibiotics during that time. Multiple courses in early childhood were found to bump risk higher, with an increase in risk of 16 percent with each course of antibiotics taken before the age of 1.

One approach to treating existing allergies is to allow colds, flus, and other acute infectious illnesses to run their course whenever possible, without using medications to suppress symptoms. This can be a delicate balance to strike with children, and it requires careful attention and lots of tender loving care, including staying warm, getting plenty of liquids, and using herbal, homeopathic, and nutritional remedies that support the immune system rather than suppress it. We'll give you specifics later in this chapter.

Once our immune system decides that a particular allergen is a hostile invader, it becomes "sensitized" to it and begins to react by creating allergy symptoms caused by the release of histamines. In the process of attacking the invaders, the histamines cause inflammation and even damage tissues. Allergic sinus congestion can cause headaches and mental fogginess. Irritated sinuses bring on fits of sneezing, mucus running down the back of the throat causes sore throat, and an overload of irritants and mucus can trigger bronchial spasms, also known as asthma. If the body tries to rid itself of the invaders via the skin, rashes, eczema, and hives may result.

Allergy drugs work to suppress symptoms rather than treat the cause of the allergy. The consequences of this type of treatment are generally unpleasant side effects and often a rebound effect where the symptom is worse if the medication starts to wear off or treatment is stopped.

Treating Asthma

More than 16 million American adults and more than 6 million American children have asthma, which constricts the bronchial tubes leading to the lungs, reducing airflow. Wheezing, coughing, labored breathing, and coughing up mucus from the lungs are the classic symptoms of asthma. If an attack is allowed to progress untreated for long enough, it can kill as the airways constrict and fill with mucus. Left untreated, even less severe asthma symptoms can cause chronic inflammation that damages and scars the lungs. While most asthma attacks are precipitated by an allergen, they can also be caused by emotional stress, exercise, and infections.

Severe attacks can happen suddenly, but more often the asthma sufferer's condition deteriorates slowly, so he or she delays getting medical help. You can do a lot to naturally relieve asthma symptoms, but if you have any suspicion that you might be in trouble, take whatever actions are necessary to open up your airways.

Asthma Medications: Is the Cure Worse than the Disease?

If you have ever been around somebody with poorly controlled asthma, you're well aware that it can be a scary, severely limiting illness. The number of people in the United States with asthma has risen steadily since the 1970s, with a 50 percent increase just since 1990. Asthma is a major reason behind emergency room visits and hospitalizations in the United States. Death rates rose rapidly for a while in the 1990s and have stabilized in this decade—probably due to better medical treatments and prevention. Still, far too many are dependent on medications that they might be able to reduce or eliminate with appropriate natural interventions.

Although asthma medications have saved many lives, they temporarily stop symptoms without addressing underlying problems and can worsen the problem over time. Most physicians treat asthma with bronchodilators that open up the airways, or treat the underlying inflammation of the lungs with corticosteroids. The list of dangerous side effects of these two types of drugs is as long as your arm. Some of the most commonly used asthma drugs have earned black-box warnings prominently displayed cautions about risk of death with these medicines—because of rare but potentially deadly side effects.

The rising number of asthma diagnoses and deaths is a very good indication that these medications aren't working and may be doing more harm than good. The adverse effects of these drugs seems to go beyond escalating the severity of asthma attacks: a Johns Hopkins study published in the *American Journal of Epidemiology* suggests a link between beta-agonists, a very

Cleaning Products and Childhood Asthma

Children with higher levels of exposure to volatile organic compounds (VOCs) appear to have *four times* the risk of developing asthma compared to children who are minimally exposed. These airway-irritating chemicals, many of which are also carcinogenic, are found in solvents, paint, cleaning products, floor adhesives, carpets, room fresheners, car exhaust, and polishes.

Krassi Rumchev and her coworkers at the School of Public Health at Curtin University of Technology in Perth, Australia, evaluated the histories of 88 children who were treated for asthma attacks in the emergency room at the Princess Margaret Hospital in Perth. The asthmatic children were compared with a control group (children who didn't have asthma), based on detailed interviews with family members and measurements of 10 common VOCs (out of about 900 that have been identified) and allergens in the children's homes. Indoor air can contain up to 1,000 times the concentration of VOCs as outdoor air. They found that at VOC levels above 60 micrograms per cubic meter, the child's asthma risk quadrupled in comparison to children in homes with VOCs well below this threshold.

Keep VOCs out of your home by minimizing your use of commercial cleaning products and personal care products. That smell of chemically scoured bathrooms and air fresheners is bad for your family's respiratory systems. Choose cleaning products made from natural ingredients. A simple mix of white vinegar and water in a spray bottle effectively cleans and disinfects most surfaces. If you replace carpets or paint, seek out low-VOC varieties, and if you can't use them, keep the newly carpeted or painted room well ventilated and keep windows open whenever possible. Be sure that car exhaust is vented away from the house. And of course, don't ever smoke around children. Tobacco smoke is a primary source of VOCs.

---

popular type of asthma drug, and an increased risk of heart disease.

We've already looked at a few theories as to why the rate of asthma is rising so fast: food additives, immune systems compromised in childhood by repeated doses of antibiotics and vaccines, and indoor and outdoor air pollution.

One example of a food additive often linked to asthma is tartrazine (yellow dye no. 5). This yellow food coloring is used in some 60 percent of prescription and over-the-counter drugs, as well as in hundreds of processed foods such as cakes, cookies, cereals, soft drinks, ice cream, gelatin, pudding, and pasta. It is well-known to be a potent allergen in many people, com-monly provoking breathing difficulties and asthma attacks. If you are allergic to aspirin, you are probably allergic to tartrazine. Children are especially susceptible to tartrazine, and there's a good chance it's responsible for many cases of childhood asthma in homes where processed foods are a dietary staple. Consumer groups tried for years to have tartrazine banned from food and drugs, but the food industry lobbyists won. Efforts to remove tartrazine from asthma and allergy drugs have also been unsuccessful. For more about drugs containing tartrazine, see the sidebar "Are You Sensitive to Tartrazine?"

In adults, asthma is more common in women, which gives us a clue that some part of it is hormonally related. Excessive estrogen, especially when not balanced by progesterone (not the synthetic progestins), can aggravate an existing asthma problem or even bring it on. Although natural progesterone tends to improve asthma symptoms, the synthetic progestins can cause or aggravate asthma. We highly recommend that you read *What Your Doctor May Not Tell You About Menopause*, by John R. Lee, M.D., for detailed information on natural versus synthetic hormones.

Many premenopausal women also suffer from tired adrenal glands and are unable to produce the necessary steroid hormones such as cortisol and adrenaline that the body would naturally produce to ward off asthma.

Drugs for Asthma

Bronchodilating inhalers are popular among asthma sufferers because they are very quick and effective at relieving the symptoms of an asthma attack and opening up the bronchial tubes for four to six hours. A sympathomimetic drug mimics the action of the sympathetic nervous system, which is responsible for the fight-or-flight reaction. They work on the same receptor sites as the body's natural hormone adrenaline, a substance released when you are under severe stress. Beta-agonist drugs work through one aspect of the fight-or-flight system, so they are classified as sympathomimetic drugs. While not all sympathomimetic drugs are beta-agonists, the most commonly used of these medications belong to this subclass. You will learn more about the beta-agonists in coming sections.

Sympathomimetics increase heart rate and blood pressure, and can cause anxiety, restlessness, and insomnia. Bronchodilators are meant to be used occasionally to relieve "mild acute" asthma attacks. The reality of how they are used is far dif-

Drugs That Can Cause or Aggravate Asthma

ACE inhibitors such as lisonopril (Zestril) and enalapril (Vasotec)

Antiarrhythmia drugs for the heart such as the beta-blockers (e.g., propranolol, timolol) and moricizine

Antinausea drug dimenhydrinate (Dramamine, Dimetabs)

Anti-Parkinson's drugs

Antipsychotic drugs such as the phenothiazines and lithium

Antiviral drugs mainly used to treat HIV such as cidofovir and protease inhibitors

Aspirin

Barbiturates

Benzodiazepines, antianxiety drugs (Valium, Dalmane)

Cephalosporin, sulfonamide antibiotics

Cholinesterase inhibitors used to treat Alzheimer's

Drugs to lower blood pressure such as guanethidine (Ismelin)

Ibuprofen-related family of nonsteroidal anti-inflammatory drugs (NSAIDs)

Narcotics

Over-the-counter sleeping pills such as diphenhydramine (Nytol, Sleep-Eze, Sominex, Tylenol PM)

Selective serotonin reuptake inhibitors (SSRIs), antidepressants such as fluoxetine (Prozac), fluvoxamine (Luvox), and paroxetine (Paxil)

Tricyclic antidepressants

Weight-loss drugs such as dexfenfluramine

ferent: many asthmatics come to depend on them, using them many times a day. This is dangerous, because they become less effective over time, and the risk of serious side effects is increased.

At an annual meeting of the American College of Allergy, Asthma and Immunology, it was acknowledged that misuse of one class of bronchodilator drug, the beta-agonists, may actually worsen asthma control and may even be responsible for the increase in asthma and asthma-related deaths. A large Canadian study confirmed this view. Overuse of these inhalers decreases the body's ability to respond to their bronchodilating effects. Over time, too-frequent puffing on beta-agonist inhalers can send asthma sufferers into a downward spiral that ends up putting them in the emergency room with a severe attack.

Examples of Beta-Agonists

Short acting: albuterol (Proventil, Ventolin, Repetabs, Volmax, Airet), bitolterol mesylate (Tornalate), isoetharine (Arm-a-med Isoetharine, Beta-2, Bronkosol), isoproterenol (Isuprel Glossets, Isuprel, Medihaler-Iso, Dispos-a-Med), levalbuterol (Xopenex), metaproterenol sulfate (Alupent, Metaprel), pirbuterol acetate (Maxair Inhaler, Maxair Autohaler), terbutaline sulfate (Brethine, Bricanyl)

Long-acting: arformoterol (Brovana), bambuterol (Bambec, Oxeol), formoterol (Foradil, Peforomist, Oxis), salmeterol (Serevent)

What Do They Do in the Body? The beta-agonist bronchodilating drugs work by stimulating receptors that cause opening of the bronchial tubes that lead to the lungs. Beta-agonists inhibit the release of histamine from mast cells in the airways and increase the movement of the tiny cilia that help propel allergens out of the lungs. Short-acting versions have more intense, less persistent effects; long-acting versions aren't effective for stopping an acute attack but are used prophylactically on a regular schedule, usually twice a day, to maintain open airways and prevent attacks.

What Are They Used For? Beta-agonists reverse the constriction of the bronchial

---

Using an Inhaler for Asthma

If you regularly use fast-acting inhalers to control your asthma, keep track of your usage. If you find yourself needing to use your inhaler more and more frequently to feel like your symptoms are controlled, heed it as a warning. Many studies have shown that more frequent inhaler use leads to a downward spiral of worsening bronchoconstriction and possibly a life-threatening attack.

Using your inhaler properly when you do have to use it will enable you to get the optimal dosage of your medicine and to get it where it needs to go. Have your doctor show you exactly how to get the medication into your airways efficiently, and ask him or her for a spacer—a long plastic canister that you attach to your inhaler that helps distribute the medication so that it goes into your lungs rather than onto the back of your throat.

Are You Sensitive to Tartrazine?

In the United States, any product that contains tartrazine has to say so on the label. Avoid drugs containing tartrazine for respiratory problems, and choose an alternative that does not contain this allergenic dye. Also avoid pills that have red coloring in them. Both red dyes and the iron oxides used to color some pills can cause allergic reactions.

tubes that occurs during an asthma attack, exercise-induced asthma, chronic bronchitis, emphysema, and other chronic obstructive pulmonary diseases (COPDs). Short-acting beta-agonists are used alone, as needed, for mild, well-controlled asthma; they are also known as "rescue inhalers." Long-acting beta-agonists (LABAs) are used long-term for symptoms that prove more difficult to control. In more severe cases, beta-agonists may be taken as a pill or inhaler along with another anti-inflammatory drug such as theophylline or cromolyn sodium. The popular drug Advair pairs a long-acting beta-agonist, salmeterol, with an inhaled steroid, fluticasone propionate; Symbicort is a similar combination, with the steroid budesonide and the LABA formoterol. More on these combinations later.

What Are the Possible Side Effects/Adverse Effects? All beta-agonists stimulate the central nervous system, which can give you a case of the "jitters," as if you've had too much coffee. Mood swings, increased appetite, fatigue, nightmares, and aggressive behavior are other possible side effects. Bronchitis, nasal congestion, increased secretion of saliva, nosebleed, muscle cramps, conjunctivitis, or discoloration of the teeth may occur.

The most common side effects of the long-acting beta-agonists are shakiness, nervousness, tension, inflammation of the nasal passageways and throat, sinus problems, and upper and lower respiratory tract infection. Others include palpitations, rapid heartbeat, chest tightness, angina (heart pains), tremor, dizziness, vertigo, headache, nausea, vomiting, diarrhea, joint and back pain, muscle cramping, generalized muscle aches, giddiness, susceptibility to flu virus and viral gastroenteritis, itching, dental pain, fatigue, rash, menstrual irregularities, nasal allergies, runny nose, laryngitis, bronchitis, dry mouth, and cough.

CAUTION!

Think Twice About Taking These Drugs If . . .

- You have ever had any kind of dangerous cardiac arrhythmias or heart blockage. If you have had arrhythmias or heart blockages due to use of digitalis, you will want to be especially cautious about using LABAs.
- You have narrow-angle glaucoma.
- You are going to have surgery. Tell your physician that you use this drug. Beta-agonists can interact dangerously with general anesthesia.
- You have diabetes, high blood pressure, heart disease, history of stroke, congestive heart failure, or hyperthyroidism; are elderly; or have a history of seizures or psychoneurotic illness. Dosages may need to be adjusted.

Diabetics who use beta-agonists should be aware that the jittery feeling they get when blood sugar is too low is hard to distinguish from the side effects of the drug.

With repeated, excessive use of short-acting beta-agonist inhalers, your body may begin to respond with what's known as paradoxical bronchoconstriction. Instead of opening your airways, use of the inhaler causes them to constrict even further. If you think this is happening to you, or if you find yourself using your rescue inhaler more than twice a week, see a doctor as soon as possible. Your asthma may be spiraling out of control.

With short-acting beta-agonists, tolerance may occur; temporary discontinuation should bring back the drug's original potency. Lower doses may be required for elderly people because of heightened sensitivity to nervous system stimulation.

Although the LABAs are good at controlling asthma symptoms, studies show a small increase in risk of death and hospitalization due to asthma-related breathing problems with salmeterol (Serevent) and formoterol (Foradil), when they are used alone. They are almost always prescribed as combination drugs, with each dose containing a LABA and a corticosteroid drug. Two such combination drugs are Advair and Symbicort. The danger of a life-threatening attack with LABAs alone has earned these drugs, as well as Advair and Symbicort, black-box warnings. The risk is small, but it does appear that some people have a paradoxical reaction to the LABAs, in which their airways constrict instead of opening in response to the medication. In 2008, the Food and Drug Administration (FDA) ordered that a new safety review be conducted into the LABAs.

An inhaled steroid drug alone is the best alternative for long-term control if short-acting beta-agonists don't do the trick; if this approach doesn't work, then a combination drug like Advair or Symbicort may be your doctor's next recommendation. Monitor yourself carefully and see your doctor right away if you suspect your asthma symptoms are worsening while you are on these drugs. You'll learn more about these combination drugs later in this chapter.

LABAs are not for treatment of an acute asthma attack. They are meant to be taken twice a day on an ongoing basis. Increasing the dose on your own to try to alleviate worsening symptoms is dangerous. Keep albuterol, epinephrine, or another fast-acting inhaler with you to open airways during an attack. If you find that your need for these fast-acting drugs is increasing despite your continued use of your long-acting beta-agonist, see your doctor as soon as possible.

Beta-blocking drugs typically used to control blood pressure should not be taken with beta-agonist drugs, as their actions directly oppose one another in the body. In fact, a person with asthma should not take beta-blockers unless absolutely necessary, as research shows that these drugs can actually bring on an asthma attack.

Taking nonpotassium-sparing diuretics with beta-agonists can deplete potassium in the body, possibly leading to changes in heart rhythm—especially if the beta-agonist is overused.

Examples of Epinephrines

Epinephrine (Adrenalin Chloride, AsthmaNefrin, microNefrin, Nephron, S-2, Vaponefrin, AsthmaHaler Mist, Bronitin Mist, Primatene Mist, Bronkaid Mist, Sus-Phrine)
Ephedrine sulfate
Ethylnorepinephrine (Bronkephrine)

What Do They Do in the Body? Like albuterol, the epinephrines are bronchodilating drugs that work quickly by stimulating receptors that cause opening of the bronchial tubes that lead to the lungs. They also work as nasal decongestants when inhaled through the nose.

What Are They Used For? Epinephrines are mainly used in inhalers but may be used in an injection to offset a severe allergic reaction. Inhalers are useful for treatment of an acute asthma attack or nasal congestion, while the injectable form is only for emergency situations where there is threat of complete closure of the bronchial tubes due to asthma attack or anaphylaxis (a life-threatening allergic reaction that involves swelling of the airways).

What Are the Possible Side Effects? These are extremely potent stimulant drugs that can cause sharp increases in blood pressure and heart pains. Rupture of the blood vessels in the brain and rupture of blood vessels around the heart have been reported in people using epinephrines. Heartbeat irregularities develop in some people even with low doses. Epinephrines have caused permanent electrocardiogram changes in healthy people, indicating some very significant effects on the conduction system that keeps the heart beating.

Bronchial irritation, nervousness, restlessness, and sleeplessness may be signs that you need to have your dosage of epinephrine reduced. If you do not feel your asthma symptoms have been relieved within 20 minutes after your usual dose, don't keep taking it. Seek medical assistance immediately.

The following are side effects specific to the form of epinephrine:

• **Inhaled form.** Palpitations, anxiety, fear.

• **Injected form.** Cerebral hemorrhage caused by rapid rise in blood pressure, especially in elderly people with diseased arteries in the brain. Agitation, disorientation, memory impairment, assaultive behavior, panic, hallucinations, suicidal or homicidal tendencies, and other serious psychological disturbances can be a result of epinephrine injection. Children may faint after being injected. Fatal arrhythmias, spasm of the arteries that feed the retinas of the eyes, and shock have also been reported. Other side effects may include pain, itching, hemorrhage, or raised red welt at injection site.

What Are the Interactions with Food? Foods rich in the amino acid tyramine, such as aged cheeses, wine, and chocolate, can interfere with enzymes needed to metabolize sympathomi-metic drugs such as epinephrines. Side effects of mixing these foods with epinephrines in sensitive people can include severe high blood pressure, intracranial bleeding, severe headache, chest pain, sweating, palpitations, changes in pulse rate, vision problems, breathing difficulties, and even coma.

Examples of Xanthine Derivatives

Aminophylline (Phyllocontin, Truphylline)
Dyphylline (Dilor, Lufyllin)
Oxtriphylline (Choledyl)
Theophylline (Theo-Dur, Slo-Phyllin, Theolair, Quibron-D Dividose, Bronkodyl, Elixophyllin, Aquaphyllin, Theoclear, Theostat, Accurbron, Asmalix, Elixomin, Lanophyllin, Aerolate, Slo-Bid Gyrocaps, Theo-24, Theospan-SR, Theovent, Theochron, Quibron-T/SR Dividose, Respbid, Sustaire, Theo-Sav, Theo-X, T-Phyl, Uni-Dur, Uniphyl)

What Do They Do in the Body? These are a class of drugs known as the xanthine derivatives or methylxanthines, which relax the smooth muscle that lines the blood vessels of the bronchial tubes and lungs. These drugs also stimulate the central nervous and respiratory systems, induce water loss (diuresis), decrease the tone of the lower esophageal sphincter, and inhibit uterine contractions.

What Are They Used For? Relief of symptoms and prevention of bronchial asthma or other bronchospasm associated with COPD. Regular use may improve lung function and shortness of breath in COPD patients. Xanthine derivatives are rarely used today to treat asthma, as they have high potential for toxicity and interact harmfully with a very long list of other drugs and foods. These medicines are used more often for COPD.

What Are the Possible Side Effects? If theophylline clearance from the body is reduced, harmful levels of the drug can accumulate in the body. Carefully consider any potential for interactions with other drugs, and don't take anything sold over-the-counter without consulting your physician or pharmacist.

At even slightly elevated blood levels of this drug, you're likely to experience nausea, vomiting, diarrhea, headache, insomnia, and irritability. In some people, the first signs of dangerous levels of theophylline in the body may be more severe. Moderately high blood levels lead to high blood sugar, low blood pressure, irregular heart rhythms, seizures, brain damage, and even death.

Other potential adverse effects at normal blood levels of theophyllines include fever, flushing, high blood sugar, oversecretion of antidiuretic hormone (which can cause fluid and electrolyte imbalances), rash, hair loss, irritability, restlessness, headache, insomnia, overexcited reflexes, muscle twitching, convulsions, nausea, vomiting, stomach pains, vomiting of blood, diarrhea, heartburn (gastroesophageal reflux) during sleep, life-threatening heart rhythm abnormalities, circulatory failure, changes in breathing patterns, respiratory arrest, protein in the urine, and rapid loss of fluid through the urine.

CAUTION!

Think Twice About Taking These Drugs If . . .

- You have peptic ulcer.
- You have an underlying seizure disorder that is not being treated with anticonvulsant medication.
- You have heart disease, low blood oxygen levels, liver disease, high blood pressure, or congestive heart failure, are elderly, or are or have ever been an alcoholic.
- You are a man over 55 years of age.
- You have heart failure.
- You are suffering from a sustained high fever.

In an acute episode of asthma, don't rely on theophylline to open your airways. Keep albuterol or another fast-acting beta-agonist inhaler around just in case.

Drug Interactions to Be Aware Of. Theophylline is one of the most dangerous drugs to combine with other drugs. The list of drugs it interacts with could go on for pages. If you're taking any type of theophylline drug, do not take any other drug or natural remedy without checking with a pharmacist or the drug information sheet first. Here are some lesser-known theophylline interactions:

- Theophylline can reduce the effectiveness of benzodiazepines (sedatives such as Ativan, Valium, and Xanax).
- Halothane and theophylline used together may lead to heart rhythm irregularities.
- Ketamine and theophylline used together may lead to seizures.
- Blood levels of lithium (used for depression and manic-depression) may be reduced by theophylline.
- The use of tetracycline along with theophylline increases the likelihood of side effects.

What Are the Interactions with Food? Theophylline has a shorter duration of action when you consume a low-carbohydrate, high-protein diet.

On the other hand, the drug stays in the body longer with a high-carbohydrate, low-protein diet.

Charcoal-broiled beef is high in polycyclic carbon, which diminishes the effectiveness of theophylline. Avoid large amounts of cocoa, tea, coffee, or other caffeinated drinks. Be aware that chocolate contains caffeine, too.

Hot pepper sauces, such as Tabasco sauce, can increase blood levels of theophylline, but this hasn't been demonstrated to be dangerous.

To avoid toxicity that results when sustained-release capsules empty into the body too quickly, take theophylline on an empty stomach. If you aren't using sustained-release tablets, you can take them with food, but less of the drug may be absorbed.

Eaten in large amounts, cruciferous vegetables such as broccoli, cauliflower, cabbage, and brussels sprouts increase the rate at which your body metabolizes theophylline.

Foods that acidify the urine cause the drug to be emptied more quickly from the bloodstream, while foods that alkalinize the urine have the opposite effect. Meat, chicken, fish, eggs, and grains tend to acidify the urine. Vitamin C and cranberries also acidify the urine. Foods that alkalinize the urine include most fruits (exceptions are cranberries, plums, and orange juice), dairy products (except cheese), and vegetables.

What Else to Take If You Take These Drugs. Studies have shown that asthmatics tend to be deficient in the mineral magnesium and that the body's ability to cope with stressful situations is compromised when low on this mineral. Daily use of beta-agonists such as albuterol, salmeterol, and epinephrine, as well as the use of theophylline, can further deplete the body's magnesium stores. Supplement with one of the following forms of magnesium: malate, citrate, gluconate, or glycinate, 500 mg a day in divided doses.

Examples of Leukotriene Receptor Drugs

Montelukast sodium (Singulair)
Zafirlukast (Accolate)
Zileuton (Zyflo)

What Do They Do in the Body? These relatively new drugs block or inhibit leukotriene receptors. Leukotrienes are one of the inflammatory substances produced during an allergic reaction. Levels of leukotrienes shoot up during an allergic asthma attack and montelukast sodium, zafirlukast, and zileuton block the swelling of the airways that results.

What Are They Used For? Prevention and treatment of asthma in people above the age of 12. These are not widely used, because they aren't as effective as other asthma drugs. A meta-analysis of 13 studies comparing leukotriene inhibitors to inhaled steroids for control of mild to moderate asthma found that the steroids were substantially more effective. Other studies show that patients who need to add a drug to their inhaled steroids to control their symptoms are better off with LABAs than with leukotriene inhibitors.

These drugs are not suitable for treating an acute attack. Keep a fast-acting beta-agonist or epinephrine inhaler with you to serve this purpose.

What Are the Possible Side Effects? People over the age of 55 who took leukotriene inhibitors reported more frequent respiratory infections, especially when they also used corticosteroids.

• **Montelukast sodium.** The FDA is investigating a possible association between the use of Singulair and behavior or mood changes that include suicidal thinking and behavior, and actual suicide. Please take this warning seriously! Other possible side effects include headache, dizziness, stomach infections, acid indigestion, increased incidence of flu, cough, nasal congestion, abdominal pain, fatigue, and fever.

• **Zafirlukast.** Headache, dizziness, nausea, diarrhea, abdominal pain, vomiting, infection, generalized pain, weakness, muscle aches, fever, back pain, and stomach discomfort.

• **Zileuton.** Headache, abdominal pain, weakness, lowered white blood cell counts, and muscle pain. Side effects frequently cause people to stop taking zileuton.

The most serious side effect that occurs with these drugs is elevation of liver enzymes, which indicates that there may be liver damage. Your physician should check your liver enzyme levels regularly, especially if you are 65 or older.

CAUTION!

Think Twice About Taking These Drugs If . . .

You have liver disease or transaminase elevations that are three or more times the upper limit of normal. This is an indication that your liver cells are being damaged by something and you shouldn't risk further harm to this vital organ by taking these drugs. Leukotriene antagonists aren't cleared from the body as well when the liver isn't doing its work properly.

Examples of Corticosteroid Inhalers

Beclomethasone (Beclovent, Vanceril, Vancenase)
Budesonide (Pulmicort, Rhinocort)
Flunisolide (AeroBid)
Fluticasone (Flovent, Flovent Rotadisk)
Triamcinolone (Azmacort)

What Do They Do in the Body? These drugs belong to a class of drugs called corticosteroids. Steroid drugs are usually given to reduce inflammation. These inhaled corticosteroids minimize the systemic side effects commonly seen with versions taken in pill form.

What Are They Used For? Control of asthma symptoms not adequately controlled by other means.

What Are the Possible Side Effects? The side effects of these medications make the choice to use inhaled steroids a tough one. It can seem so much easier to puff on an inhaler than to enact the lifestyle overhaul that may be necessary to address asthma symptoms at their root—until you understand how those drugs may be adversely affecting your body. No matter what you choose to do, it is essential to control airway inflammation and shortness of breath in a proactive way. Letting asthma symptoms persist without doing anything about them can lead to permanent respiratory damage.

Some research suggests that dosages of steroid inhalers are often higher than necessary for symptom control. To minimize side effects, talk with your doctor about finding the minimum effective dose.

The classic signs of long-term excess steroids in the system are puffy cheeks, weight gain, unstable blood sugar, and thin skin that breaks and bruises easily.

Inhaled corticosteroids may increase your risk of open-angle glaucoma, an eye disease that causes blindness, by up to 50 percent. Solid evidence also exists that long-term use can lead to loss of bone mass. This may not seem significant in a young person, but the more bone mass you build in your youth, the more you can afford to lose as you age before you end up with symptomatic osteoporosis. Many people who use inhaled steroids use them for years and years, so this can be a very real risk. If you must use inhaled steroids, do all you can to keep bones strong by following our recommendations in Chapter 20 for calcium, magnesium, vitamin D, and weight-bearing exercise.

Fungal yeast (candida) infections of the throat are a common side effect of inhaled corticosteroid use. This can cause irritation or hoarseness, rash, wheezing, and swelling of the face.

Even inhaled steroids can cause side effects throughout the body. Dozens of side effects may occur, including weight gain, water retention, increased susceptibility to infection (especially in the upper respiratory tract), high blood pressure, imbalances of minerals such as potassium and calcium, decreased growth in children and adolescents, and protein loss.

Other side effects may include hypersensitivity (allergic) reactions, bronchospasm (the very problem it's given to treat), acne, bruising, itching, wheezing, cataract, light-headedness, unpleasant tastes or smells, loss of senses of taste and smell, nausea, vomiting, dizziness, agitation, depression, mental disturbances, fatigue, insomnia, migraine, eczema, rash, skin discoloration, coughing, nasal congestion, abdominal pain, dry mouth, digestive problems, rapid heartbeat, palpitations, nervousness, shakiness, menstrual disturbances, and headache.

CAUTION!

Think Twice About Taking These Drugs If . . .

- You are having an acute attack of asthma. Corticosteroids don't work fast enough to help under these circumstances. Always keep a fast-acting inhaler on hand just in case.

- You have any kind of systemic fungal infection, including candida, a very common problem that can be made much worse by taking steroid drugs.

The full impact of long-term use of inhaled corticosteroids won't be completely understood

Use Caution Withdrawing from Steroid Drugs

If you have asthma, you are particularly vulnerable to a life-threatening attack while you are withdrawing from steroids taken by mouth (oral steroids), such as prednisone or hydrocortisone, or high doses of inhaled steroids. Taking large doses of steroids may cause your adrenal glands to shut down or greatly decrease their production of these substances. If you have been taking steroids regularly for a long period of time, your endocrine system may take several months to recover. In older people, the adrenal glands may never recover, and they may end up dependent on steroid drugs for life.

Anyone who is taking or has recently stopped taking oral corticosteroids or large doses of inhaled steroids over a long period of time should carry a warning card with this information on it. If you have an acute attack of asthma during this time or are under a lot of stress, resume the systemic steroid immediately and see your doctor.

One way to minimize the risk of dependency while taking oral steroids is to use the smallest possible dose of hydrocortisone, the natural form of cortisone, rather than the more potent synthetic drugs such as prednisone.

Even inhaled steroids should not be stopped suddenly. You could end up having a severe attack. Stop using one only under the guidance of a physician.

for some time. These are relatively new drugs that many people will end up taking for years or decades. With what is known at this juncture about the effect of these drugs on bone health and immune function, however, we suspect that allopathic medicine is underplaying the long-term risks. Although your physician may tell you that inhaled steroids are essentially free of the side effects of systemic versions, some people who use them for extended periods may experience weight gain, mood swings, or even adrenal suppression, and recent studies indicate that inhaled steroids may cause systemic side effects—including osteoporosis—more quickly than anyone suspected.

Lesser-Known Interactions to Be Aware Of. Corticosteroids interact with many other drugs, and you should check with your pharmacist or the drug information sheet before taking any additional drug or natural remedy. The following are some of the lesser-known interactions with corticosteroids:

- If you are taking oral anticoagulant drugs and corticosteroids, your physician may have to adjust the anticoagulant dose; in some cases, corticosteroids cause the anticoagulant to be less effective.
- Theophylline and corticosteroids used together may result in some alteration of the effects of either or both.
- Alcohol can add to the stomach irritation that can be a side effect of corticosteroid use.
- Use salt in moderation if you are using a steroid drug. The two together can cause stomach irritation, and fluid and sodium retention.

What Else to Take While Taking This Drug. Corticosteroids cause increased excretion of potassium, calcium, zinc, and magnesium, and this can result in depletion of these important minerals. Use supplements of each mineral.

Your need for the vitamins B_6, C, and D is increased during corticosteroid therapy.

Use extra probiotics to help maintain healthy intestinal flora, and be sure to rinse your mouth thoroughly (without swallowing the water) after each inhaled dose to prevent candida infection in the mouth and throat.

With oral administration of steroid drugs, high-fat meals cause increased drug absorption, appetite is increased, and foods in general are better absorbed, so weight gain can result. The body can absorb enough of the inhaled form to cause these side effects.

Examples of Combination Long-Acting Beta-Agonists (LABAs) and Inhaled Steroids

Fluticasone propionate/salmeterol (Advair)
Budesonide/formeterol (Symbicort)

What Do They Do in the Body? Advair and Symbicort are combination drugs. They contain an inhaled steroid and a long-acting bronchodilator. Advair is prescribed far more often.

What Are They Used For? Long-term maintenance treatment of asthma.

What Are the Possible Side Effects? Headache; cough; diarrhea; nausea; vomiting; dizziness; dry mouth; mouth, throat, and sinus irritation; sinus infection; muscle pain; stomach pain; and weight gain.

CAUTION!

Think Twice About Taking These Drugs If . . .

You have any history of heart problems, liver problems, diabetes, high blood pressure, cataracts, glaucoma, depression, recent infections, or low thyroid activity (hypothyroidism).

What Else to Take While Taking This Drug. Follow the guidelines for salmeterol and inhaled steroids.

Miscellaneous Asthma Drugs

Ipratropium bromide (Atrovent)

What Does It Do in the Body? Inhibits the body's overreaction to asthma triggers by blocking the action of the excitatory neurotransmitter acetylcholine. It also has antisecretory effects, helping relieve the discomfort of a runny nose.

What Is It Used For?

- **Bronchial inhalers.** Reversal of bronchospasm caused by asthma, emphysema, or other cardio-pulmonary diseases.

- **Nasal inhalers.** Relief from nasal allergies and common cold symptoms.

What Are the Possible Side Effects? Headache, nausea, flulike symptoms, back and chest pain, dizziness, dry mouth, constipation, coughing, shortness of breath, bronchitis, paradoxical bronchospasm, increased production of sputum, upper respiratory infection, inflammation of the pharynx, runny nose, and inflammation of the sinuses.

CAUTION!

Think Twice About Taking This Drug If . . .

- You are sensitive to the drug atropine, soy lecithin (commonly found in processed foods and chocolate), soybeans, or peanuts.
- You are trying to treat an acute asthmatic episode; it won't work quickly enough.

Use caution if you have narrow-angle glaucoma, enlarged prostate, or bladder neck obstruction.

When using Atrovent, be very careful not to get it in your eyes.

Nedocromil (Tilade)
Cromolyn (Intal)

What Do They Do in the Body? These drugs are mast cell stabilizers, which means that they suppress the release of inflammatory chemicals like histamine in the airways. They don't work as well as inhaled steroids but have less severe side effects. Mast cell stabilizers have been in use for a very long time, but almost no research has been done on them since the 1980s.

What Are They Used For?

- **Bronchial inhaler.** To prevent asthma attacks.

- **Nasal inhaler (Nasalcrom).** Relief from nasal allergies.

What Are the Possible Side Effects? Sore or dry throat, bad taste in the mouth, wheezing, nausea, cough, nasal congestion, sneezing, worsening asthma, allergic reaction, drowsiness, itchy nose, nosebleeds, burning nose, stomachache, dizziness, painful or frequent urination, joint pain or swelling, watery eyes, headache, muscle pain.

Omalizumab (Xolair)

What Does It Do in the Body? This drug is a monoclonal antibody made with recombinant DNA technology. It reduces the body's asthmatic response to allergic triggers. Because it is relatively new, and thus relatively untested, we don't recommend it at this time.

What Is It Used For? Xolair is only administered by injection in people with allergic asthma for whom other asthma medications don't control their attacks well enough. A blood test for response to allergic triggers is performed by the doctor to determine whether this drug is suitable. It takes up to 17 weeks of once or twice monthly injections to reduce asthma symptoms.

What Are the Possible Side Effects? Anaphylaxis (bronchospasm, fast drop in blood pressure, fainting, rash, fluid collecting around the heart) is a significant risk with this injected drug, even if you have been using it for a while. When it's given in the doctor's office, your doctor should be at the ready with epinephrine to treat this kind of reaction. Other possible side effects include injection site reaction, viral infection, upper respiratory tract infection, sinusitis, headache, and throat inflammation.

CAUTION!

Think Twice About Taking This Drug If . . .

- Please think twice about taking this drug, period. This drug was issued a black-box warning by the FDA due to the risk of anaphylaxis previously mentioned. This is the FDA's most serious warning.
- You have ever had an anaphylactic reaction to this drug.
- You are trying to treat an acute asthmatic episode; it won't work quickly enough.

Drugs for Allergies

Examples of Antihistamines

Azatadine maleate (Optimine)
Azelastine (Astelin)
Brompheniramine maleate (Dimetapp)
Cetirizine (Zyrtec)
Chlorpheniramine (Chlor-Trimeton, Aller-Chlor)
Clemastine fumarate (Antihist-1, Tavist)
Cyproheptadine (Periactin)
Desloratidine (Clarinex)
Dexchlorpheniramine maleate (Polaramine)
Diphenhydramine (AllerMax, Benadryl, Banophen, Diphenhist)
Fexofenadine (Allegra)
Levocetirizine (Xyzal)
Loratadine (Claritin)
Phenindamine (Nolahist)
Promethazine (Phenergan, Allergan)
Pyrilamine maleate
Tripelennamine (PBZ)

There are dozens of prescription and over-the-counter varieties of antihistamines. Because histamine is only one of many substances that cause allergy symptoms, these drugs work only 40 to 60 percent of the time. They are most effective at relieving sneezing and itching but don't have much effect on nasal congestion.

You may notice that several of these drugs seem similar to others in their class: Claritin (loratadine) and Clarinex (desloratidine), for example, or cetirizine (Zyrtec) and levocetirizine (Xyzal). The latter in each pair is a "me-too" drug—a chemical that was developed and sent through the FDA approval process not to create a better drug but to maintain patent protection or compete with other similar drugs from other drugmakers. We're not aware of any research showing that you will better control your symptoms with big-bucks, brand-name Clarinex or Xyzal than with generic, over-the-counter versions of loratadine or cetirizine.

All antihistamines have the potential to adversely affect heart rhythms; terfenadine (Seldane) and astemizole (Hismanal), which were finally pulled off the market, can cause a very rare and potentially fatal arrhythmia. If you still have these drugs in your medicine cabinet, please throw them away.

Fexofenadine (Allegra) is chemically similar to terfenadine but has not been found to cause this rare arrhythmia. Allegra's most common side effects are nausea, vomiting, weakness, and sleepiness. It should not be used by those taking monoamine oxidase inhibitors (MAOIs) or by anyone with urinary retention, narrow-angled glaucoma, high blood pressure, or heart disease. Allegra-D and Claritin-D are combinations of an antihistamine and the decongestant pseudoephedrine, which is described later in this chapter.

Some other antihistamine combinations include an analgesic (painkiller) such as acetaminophen, an expectorant such as guaifenesin, or an antitussive (anticough) such as menthol, codeine, or dextromethorphan. Well-known brand names of such combinations include Actifed, Advil Cold & Sinus, Alka-Seltzer Plus, Naldecon, Benylin, Chlor-Trimeton, Comtrex, Robitussin, Sudafed, Contac, Vicks, Dimetapp, Tylenol, and Dristan. Read labels carefully, and be aware of possible side effects and interactions of all of the drugs in these combinations, should you end up using them.

Ethylenediamines (pyrilamine maleate, tripelennamine) are associated with more digestive system side effects than other antihistamines, and cyproheptadine (Periactin) appears to cause more pronounced increases in appetite and weight gain than other drugs in this class.

Most antihistamines cause drowsiness, even so-called nonsedating versions, and other sedating drugs will have an additive effect, so don't combine them with alcohol or antianxiety drugs such as Ativan, Librium, Xanax, or Valium.

Fiorinal (a drug for tension headaches), tricyclic antidepressants, antiseizure drugs, prescription pain relievers, and muscle relaxants can also make you sleepy when taken with most antihistamines.

Don't use any antihistamine without a doctor's supervision if you have high blood pressure, cardiovascular disease, diabetes, enlarged prostate, or hyperthyroidism.

What Do They Do in the Body? These drugs compete with histamines at specific receptor sites, blocking allergic symptoms.

What Are They Used For? Relief of symptoms associated with seasonal allergies or the common cold, including runny nose; watery, itchy eyes; sneezing; and itchy rash. Claritin and Allegra don't cause drowsiness.

What Are the Possible Side Effects? Some people are allergic to antihistamines. Fluid retention (edema) in the extremities, throat, or even around the heart can occur. Other signs of allergy to antihistamines include dermatitis, asthma, lupuslike symptoms, rash, increased sensitivity to light, or even life-threatening anaphylaxis.

Other side effects that have been observed include precipitous dips in blood pressure when moving from sitting to standing or from lying down to standing, palpitations, heart rhythm irregularities (ranging from merely uncomfortable to life threatening), faintness, blood pressure changes, and changes on electrocardiogram (ECG) readings.

Drowsiness, sedation, dizziness, disturbances in coordination, headache, and irritability are among the more common side effects.

Also reported are stomach distress; anorexia; weight gain; nausea; vomiting; diarrhea; constipation; urinary problems (difficulty urinating or too-frequent urination); breast development in males (gynecomastia); spontaneous lactation in women; decreased libido; impotence; thickening of bronchial secretions; chest tightness; wheezing; nasal stuffiness; dry or sore mouth, nose, or throat; depressed respiratory function; tingling; feeling of heaviness; weakness of hands; easy bruising; jaundice; skin redness; stomach inflammation; high or prolonged glucose tolerance curves; increased levels of glucose in the urine (a symptom of diabetes); changes in blood cell and spinal fluid protein counts; increased blood cholesterol levels; excessive perspiration; chills; hair loss; vision disturbances; cough; menstrual disturbances; nightmares; mild to moderate transaminase elevations (indicating liver damage); and anemia.

CAUTION!

Think Twice About Taking These Drugs If . . .

- Do not give these drugs to children under the age of 2 without a specific recommendation from a physician. The FDA reports that Phenergan (promethazine) has caused deaths in children under the age of 2 and that it is dangerous in older children. Even if a doctor does prescribe this drug for your child, be aware that it's dangerous and could be fatal.
- You are taking MAOIs.
- You have sleep apnea. In people with this disorder, the sedative effects of antihistamines can cause respiratory depression.
- Don't use these drugs if you have narrow-angle glaucoma, stenosing peptic ulcer, symptomatic enlarged prostate, bladder

neck obstruction, pyloric (stomach) or duodenal (small intestine) obstruction, or liver disease.

Taking the drugs erythromycin, ketoconazole, or itraconazole can prompt life-threatening arrhythmias if taken with Claritin.

Taking antihistamines during a bout of lower respiratory tract disease (such as asthma, emphysema, or chronic bronchitis) can thicken bronchial secretions, making them more difficult to cough up.

People over the age of 60 are more likely to experience dizziness, sedation, fainting, confusion, and dipping blood pressure.

Be sure to tell your doctors that you use an antihistamine if you require general anesthesia. The activity of anesthetic drugs is increased by antihistamines, and the anesthesiologist will need to reduce the dosage.

Children using these drugs may become less mentally alert or become very excited. Overdoses in children can lead to hallucinations, convulsions, or even death.

It's a good idea to stay out of the sun while taking loratadine. It can make you more sensitive to ultraviolet light.

These drugs will not work to reverse the bronchospasm that occurs during an acute asthma attack.

Be Aware of Alcohol and Antihistamine Interactions. Alcohol and other central nervous system depressant drugs can have an additive effect when taken with antihistamines. Your ability to drive may be impaired by very small amounts of alcohol when you take antihistamines.

What Are the Interactions with Food? Citrus and other acidic juices can cause decreased drug activity when mixed with antihistamines.

Vitamin C can help your kidneys clear antihistamines from the body.

Drugs for Colds, Coughs, and Allergies

Examples of Expectorants

Guaifenesin (Guiatuss, Anti-Tuss, Genatuss, Glyate, Halotussin, Mytussin, Robitussin, Siltussin, Scot-Tussin Expectorant, Tusibron, Uni-Tussin, Diabetic Tussin EX, Organidin NR, Naldecon Senior EX, Breonesin, GG-Cen, Hytuss 2X, Gee-Gee, Glytuss, Duratuss-G, Guaifenex LA, Fenesin, Humibid LA, Liquibid, Monafed, Muco-Fen-LA, Pneumomist, Respa-GF, Sinumist-SR Capulets, Tonro EX)

What Does It Do in the Body? Guaifenesin is an expectorant. It enhances the output of lubricating fluid in the respiratory tract so that mucus is easier to expel by coughing. Coughs are less frequent and more productive.

What Is It Used For? Relief of dry, nonproductive cough and respiratory conditions where mucus is present.

What Are the Possible Side Effects? Nausea, vomiting, dizziness, headache, and rash.

CAUTION!

Think Twice About Taking This Drug If . . .

Your cough is caused by asthma, smoking, or emphysema, or you have excessive mucus in your respiratory tract.

A cough that won't go away may be an indication of a serious medical condition. If it persists for more than one week or if you seem to have recurrences frequently, see a health professional for evaluation. If the cough is accompanied by a rash or a headache that won't go away, you should also consult with your doctor.

According to the American College of Chest Physicians (ACCP), over-the-counter cough medicines don't help recovery from coughs, because they don't contain high enough doses of cough suppressants and expectorants. Trying to use these medicines to suppress coughs can delay diagnosis of something that urgently requires medical treatment, such as whooping cough or bronchitis that could turn into pneumonia. The ACCP's recommendation: if you are going to use over-the-counter medications to treat a cough, try antihistamines or decongestants to dry up mucus. But keep in mind that a cough is designed to eliminate disease-causing substances from your body. Let it run its course when possible, using natural methods (described later in this chapter) to help the cough do its job.

Over-the-counter cough medicines can be hazardous to children's health. They are a common drug of abuse in the 12-to-25 set in the United States. In this age bracket, cough syrups and decongestants are used for the purpose of getting high, roughly as often as LSD, Ecstasy, and methamphetamine. To get high, all a teen needs to do is guzzle a bottle of cough syrup that contains dextromethorphan (DMX) or codeine. Second, parents who unintentionally give too many over-the-counter cough and cold medications to their young child can easily cause harm. What kind of harm? Even recommended doses of these medications can cause damage. These drugs were approved back in the 1970s and were never adequately tested in pediatric populations.

Children under the age of 2 are most at risk for harm from over-the-counter cough and cold medications. If you are a parent, know that it's easy to overdose a very young child, and that combining drugs with multiple ingredients (decongestant, pain medication, cough suppressant) can lead to dangerous interactions or overdoses. In 2007 the Centers for Disease Control and Prevention (CDC) issued a warning that cough medicines given to children under the age of 2 can cause serious illness and death. One of the common causes of these reactions is giving adult doses of medication to children.

Examples of Decongestants

Epinephrine (Adrenalin Chloride)

Naphazoline (Privine)

Oxymetazoline (Afrin, Allerest, Dristan 12-Hour Nasal)

Phenylephrine (Alconefrin, Neo-Synephrine, Rhinall, Sinex)

Pseudoephedrine (Afrin, Drixoral Non-Drowsy Congestion Relief, Genaphed, Halofed, Pseudo-Gest, Sendotabs, Sudafed, Sudex, Cenafed, DeFed-60, Efidac/24, Allermed, Triaminic AM, Decofed Syrup, Cenafed Syrup, PediaCare Infants')

This class of drugs works by constricting blood vessels. Decreased blood flow to the nasal passageways and sinuses helps reduce swelling and mucous congestion. They are often used along with antihistamines and are available in oral and topical (nasal spray and eyedrop) versions.

After three to five days' use of topical decongestants, rebound congestion often occurs. Despite repeated use, nasal congestion is no longer relieved with the drug. If this happens to you, gradually wean yourself from the medication and allow one to two weeks for things to get back to normal.

When taken orally, decongestants cause central nervous system stimulation. Nervousness, irritability, insomnia, elevations in blood pressure and heart rate, irregular heartbeats, headache, pupil dilation, and palpitations can result. If you use a beta-agonist asthma medication (albuterol, salmeterol) and add a decongestant, the two drugs can have additive effects, making you feel as though you've had a few too many cups of coffee. This effect can be dangerous in people with high blood pressure and other types of heart disease.

What Do They Do in the Body? Swollen mucous membranes in the nose and eyes are a hallmark of seasonal allergies, colds, and flu. These over-the-counter drugs counter this inflammation by causing constriction of mucous membranes.

What Are They Used For? Hay fever, nasal allergies, sinusitis, common cold symptoms, and relief of congestion in the middle ear caused by infection. Inhaled through the nose, some can work directly on nasal inflammation or relieve ear blockage and pressure during air travel.

Pseudoephedrine and phenylpropanolamine are mixed-acting agents, which means they have a more generalized effect on the body, while epinephrine is a direct-acting agent with very specific effects on the airways.

What Are the Possible Side Effects? With topical use as a nasal spray: burning, stinging, sneezing, dryness, local irritation, and rebound congestion after stopping the drug. When taken internally: fear, anxiety, tension, restlessness, headache, light-headedness, dizziness, drowsiness, tremors, insomnia, hallucinations, psychological disturbances, convulsions, central nervous system depression, weakness, heart rhythm

Phenylpropanolamine: Avoid This Drug!

Phenylpropanolamine (PPA), once an ingredient in decongestants and diet drugs, increases stroke risk significantly, especially in women between the ages of 18 and 49. It may be responsible for hundreds of strokes in people under the age of 50. The FDA has released consumer advisories to tell the public that PPA is not a safe drug and has told drugmakers not to put it into their products anymore. You may still find it on store shelves in decongestants and diet pills. Toss older products that contain PPA in the trash, and avoid buying products that contain PPA in the future.

abnormalities, low blood pressure connected with cardiovascular collapse, transient high blood pressure, nausea, vomiting, paleness, difficulty breathing, loss of tone in the muscles of the face and mouth, sweating, urinary problems, twitching of the eyelids (blepharospasm), eye irritation or tearing, and heightened sensitivity to the sun (photosensitivity).

CAUTION!

Think Twice About Taking These Drugs If . . .

- You are taking MAOIs.
- You are hypersensitive to stimulating drugs. Some people's bodies respond very strongly to small doses. If you are experiencing dizziness, weakness, tremor, and heart arrhythmias, you may be getting too high a dose.
- You have glaucoma. If you are using the ophthalmic decongestant naphazoline, don't use nasal sprays containing these drugs.

Powerful stimulation of the central nervous system by these medications can lead to convulsions or cardiovascular collapse. Don't take internally if you have severe hypertension or heart disease. Use with caution if you have any of the following conditions: hyperthyroidism, diabetes, any kind of cardiovascular disease, elevated intraocular pressure (often a warning sign of glaucoma in its early stages), or enlarged prostate. Consult with your doctor if you have high blood pressure and want to use an over-the-counter decongestant.

There is some potential for addiction to phenylpropanolamine and pseudoephedrine. Use only when necessary, and discontinue as soon as you can.

In elderly people, long-term, high-dose therapy can lead to toxicity and psychosis more easily than in young people.

Beware of rebound congestion, particularly with nasal sprays. Don't fall into a pattern of increasing doses to compensate. Even the nasal inhaler can deliver enough drug to your system to cause toxicity.

Be Aware. Theophylline and nasal decongestants taken together can lead to theophylline toxicity. Dangerous heart arrhythmias can result.

Beta-blockers increase levels of epinephrine in the bloodstream when they are taken together. A hypertensive episode followed by slowed heartbeat can result. Diabetics may need to use higher doses of insulin or oral hypoglycemic drugs while using epinephrine.

Examples of Steroid Nasal Decongestants

Beclomethasone dipropionate (Beconase AQ, Vancenase, Qvar)
Budesonide (Rhinocort Aqua Nasal Spray)
Ciclesonide (Omnaris)

Flunisolide (Nasalide)
Fluticasone propionate (Flonase, Flounce)
Mometasone furoate (Nasonex)
*Triamcinolone acetonide (Nasacort, Tri-Nasal
    Spray)*

What Do They Do in the Body? When inhaled through the nose, these steroid preparations have an anti-inflammatory effect on nasal mucous membranes. As with the steroid inhalers used for asthma, inhalation somewhat decreases the risk of the adverse effects commonly seen with steroid medications.

What Are They Used For? Relief of symptoms of nasal allergies.

What Are the Possible Side Effects? Mild inflammation of the nose and throat, burning, stinging, dryness, and headache are most common. More rarely occur light-headedness, nausea, nosebleed, bloody mucus, rebound congestion, bronchial asthma symptoms, occasional sneezing attacks, decreased sense of smell, loss of or unpleasant taste in the mouth, throat discomfort, ulceration or deterioration of the mucosa that lines the nasal passages, watery eyes, sore throat, vomiting, *Candida albicans* infection in the nose or throat, and reduced resistance to infection.

Steroids are powerful medicines and can have long-term adverse effects even when used intranasally. Children who use nasal steroid sprays long-term have been found to have slight (half an inch) reduction in growth during the time the sprays are used. Other potential side effects of long-term nasal steroids include wearing through of the septum that separates the nostrils, raised intraocular pressure (which can lead to glaucoma), cataract, hypercorticism (known as Cushing's syndrome) including swelling of the face and weight gain around the middle of the body, and osteoporosis.

CAUTION!

Think Twice About Taking These Drugs If . . .

- You have an untreated infection of the nasal mucous lining. Don't use intranasal steroids.
- You are already using systemic steroid drugs such as prednisone. Adding a nasal steroid inhaler can increase the likelihood of suppression of the body's natural production of steroid hormones. If your doctor is weaning you off of systemic steroids and onto inhaled versions, look out for signs of adrenal insufficiency (joint and muscle pain, lack of energy, depression).
- You have been using intranasal steroids long-term. You should have regular exams to be sure your nasal passages don't suffer permanent damage.

Some people who are sensitive to these medications may develop acne, menstrual irregularities, swelling of the face, weight gain, or other symptoms of elevated levels of steroid hormones.

Use these drugs cautiously if you have tuberculosis; an untreated fungal, bacterial, or systemic viral infection; or herpes of the eye, or if you are recovering from an ulcerated nasal septum, or nasal surgery or trauma, as healing is slowed by steroid drugs.

Avoid exposure to chicken pox or measles while using these drugs.

Other Tips on These Drugs. If your nose is very runny, you may want to use a topical nasal decongestant for the first couple of days you use intranasal steroids. This will dry things up a bit so that the nasal steroid isn't simply flushed out of your nose without being absorbed.

Examples of Cough Suppressants

Codeine (Codeine sulfate)

What Does It Do in the Body? Suppresses cough (at low doses), blocks pain response (at higher doses).

What Is It Used For? Relief of symptoms of cough caused by respiratory tract irritation or relief of mild to moderate pain.

What Are the Possible Side Effects? Codeine is an addictive narcotic and should not be used unless absolutely necessary. Nonaddicting drugs with similar actions are available.

Nausea, vomiting, sedation, dizziness, and constipation are the most common side effects. Other side effects can include allergic reactions, central nervous system depression, light-headedness, euphoria, restlessness, weakness, headache, hallucinations, disorientation, vision disturbances, convulsions, biliary tract spasm, heart rhythm irregularities, fainting, decreased urinary output and other urinary problems, water retention, and rapid blood pressure changes when moving from lying to sitting or from sitting to standing.

CAUTION!

Think Twice About Taking This Drug If . . .

- You have recently had a head injury or if you have known intracranial lesions or elevated pressure of the fluid surrounding the brain and spinal cord. Codeine is more likely to have dangerous side effects in these cases. Drowsiness, dizziness, and other symptoms of head injury are also side effects of codeine, so you should avoid taking any medications containing this drug until you've been thoroughly evaluated. The same goes for acute abdominal conditions.

- You have asthma or other COPDs. Codeine can depress respiratory function.
- You are prone to drug dependency. Addiction can occur. Use only when absolutely necessary. Don't use this drug for more than a few days at a time.

Be Aware. Central nervous system depressants (opiates, general anesthetics, phenothiazines, tricyclic antidepressants, tranquilizers, and alcohol) and codeine have additive effects, meaning they increase the effects of the other drugs and can impair your ability to drive or perform other tasks.

Hydrocodone combinations

What Does It Do in the Body? Hydrocodone is a narcotic cough suppressant and analgesic (pain reliever) that works by blocking receptors that transmit pain impulses and by suppressing the cough reflex. It causes euphoria, sedation, and general physical depression. It is used in combination with other painkiller drugs such as acetaminophen and the ibuprofen-type drugs.

What Is It Used For? Relief of moderate to severe pain, and for relief of cough. It is also used before and during surgery to enhance the effects of anesthesia. A few over-the-counter drugs contain hydrocodone in very small amounts. It's a very potent narcotic analgesic, it's addictive, and it was the most-prescribed drug in the United States in 2001. If anybody at the FDA was paying attention, it might have occurred to them that when an addictive drug is found among the top 10 prescribed drugs in the country, we must have an abuse problem with that drug on a national scale. Please be aware that hydrocodone drugs found in family medicine cabinets are commonly abused by teens.

What Are the Possible Side Effects? The FDA has issued a warning that Tussionex, a combination of hydrocodone and the antihistamine chlorpheniramine, can cause life-threatening breathing problems and death when given above or more frequently than the recommended dose and says that Tussionex should not be used in children less than 6 years old.

Most frequent side effects include light-headedness, dizziness, sedation, nausea, vomiting, and sweating. Also, respiratory depression or arrest, apnea (irregular breathing), circulatory depression, coma, shock, cardiac arrest, drastic mood swings, delirium, insomnia, agitation, disorientation, drowsiness, sedation, lethargy, physical impairment, headache, mental cloudiness, vision changes, increased intracranial pressure, pupil dilation, cramps, abdominal pain, taste alterations, dry mouth, loss of appetite, constipation, spasm of the biliary tube (where bile passes from the gallbladder into the intestines), facial flushing, chills, faintness, heart rhythm irregularities, dramatic blood pressure fluctuations, urinary problems, and reduced libido. Other possible side effects include bronchospasm, depression of the cough reflex (although hydrocodone may be administered for this purpose, complete suppression of coughing may do more harm than good), interference with the body's ability to regulate its temperature, muscular rigidity, and tingling in the extremities. Those who are hypersensitive to narcotic analgesics may have rash, itching, profuse sweating, spasm of the larynx, or fluid retention.

CAUTION!

Think Twice About Taking This Drug If . . .

- You are hypersensitive to narcotics.
- You are having an asthma attack.
- You have diarrhea caused by poisoning. The toxic material should be eliminated from the system completely before you use any narcotic-containing drug.

- You are prone to depression or addiction. This is good reason to stay away from this drug completely. Hydrocodone is addicting. OxyContin and Vicodin, prescription versions of this drug, are major drugs of abuse in the United States.
- You have had a head injury, or have a brain tumor or any other kind of brain lesions. These conditions make hydrocodone an unsafe choice for you.

Use any narcotic-containing drug with extreme caution if you are elderly or debilitated. Those with cardiovascular disease, convulsive disorders, raised eye pressure (which can lead to glaucoma), alcoholism, delirium tremens, hardening of the arteries in the brain, ulcerative colitis, fever, emphysema, severe obesity, hypothyroidism, Addison's disease, enlarged prostate, urinary problems, gallbladder disease, or recent gastrointestinal or urinary tract surgery are at special risk when using narcotics.

Those with asthma or another COPD should use extreme caution when taking this drug. It significantly depresses respiratory function, decreasing both the depth and frequency of breaths.

If you are prone to low blood pressure, you should know that hydrocodone can cause blood pressure to dip further.

Kidney or liver impairment can cause this drug to accumulate in the bloodstream, making adverse effects more likely.

This drug may cause you to become constipated. Those with ulcerative colitis should be aware that narcotics can cause diarrhea or toxic dilation of the colon.

Be Aware. The following drugs may prolong the effects or increase the potency of hydrocodone: alcohol, barbiturate anesthetics, chlorpromazine, and cimetidine (adverse effects more likely).

Examples of Drugs for Flu

Oseltamivir phosphate (Tamiflu)
Zanamivir (Relenza)

What Do They Do in the Body? Both drugs are neuraminidase inhibitors. They inhibit enzyme activity in flu viruses, which in turn inhibits their growth and spread. Relenza is inhaled, and Tamiflu is taken as a pill. They have to be taken within 36 to 48 hours of the onset of flu symptoms to be effective. Even when taken within this time frame, studies show only a one- to a one-and-a-half-day shortening of the illness's duration on average. Keep in mind that these medications do not prevent you from passing the flu on to others.

Some studies have looked at the use of Tamiflu for flu prevention in people who don't have flu symptoms but who stand at risk of catching the disease. Most of these studies suggest only a small benefit of neuraminidase inhibitors for prevention, if any at all. With the adverse-effect profiles of these drugs, it's unlikely that they will ever be used widely for prophylaxis.

What Are They Used For? Treatment or prevention of influenza.

What Are the Possible Side Effects? The following are drug-specific side effects:

• **Tamiflu.** Nausea, vomiting, insomnia, and vertigo. Rarely, unstable angina, anemia, colitis, pneumonia, and tonsil abscesses have occurred. Additional side effects have been reported in children, including abdominal pain, nosebleed, ear disorders, and conjunctivitis.

• **Relenza.** Malaise, fever, abdominal pain, muscle pain, joint pain, itching, and dizziness. In children without the flu who received the drug as a preventive, far more adverse effects were reported, including nasal symptoms, throat or tonsil discomfort or pain, and cough.

A few years after their approval by the FDA, 25 people under the age of 21 had been reported to have died while using Tamiflu. Around 600 reports came in about abnormal behavior, hallucinations, and convulsions in people between the ages of 10 and 19 who were taking this oral neuraminidase inhibitor. (Most of these took place in Japan, where these medicines are much more widely used.) In two separate instances, a 12-year-old and a 13-year-old jumped out of a second-floor window after taking Tamiflu; others fell from windows or balconies or ran into traffic. Relenza, the inhaled version, has been the subject of at least 115 reports of psychiatric side effects as well.

CAUTION!

Think Twice About Taking These Drugs If . . .

• You have been symptomatic for more than 40 hours. No studies have shown that neuraminidase inhibitors work once flu has progressed this far.
• You have asthma or other chronic lung disease. In some asthmatics, zanamivir caused their airways to constrict. Adverse events are more common in people with pulmonary disease, and the drug has not been shown to help them.

Some strains of flu are resistant to these drugs. If you happen to be infected with one of these strains, the drugs will not be effective.

Should You Get a Flu Shot?

At this writing, the flu vaccine is recommended for children 6 months of age to 5 years of age;

anyone over 50; people with chronic health conditions, including asthma, diabetes, coronary artery disease, or HIV; and any health care practitioners or others who come into regular contact with people at high risk of having the flu. The general buzz is that everyone should probably have a flu shot. After all, who wants to end up with the flu? Even when it's not life-threatening, it keeps us home from work and school and makes us miserable. Better safe than sorry . . . right?

The flu can be deadly. According to government statistics, pneumonia and influenza (P&I) deaths are among the top 10 causes of death in the elderly. However, these statistics combine deaths from two very different disease conditions that are common in the elderly, which makes it hard to know the true mortality rate from influenza alone. And wouldn't it be wonderful if flu shots were the magic bullet they're made out to be? But deaths from flu are increasing in spite of flu shots. According to statistics released by the CDC, even adjusting for the fact that there are increasing numbers of people over the age of 65, who are more susceptible to death from the flu, P&I deaths have increased by 44 percent among people 65 and older since 1979.

Let's put aside continuing uncertainty about the actual number of influenza deaths versus pneumonia deaths and figure that deaths from both of these conditions are increasing at roughly the same rate. If flu vaccinations are working so well, why is this happening? One reason is that as you age, which is when you need the most protection from flu, your body's ability to create antibodies in response to the vaccine deteriorates. It is known that only about half of the elderly who receive flu shots can mount an antibody response strong enough to be protective. A study from the Netherlands showed that among two groups of elderly people, one that received flu shots and one that received a placebo, the group receiving the flu shot had only a 1 percent lower incidence of flu than the placebo group!

Research published in the journal *Lancet*, which used Great Britain's socialized medicine database, found that while flu shots in the elderly did help protect against some strains of flu, overall flu shots did not reduce the risk of dying.

The strains of flu that sweep through North America are different every year, and to get vaccines made and distributed in time, the CDC have to make an educated guess at which strains to include in the vaccine well before flu season hits. The antibody response is less protective if the manufacturers of the vaccine pick the wrong flu virus. In the 2007–2008 flu season in the United States, researchers chose the wrong strains, and the vaccine was only half as protective as it would have been if the right strains of the virus had been used. A well-matched vaccine in young, healthy adults or children reduces chances of catching the flu by 70 to 90 percent. The vaccine is less effective in very young children, whose immature immune systems are not yet ready to mount an adequate antibody response. The 2007–2008 vaccine only reduced those chances by 44 percent. In other words, a lot of people who got the jab also got the flu.

Researcher Tom Jefferson, M.D., of the Cochrane Vaccines Field centered in Rome, Italy, has published a review of available research studies in the vaunted *British Medical Journal*, and the results of that study strongly suggest that (in Dr. Jefferson's words) "we've got an exaggerated expectation of what vaccines can actually do." In his analysis of studies of the effectiveness of flu vaccines, he found that:

• Flu vaccines are only mildly effective in the elderly; their immune response to the vaccine tends to be much weaker than that of younger, healthier people.

• There is no good science whatsoever upon which to base prescribing this vaccine to children under the age of 2—who are already being jabbed with more than 10 different vaccines, often starting with the first shots at birth or within weeks of birth. Many experts believe this practice plays an important role in the dramatic increase in allergic (including asthma) and autism-related disorders in our children, and in their overall lack of resistance against infectious diseases against which we do not vaccinate.

• Flu vaccination has little to no effect on hospital stays, time off from work, or death from or complications from the flu.

Other points worth considering:

• High numbers often quoted regarding flu mortality—usually in the neighborhood of 36,000 deaths per year—are likely overinflated. Unless a nasal swab is performed on a person with respiratory symptoms, there's no way to be certain whether the illness is actually the flu. Any illness that resembles the flu is often reported to be influenza, and the number of cases is probably inflated—and this also leads to exaggerated expectations of what the flu vaccine is capable of preventing.

• Some research finds little to no difference in risk of developing flu between vaccinated and unvaccinated people. Those who say the vaccine is "effective" are usually referring to the effect of the vaccine on immune parameters, measurable in the blood after the shot is given. If those immune parameters are boosted following the shot, the consensus is that it's effective—but this does not mean it always prevents the illness or even that it prevents the illness more often than a placebo.

Dr. Jefferson rightly points out that "there's a huge gap between policy and evidence" when it comes to the widespread use of the flu vaccine. The risks of getting the shot are quite small—but they are not without side effects. Studies have shown that as many as 1 in 10 people who get a flu shot experience flu symptoms within a week.

One supplement that has been found to help older people marshal a better immune response to flu shots is the steroid hormone DHEA. In studies of elderly mice and elderly humans, small doses of this hormone significantly improved immune response to the flu vaccine. We don't recommend using DHEA if you are under 40 years old, though.

If you feel it's important to follow your physician's orders and get a flu shot, by all means do it, but please don't fool yourself into thinking that this shot is highly protective and that you don't need to take care of yourself to prevent the flu.

Natural Alternatives for Colds and Allergies

Prevention is by far the easiest way to deal with colds, flus, and allergies. How well your immune system is working has a lot more to do with whether you get the flu than whether you're exposed to it or have had a flu shot. In other words, it's about you, not about the germ! The Six Core Principles for Optimal Health provide the groundwork for prevention. In the rest of this chapter, we'll cover other steps you can take.

Controlling Allergies

To control allergies, take the necessary steps to allergy-proof your home, car, and workplace; to consciously manage the stress in your life; and to get plenty of rest, good nourishment, and exercise.

You can find out what you're allergic to by noticing when you sneeze and wheeze. Is it when you dust or clean out your closets? Is your asthma at its worst when you wake up in the morning with your face buried in your pillow? When you hug your beloved cat, dog, or rabbit, are you rewarded with several sneezes in succession or tightening in your bronchial tubes? Does the heavily perfumed woman in the elevator make your nose run and your eyes itch? Does mowing the lawn give you itchy eyes and a rash? If so, you are probably one of the scores of people who react to dust mites, pollens, pet danders, molds, synthetic perfumes, and other airborne allergens.

If you fall into this category, environmental controls are the first step you need to take to control allergy symptoms. If you're allergic to dust, try to keep closets, carpets, shelves, and drapes as dust-free as possible, and wear a dust mask while you do housework. Buy dust-mite-proof covers for pillows and mattresses, and wash bedding in hot water once a week.

If you're allergic to your pets but can't bring yourself to give them away, keep them well groomed and don't let them sleep on your furniture or in your bedroom.

If you're allergic to pollens, learn what times of day pollen counts are high in your area and try to stay indoors during those times.

Be Aware of Fakegrances

Fake fragrances, or fakegrances as we call them, are almost totally unregulated in the United States and are made primarily from a toxic brew of chemicals. The justification for this is that the toxins are present in very small amounts, but fakegrances are everywhere these days, from laundry soaps, fabric softeners, and dry cleaning to garbage bags, cleaning products, and per-

fumes. Some experts believe that fakegrances may be one of the leading causes of asthma and allergies, especially among children.

If you have asthma or allergies, one of your first steps should be to eliminate all sources of fakegrances from your home, car, and office. Throw away the so-called air fresheners and scented candles, stop using perfume unless it's made from essential oils, and buy "fragrance free" laundry detergents and fabric softeners.

If you find yourself sniffling and sneezing when you're driving, try to determine whether you are reacting to exhaust from other cars or something inside your own car. Many plastic fabrics give off fumes that can be allergenic. If you find you're allergic to car exhaust, set up your life so that you avoid exposure to it as much as possible. Running or bicycling for exercise along streets with heavy traffic, inhaling toxins with every breath, is just asking for trouble. If you live in the city, go to a gym to work out.

Of course, do your best to avoid being anywhere near cigarette smoke—especially if you have asthma. Secondhand smoke is a nose, throat, and lung irritant and carcinogen even if you're not allergic to it.

Check Your Ventilation System

Most of us who live in hot and humid summertime climates wouldn't think of going without air-conditioning. Not only can it bring relief from stifling heat and humidity, it can filter out the summer pollens that give 1 in 13 Americans hay fever. But if you're suffering from lung- and sinus-related illnesses in spite of being snug in your air-conditioned house or office, be sure your cooling system is putting out clean air. Studies have shown that cooling systems can make bronchial and sinus problems such as asthma, bronchitis, allergies, and summer colds either better or worse, depending on whether the air is clean.

Here is a very sophisticated way for you to check your air-conditioning filter—pull it out and look at it. If it looks dirty, wash it, vacuum it, or replace it, depending on the type.

If you have a forced-air cooling and ventilation system, pay attention to whether the ducts are clean, where the outside air source is, whether the air is recycled, and where the intake duct is. Be sure your air sources are clean. Be aware that an expensive professional duct cleaning won't do you any good if the whole house isn't cleaned immediately afterward. A duct cleaning stirs up dust and mold, spreading it through the house. If you don't clean your house at the same time, it will just end up back in the ducts.

Natural Allergy Remedies

Treating allergies with antihistamines is a temporary stopgap measure that doesn't address the underlying problem. These drugs shouldn't be used for more than a few weeks at a time. If you've tried everything and your allergy symptoms are still affecting the quality of your life, look into desensitization (allergy shots). Minuscule amounts of allergens are injected in gradually increasing amounts so that your body can learn not to respond with an allergic reaction. Treatment can be expensive and take up to three years, and it doesn't work for everyone. Carry allergy-fighting supplements with you so that as soon as you feel an allergic reaction coming on, you can nip it in the bud.

Some cases of hay fever or allergic sinusitis can be greatly improved when food allergens are identified and eliminated. Decreasing the total allergic load the body has to cope with can help you become less sensitive to allergens in general. Refer to the section "Beat IBS and Treat Food Allergies Naturally" in Chapter 11 to find out how to identify foods that might be causing problems for you.

Elimination of white flour, refined sugar, and any foods containing chemicals (additives, preservatives, and dyes) is another simple but helpful step you can take before deciding you need drugs to get through hay fever season. Tartrazine, or yellow dye no. 5, is well-known to provoke allergic responses, and for some people, just cutting out the processed foods that contain yellow dye is enough to control their allergy problems. Tartrazine is contained in some 60 percent of commercial medications as well as the majority of processed foods. See the section "Asthma Medications: Is the Cure Worse than the Disease?" and the sidebar "Are You Sensitive to Tartrazine?" for more details on tartrazine.

Next time you feel sinus congestion coming on—whether from allergy, cold, or flu—you might want to try humming your favorite tune instead of turning to decongestants, nasal steroids, or antibiotics. In a study recently published in the *American Journal of Respiratory and Critical Care Medicine,* a group of Swedish scientists discovered that the simple act of humming can help keep sinuses clear. In 10 men ages 34 to 38, researchers measured the speed of air exchange between nose and sinus cavities before and during a bout of humming, and found that air exchange increased. So did, in those areas, the production of the natural anti-inflammatory nitric oxide—fifteenfold!

Quercetin

Quercetin is arguably the most powerful and effective natural remedy for allergies. In most people it effectively dries out the mucus membranes and helps quiet the inflammation that can irritate nasal passages. Quercetin is a powerful antioxidant flavonoid (found naturally in red wine, onions, apples, black tea, buckwheat, citrus, and eucalyptus) that inhibits the release of histamine from mast cells. It has potent anti-inflammatory and cancer-inhibiting activities as well. The typical dose is 500 mg, but if it dries you out too much, reduce the dose.

Other important bioflavonoids include those found in grapeseed extract (proanthocyanidins) and green tea.

Vitamin C

Vitamin C is a well-known natural remedy for allergies. This essential vitamin, which most Americans aren't getting in optimal amounts, directly lowers histamine levels in the body, supports the adrenal glands that produce allergy-fighting hormones, and supports the immune system in many ways. The Six Core Principles for Optimal Health recommend 2,000 mg of vitamin C for everyone as part of a daily regimen. During allergy season, you can take an additional 1,000 mg to 2,000 mg throughout the day. If your symptoms continue or worsen, increase the dosage to 1,000 mg every two or three hours. If you get diarrhea, back off on the dose until it stops. Your tolerance for vitamin C can increase dramatically when you have allergies, a cold, or a flu. Some people can't tolerate vitamin C except in food. If this applies to you, try some of the other remedies we recommend.

Defensive Herbs

We have many herbs at our disposal that effectively strengthen and support the immune system without encouraging it to overreact. You can try a regimen of two weeks of the herb echinacea or astragalus. For some people, stinging nettle (*Urtica dioica*) works wonders to allevi-

ate allergy symptoms. Follow directions on the container.

Some people are allergic to echinacea and other herbs. If taking an herb makes your symptoms worse, stop taking it!

The Chinese, who have had thousands of years of practice, have created some effective natural allergy remedies that have few to no side effects. Be sure to use a reputable brand. You'll find recommendations in the Resources and Recommended Reading section at the back of this book.

Culinary herbs like ginger and turmeric have long been used in Asian and Middle Eastern traditional medicine as natural remedies for asthma and allergy. Research from this millennium suggests a few reasons for the effectiveness of these herbs at reducing allergy and asthma symptoms. One explanation is that ginger and turmeric—along with cumin, anise, fennel, rosemary, garlic, and pomegranate—reduce the activation of an inflammatory pathway linked to allergy and asthma. Even if adding these herbs to your meals doesn't improve symptoms, it will make them taste great!

Pantothenic Acid (Vitamin B₅)

Pantothenic acid can be helpful in treating allergies, especially when they are aggravated by fatigue, exhaustion, or stress. Try taking 250 mg to 1 gram (1,000 mg) twice daily.

Omega-3 Fats: EPA from Fish

The omega-3 fats found in fish can be useful for treating inflammatory conditions such as allergies, asthma, and eczema. For this purpose, a specific kind of omega-3 fat called eicosapentaenoic acid (EPA) appears to work best. Although a different kind of omega-3 fat, alpha-linolenic acid (ALA), is found in flax oil, we don't recommend this type of omega-3 for people with conditions related to inflammation. Flax oil is highly unstable, which means that it becomes rancid easily, and ALA has to be converted to EPA to do this job. This conversion doesn't always happen efficiently. EPA is only found in appreciable quantities in fish oils and certain types of algae. Refer to Chapter 9 for detailed information on how to choose an omega-3 supplement.

Other fatty acids that can help with asthma and allergy, including the omega-6 fat alpha-linolenic acid, are naturally found in fresh fruits and vegetables, whole grains (such as oats), seeds, and fish, so be sure to eat plenty of these foods in addition to supplementing with EPA.

A diet rich in seafood and antioxidant-rich vegetables, fruits, and nuts—the Mediterranean diet—has been found to protect against childhood allergy and asthma. A study published in the journal *Thorax* surveyed 690 children aged 7 to 18, all of whom lived in rural Crete, a part of Greece. Those children who adhered at least moderately to the traditional Mediterranean diet had significantly less risk of asthma and allergy. More oranges, grapes, apples, and nuts in the children's diets appeared to confer more protection.

Bee Remedies

Bee pollen may give some people relief, but try just a little bit first, in case you are one of the few who are allergic to it. If you can buy fresh local honey at a farmer's market or health food store, you can try that instead. The local pollens in the honey can help desensitize your hay fever reactions.

Alternative Approaches to Treating Asthma

It's long been suspected that antioxidant supplementation could help asthmatics control their symptoms. The inflammation that springs up in the airways of asthma sufferers causes the formation of free radicals, and those free radicals in turn increase the process of inflammation. It makes sense that supplying extra antioxidants would help stop this vicious cycle from getting out of hand.

A small study published in the journal *Respiratory Medicine* demonstrates promise for vitamin C as a natural asthma remedy. Eight subjects with exercise-induced asthma (EIA) were given either 1,500 mg of vitamin C per day or a placebo for two weeks; then after a one-week period of no supplements for either group, the groups got the opposite treatment. Exercise tests showed that the vitamin C significantly reduced symptoms of EIA.

In a study published in 2001 in the journal *Archives of Environmental Health,* researchers recruited five male and 12 female asthmatics between the ages of 18 and 39. One group was given 400 IU of vitamin E and 500 mg of vitamin C before a moderately intense exercise session with exposure to ozone, a substance known to cause asthma attacks; another got a placebo. Those who took the antioxidants had a less severe episode of wheezing and chest tightness than those who didn't. If you're asthmatic, try taking your daily dose of 200 to 400 IU of vitamin E and 500 to 1,000 mg vitamin C an hour or so before your workout.

For their study published in 2004, researcher Rachel M. Rubin and coworkers at Ithaca University's Division of Nutritional Science evaluated blood nutrient levels in just over 7,500 children of ages 4 to 16. They found that higher blood levels of vitamin C and beta-carotene offered significant protection against asthma. Higher beta-carotene and vitamin C levels were associated with a roughly 10 percent reduction in asthma prevalence in children who were not exposed to cigarette smoke, and with a 40 percent reduction in kids who were exposed to smoke. Higher selenium levels had a more pronounced effect: higher levels lent 10 to 20 percent reduction in asthma prevalence in kids not exposed to smoke, and 50 percent reduction in those who were subjected to secondary smoke. It makes good sense to supplement children's diets with a high-quality multivitamin—especially if they have asthma.

Caffeine is a natural asthma remedy as well. We don't recommend that you drink more than two 8-ounce cups of coffee per day, but if you don't drink coffee normally, a cup can be used as medicine to open airways when necessary.

A number of good studies show that homeopathy can work well to control asthma. If this appeals to you, work with a certified homeopath. A substantial body of research shows that acupuncture can help with asthma as well.

Yoga exercises that include deep breathing and deep relaxation techniques have been found to be very effective in reducing the number and severity of asthma attacks. Researchers in London, England, trained 612 people with mild or well-controlled asthma in a set of breathing exercises called the Papworth method—which also includes relaxation training. The method reduced asthma symptoms by one-third and significantly reduced depression and anxiety. Breathing exercisers, gadgets into which you breathe in and out of as a sort of "strength training" for the respiratory muscles, are also widely available. Ask your asthma doctor which one he or she might recommend.

Although sudden bouts of exercise can trigger an asthma attack, for many people regular aerobic exercise is helpful because it increases the capacity of the lungs to take in oxygen and it strengthens the heart.

Drs. Jonathan Wright, M.D., and Alan Gaby, M.D.—pioneers in the use of nutrition to prevent and cure illness—swear by intramuscular vitamin B_{12} injections (1,000 mcg) for childhood asthma. Talk to your doctor; he or she should be happy to try B_{12} for any child dependent upon asthma drugs. If not, look for a naturopathic doctor.

Some studies show that vitamin B_6 is useful in treating asthma. You can try 50 mg of vitamin B_6 twice daily taken with food.

Magnesium and potassium are minerals important for good lung function. As only about 15 percent of children in the United States are

Asthmatic Moms Can Reduce Children's Risk with the Right Foods

Asthmatic women of childbearing age, take note: eating fish may protect your children against developing this condition. Frank Gilliland, M.D., Ph.D., and colleagues from UCLA gathered a large group of school-aged children from 12 school districts in southern California. They split them into two groups: one consisting of children who had been diagnosed with asthma by age 5, and the other of children who had never been diagnosed with asthma. Each child's mother filled out a detailed questionnaire about what foods she ate during her pregnancy. Mothers who had asthma and ate plenty of oily fish (including salmon, mackerel, trout, sardines, and cod) during pregnancy had 71 percent reduced risk of their children developing asthma compared to those asthmatic moms who did not eat much oily fish during pregnancy. No effect was seen in nonasthmatic mothers.

Other research has demonstrated a slight protective effect of the Mediterranean diet against asthma, atopy, and allergy in children when mothers consume it during pregnancy.

believed to get even the recommended daily allowance (RDA) for magnesium, researchers have long suspected a link between low intake of these minerals and asthma risk. At USC's Keck School of Medicine, doctors administered lung function tests to 2,566 children from ages 11 to 19 and gave them detailed questionnaires about their diets. The less magnesium these kids took in, the poorer their lung function turned out to be. Getting processed foods out of kids' lives and introducing whole foods (the richest sources of magnesium in the diet are whole grains and leafy greens) is likely to promote better lung function, as is the use of a good-quality multivitamin.

A growing body of evidence supports a hormonal link to asthma. Women are four times as likely to have an asthma attack when they are premenstrual, and hormone replacement therapy (HRT) that uses estrogens can aggravate asthma. Many women with asthma find that their symptoms improve while they are pregnant, when progesterone levels rise dramatically, and that asthma returns with a vengeance postpartum. The hormonal culprit is most likely what Dr. John Lee has termed "estrogen dominance," meaning even though estrogen levels may be low premenstrually, there is little or no progesterone in the body to balance or oppose it, causing symptoms of estrogen excess. It is very common for premenstrual asthma to clear up with the use of natural progesterone cream. (The synthetic progestins are apt to aggravate asthma.) See Chapter 19 for details on using natural progesterone.

Another intriguing theory appears in the book *Your Body's Many Cries for Water* by F. Batmanghelidj, M.D. (Global Health Solutions, 1995). Dr. Batmanghelidj's theory is based on the fact that part of the physical response the body has prior to and during an asthma attack is the release of histamines, which cause inflam-

mation. Histamine plays an important role in the regulation of water distribution in the body. He explains that when concentrated blood (a direct consequence of dehydration) enters the lungs, the body's response is to release histamines, which causes constriction of the airways in the lungs, thus reducing the need for water. Batmanghelidj also believes that long-term dehydration can cause an up-regulating of the immune system, causing it to overreact to allergens.

This theory makes a lot of sense. If you feel an asthma attack coming on, you can try drinking one or two glasses of water and see if that helps.

The Emotional Stress Factor in Asthma

Asthma has a very clear and definite link to chronic emotional stress. Hostility and anxiety both can directly impact lung function. In 2007, the journal *Health Psychology* published a study on 5,115 participants in the Coronary Artery Risk Development in Young Adults (CARDIA) study group. These young adults, aged 18 to 30, had their hostility levels measured with a standard psychological test. The more hostile the subjects were, the more likely they were to perform poorly on tests of lung function. This relationship was independent of smoking status, age, asthma diagnosis, and socioeconomic status.

Asthma inhalers using cortisone-like steroids and epinephrine are among the most effective ways to prevent and control asthma attacks. This fact should give us a major clue that asthma can be aggravated by adrenal glands that are tired and depleted because they are working overtime due to chronic stress. The adrenals are trying to produce stress hormones such as cortisol and adrenaline (which is related to epinephrine). If your body's best natural defense against an asthma attack is to pump out some adrenal hormones, and it is unable to do so because the adrenal glands are depleted, the inhaler is the next best thing as a temporary stopgap measure. But to the extent that this is a problem in a child or adult, a serious depletion is present and needs to be addressed.

What Sets Off an Asthma Attack

Once a person is predisposed to have asthma, a variety of factors can set it off. Here is a list of the best-known culprits:

Airborne allergens such as pollen

Animal dander

Carbon dioxide released by cooking or heating with gas

Drugs such as aspirin and beta-blockers

Emotional stress

Exercise

Food additives such as food dyes (especially yellow dye no. 5)

Preservatives such as sulfites and benzoates

Flavorings such as salicylates, aspartame, and MSG (often disguised as "natural flavors" and hydrolyzed vegetable protein)

Stabilizers and emulsifiers such as carrageenan and vegetable gums

Food allergies (most commonly eggs, wheat, citrus)

Fresh paint

Room deodorizers and household cleaners

Strong odors from cooking

Tobacco smoke

If you are suffering from asthma that's serious enough to compromise everyday life, your best bet is to combine some type of counseling with avoiding environmental triggers and making lifestyle changes such as managing stress and good nutrition. Tackling any one of those three causes (emotional, environmental, lifestyle) will help, but it usually takes working on all three to truly solve the problem.

Nutritional Prescription for Allergies and Asthma

1. Avoid processed foods such as chips, cakes, cookies, puddings, cheeses, canned foods, and frozen foods that contain additives, preservatives, dyes, or flavor enhancers such as MSG and hydrolyzed protein.
2. Avoid excessive sugar and refined white flour.
3. Avoid overdoing caffeine, which puts stress on the adrenal glands. Limit intake to one 8-ounce cup of coffee per day. If you can give it up all together, or switch to tea, all the better.
4. To treat asthma, you can try taking some or all of the following supplements, in addition to what is recommended in the Six Core Principles for Optimal Health:

   • Quercetin, 500 mg daily and up to twice daily.

   • Vitamin C, 1,000 to 4,000 mg, three to four times a day (has antihistamine-like activity and supports the adrenal glands).

   • Vitamin A (preformed, not as beta-carotene), up to 50,000 IU a day in divided doses for up to two weeks to help heal mucous membranes and resist infection (do not take over 10,000 IU daily if you are pregnant or if you could become pregnant).

   • Vitamin B_6, 50 to 100 mg three times a day.

   • One of the following forms of magnesium: malate, citrate, gluconate, or glycinate, 200 to 300 mg three times a day.

• Fish oil supplements daily containing 1,000 to 3,000 mg of EPA for up to three weeks when symptoms become troublesome (make sure they have a natural preservative such as vitamin E).

• N-acetyl cysteine (NAC), 500 mg two to three times a day.

• Licorice root tincture to support the adrenal glands (follow directions on the container). The glycyrrhizin in the whole plant tincture is removed in deglycyrrhizinated licorice (DGL), which we recommended for ulcer and other digestive problems, but it's this substance that helps fortify adrenal function. Don't use for more than three weeks if you have high blood pressure, and keep in mind that licorice that has not had its glycyrrhizin removed can interact dangerously with several drugs. Diuretics, especially those that don't spare potassium, and digoxin (Lanoxin) can both lead to irregular heartbeats, cardiac arrest, and dangerously high blood pressure when combined with nonglycyrrhizinated licorice extract.

• St. John's wort (Hypericum) to help control anxiety, 300 mg three times daily.

• Ginkgo biloba in a standardized extract, 60 mg one to three times daily.

Preventing and Treating Colds and Flus Naturally

We have been led to believe that we "catch" more colds in the winter because of the colder weather. But the common cold was unknown to the Eskimos before the white man went to the Arctic, bringing his refined white flour, sugar, and alcohol with him. And why do some people regularly get colds and flus while others seem immune? Maybe it has something to do with lifestyle. Bacteria and viruses are everywhere, all of the time, and those who have poor resistance because of their lifestyle choices are the ones most likely to end up sickened by them. As Louis Pasteur, the father of the germ theory, said on his deathbed: "The germ is nothing; the terrain is everything."

Busy Americans think they don't have time for a cold or a flu. They stock up on cold and flu drugs that control symptoms. Once they've managed to mask those symptoms, they consider themselves to be well again, and they go on with their lives. Truth be told, what these people are doing is not healing but suppressing symptoms. Symptom suppression bypasses the immune response to illness, essentially robbing the immune system of the opportunity to push the body through the natural healing process. Fever, the production and expulsion of mucus, cough, and fatigue are all considered nagging symptoms to be banished, but they are also natural and beneficial healing effects orchestrated by the immune system. When they are allowed to run their course as much as possible, the body is cleansed, rejuvenated, and better educated for the next bug that comes around.

To allow this process to happen, dress warmly and rest as soon as you begin to experience any symptoms. Warmth is important when you're fighting a flu or cold, because warmth accelerates the action of the immune system. If you have a fever, consider it a blessing; this is the body's way of "cooking out" the bug that has infected it. The same goes for children. Too many parents panic and pull out the Tylenol as soon as their kids' temperature hits 100, and this is counterproductive to a child's healing process. Don't suppress coughs or the flow of mucus with drugs—this will prevent you from expelling toxic material from your body. Rest and recuperate for as long as you need to. It will be well worth the extra couple of days away from work or school. That being said, never let a persistently high fever or cough get out of control. See a doctor if necessary.

When the weather turns cold, we tend to overheat our homes, creating dry, low-humidity air. Microorganisms (germs) multiply faster in your nasal passages when the humidity is low. (Didn't we just say in the section on allergy that it's good when the air-conditioning is on because it dries things out? Right—but microorganisms don't cause allergies. Drying out nasal passages reduces natural mucus production so the nose can't get rid of those bad bugs as quickly.) When the heat goes on, a humidifier should go on with it.

When you feel cold or flu symptoms, act immediately. Even a few hours can make a big difference. Get to bed early, stay warm, avoid junk food, and drink plenty of clean water and hot herbal or green tea. Too much sugar will depress your immune system, making you more susceptible to opportunistic germs.

Colds and flus are passed on from one person to another more through shaking hands than any other cause. This is a good reason to keep your hands away from your face and to wash your hands before you eat, just like your mother told you! When the Japanese have a cold or flu, they would never think of going out into a crowd without first donning a surgical mask over nose and mouth.

Another major factor that contributes to cold and flu season is the holidays. Not only do family gatherings and travel stress us out, but also we tend to overeat more during the holidays and consume more alcohol and sweets that suppress the immune system.

The number one, all-time, and most effective medicine for colds and flus is an ounce of prevention: a nutritious diet, plenty of clean water, exercise, enough sleep, and relaxed time spent with loved ones. However, since these simple guidelines are easier described than adhered to, here are some natural helpers for fending off and alleviating colds and flus. One of the most important keys to warding off a cold or flu is to start treating it early, at the first signs. If you wait until you have full-blown symptoms and feel miserable, the medicines only alleviate the symptoms somewhat.

Cold/Flu Kit for Kids

Sick kids aren't about to swallow some yucky-tasting medicine, and with their sensitive taste buds, it's easy to get a "Yuck." Fortunately, kids find most of the cold and flu essentials easy to tolerate. The Oscillococcinum tastes like sugar—no problem. Most kids like zinc lozenges, especially when they're coming down with a cold, and chewable vitamin Cs are easy to find. They'll probably hate the throat spray—it does pack a punch—but it's worth a try. A spoonful of dark, rich, sweet honey is good for soothing a cough in children over 1 year of age.

Echinacea

Taken at the first sign of a cold or flu, echinacea can help boost the immune system. Many herbalists like to combine echinacea with goldenseal and astragalus. If you feel worse after taking these herbs or any others, stop taking them, as you may be allergic to them.

Hyssop

This ancient herb has been used for at least two millennia to treat sore throats, chest colds, and laryngitis. In the 1800s, herbalist Nicholas Culpeper prescribed hyssop for ear infections and "all griefs of the chest and lungs." It's an excellent aid for getting tough mucus moving up and out of the body. You can make a hyssop tea by adding 1 to 2 teaspoons of dried herb to a cup of boiling water and allowing it to steep for 10 to 15 minutes. Drink a cup of this infusion up to three times a day. Children should take a smaller dose: ½ cup of infusion three times daily for kids ages 6 to 12 and ¼ cup for kids ages 2 to 6. Children younger than 2 can take 1 or 2 tablespoons three times a day.

Never take essential oil of hyssop internally; instead, use it for steaming out coughs, flu, bronchitis, and asthma. Put two drops of hyssop oil and one drop of peppermint oil in a small pot of water. Heat until steaming, turn off the heat, drape a towel over your head, and gently inhale the steam (be careful not to get too close to the steam). Ten drops of hyssop added to 1⅓ tablespoons of almond or sunflower oil make a soothing chest rub.

Here's a new take on the old "spoonful of sugar" scenario: Researchers from Pennsylvania State University found that 1 tablespoon of buckwheat honey worked better to calm a child's nighttime cough than dextromethorphan, the active ingredient in many commercial cough medicines. Buckwheat honey was used because its dark color reflects a high content of antioxidants, which are believed to play an important role in honey's cough-soothing properties. Never under any circumstances give honey to a child under 1 year of age, as it can cause infant botulism.

Chinese Herbs

The Chinese have dozens of tried-and-true herbal remedies called "patent medicines" that they have used for thousands of years. These are just starting to catch on in the United States. They are available at many health food stores and herb shops. Two of the most popular Chinese cold prevention remedies are Yin chiao and Ganmaoling. If you're starting to get a cough or other symptoms in your lungs, try Sangchu tablets. These herbs work very specifically to balance the body and work best if they are taken alone, without any other medication. See the Resources and Recommended Reading section for sources.

Homeopathics

Many people respond well to homeopathic medicines. Coldcalm by Boiron can work well for colds, and many people swear by Oscillococcinum for the flu. Boericke and Tafel makes a cough syrup called B & T Homeopathic Cough and Bronchial Syrup.

Herbal Teas

Quite a few tea mixtures can help with cold and flu symptoms. Chamomile tea works well, and Celestial Seasonings' Sleepytime tea contains chamomile and other soothing and relaxing herbs. The same company makes Mama Bear's Cold Care tea, which is mostly peppermint and licorice and works well for soothing a cough. For respiratory ailments, look for teas containing licorice, fennel, and horehound. For sinus ailments and headaches, look for chamomile, echinacea, goldenseal, and bayberry. Again, if your symptoms get worse, you may be allergic to the herb, so stop taking it.

Ginseng

Studies have shown that 100 mg a day of ginseng extract can significantly cut your chances of catching a cold or flu bug.

Your Natural Remedy Travel Kit

Keep preventive medicine in your desk drawers at work so that if you feel a cold or flu coming on, you don't have to wait until you get home to treat it. When you travel, always plan ahead by bringing natural remedies for colds and flus, indigestion, insomnia, and tension or stress. It's especially important to plan ahead during the holiday season, when we often combine extra-stressful travel, cold weather, too many immune-depressing sugary foods, and family tensions. Also remember to drink plenty of clean water and take your multivitamin every day. Here are suggestions for your travel kit:

• Melatonin, sublingual (under the tongue) tablets before bed for insomnia and jet lag.

• Ginger capsules or ginger tea for nausea and gas.

• Chewable papaya tablets for indigestion after a big meal.

• Echinacea, astragalus, goldenseal capsules or tincture for cold and flu prevention.

• Zinc lozenges combined with vitamin C and propolis for cold prevention. Zinc has a direct effect in boosting the immune system and may have some antiviral properties as well.

• An herbal throat spray that includes echinacea and goldenseal to prevent a sore throat from taking hold.

• White willow bark capsules or tincture to treat a headache or other types of pain.

• St. John's wort capsules, tablets, or tincture for stress and anxiety.

• Chromium picolinate tablets (200 mcg) to balance blood sugar.

• Oscillococcinum, a homeopathic remedy, to prevent the flu. Open one tube, pour it into your mouth, and suck on the contents until gone (it contains tiny sugar pellets). Since this is a homeopathic remedy, it is important not to consume caffeine, menthol, or peppermint within 30 minutes of taking it. Take every six hours. If it doesn't work after three tubes, it's probably not going to. Oscillococcinum's action is fast and dramatic when it works.

• Vitamin C in Emergen-C packets. Vitamin C supports the immune system on many levels. At the tissue level, it counteracts histamines, which cause inflammation and congestion, and is needed for tissue repair. At the cellular level, it acts as an antioxidant and is essential to the functioning of the white blood cells that fight disease. Take at least one packet every 2 hours when you feel a cold or flu coming on, for up to 12 hours.

• Elderberry syrup or extract. Sambucol, made by Nature's Way, is the one with the best clinical support for its antiviral action.

• Yin Chiao is a Chinese remedy that can be very effective in preventing colds and flu. Take at the first sign of a cold or flu.

Vitamin C

If you feel like you're coming down with a cold, you can take 2,000 mg a day of vitamin C. The esterified C type works best for a sensitive stomach. Along with its antioxidant activity, the vitamin C can lower your histamine level, giving you relief from sinus congestion, watery eyes, sniffling, and sneezing.

Zinc Lozenges

Alternative health professionals have been telling us for at least a decade to suck on zinc and vitamin C lozenges to shorten the duration of a cold, and finally a scientific study has been published in the *Annals of Internal Medicine* confirming this. Of 100 cold sufferers, half were given lozenges with zinc and half without. The group with zinc got better in an average of four days, while the group without zinc got better in an average of seven days.

If anyone tries to tell you that only one special type of zinc works, you can be assured that this is hogwash. Any type of zinc chelate will work just fine. Look for a zinc lozenge that contains at least 5 mg of zinc, and follow the directions on the container.

Beta-Glucan

Medicinal mushrooms such as shiitake, maitake, and reishi have long been revered for their immunity-boosting effects. Modern research demonstrates that their most active ingredient is a carbohydrate called beta-glucan, which is also found in oats, barley, and baker's yeast. Beta-glucan encourages the bacteria- and virus-eating potential of white blood cells, which helps the body knock out cold and flu bugs and secondary infections. An added benefit: beta-glucan has enormously promising anticancer effects. You can add beta-glucan to your diet by taking 250 mg per day of purified beta-glucan or a concentrated medicinal mushroom supplement.

Protecting Your Sinuses and Throat

Rinsing the sinuses with a saline solution is one of the most effective ways to prevent allergies and fend off a cold or flu.

Many colds and flus begin with an infection in the sinuses, which then drips down the back of the throat, infects the throat, and then moves on to the lungs. Allergic irritation and inflammation can contribute. Rinsing your sinuses with a mixture of warm water, salt, and baking soda once or twice daily will reduce congestion, rinse mucus and allergens away, and open up sinuses and nasal passages. Combine 1 cup of body-temperature warm water, ¼ to ½ teaspoon of salt, and a pinch of baking soda. You can use a neti pot, or nasal irrigator, which can be found at most health food stores and even drugstores. These look like little ceramic or plastic pitchers with a long spout that fits snugly into one nostril. Or use a rubber ear syringe, a shallow cup, or the palm of your hand.

Do this over a sink. Tip your head to one side (not back), insert the syringe into the top nostril, and gently squeeze or pour the water in, allowing it to drain out of the other nostril. If you have mucus in the throat, you can plug the lower nostril so that the solution drains into the throat, but try not to swallow it. If you're doing this with your palm, you have to gently sniff the water up the nostril—this takes a bit more finesse.

If you have a sore throat, go after the bacteria on the throat by gargling with salt water, a strong mouthwash, or an herbal spray that contains goldenseal and propolis.

Special Treatments for Viruses

Although your best defense against a virus is a strong immune system, some natural supplements will greatly aid your body in fending off viruses.

Selenium

Selenium is a trace mineral that we need only in microgram amounts, but a deficiency can make us much more susceptible to the flu. There is new evidence that taking larger doses of selenium can make a major difference in helping the body fight off a virus. A normal daily dose of selenium is 50 to 200 mcg, but if you're fighting a cold or flu, you can take up to 800 mcg daily for three days. Selenium also works well to help fight off the herpes virus, in the same dosages.

Elderberry

European black elderberries (*Sambucus nigra* L.) have been used as a folk remedy for flu, colds, and coughs for at least 2,500 years. Even Hippocrates mentioned it in his writings. If you're from the American Midwest, chances are your grandparents made elderberry wine and sipped it on winter evenings as a tonic.

From 22 pounds of elderberries that had sat for some time in her supervisor's freezer, an Israeli flu researcher, Madeleine Mumcuoglu, isolated proteins that deactivated a flu virus in the laboratory. The mechanism, she theorized, had to do with the way flu viruses find their way into living cells where they can replicate. (Viruses can't replicate on their own.) They puncture cell walls with tiny spikes called hemagglutinin and can then slip in and alter the cells' DNA.

After watching viruses and elderberry in the laboratory, Mumcuoglu found that the active ingredients in elderberry actually disarmed the spikes by binding to them and preventing them from piercing the cell membrane. The viral spikes are covered with an enzyme called neuraminidase, which acts to break down the cell wall. Research suggests that bioflavonoids, present in high concentration in elderberries, may inhibit the action of this enzyme.

Nearly a decade later, Mumcuoglu and her colleagues performed a double-blind study with a group of people suffering from the flu. Half the group were given an elderberry extract, and half were given a placebo. Within 24 hours, flu symptoms of fever, cough, and muscle pain in the elderberry group had dramatically improved in 20 percent of the patients. By day two, another 75 percent had clearly improved, and by day three, more than 90 percent of the group was better. In contrast, among those taking the placebo, only 8 percent showed any improvement after 24 hours, and the remaining 92 percent took about six days to improve. Nobody in the elderberry group complained of any side effects.

The elderberry group also had a higher level of antibodies to the flu, indicating an enhanced immune system response. If a pharmaceutical drug or the flu shot had anywhere near this type of response, everyone would have some in their medicine cabinet!

A study performed in Norway and published in 2004 enrolled 60 flu sufferers who had been sick for 48 hours or less. They were given either 15 milliliters of elderberry syrup or a placebo four times daily for five days. Symptom questionnaires revealed that elderberry syrup shaved an average of four days off of influenza A and B infections when compared to the placebo.

Other studies show great promise in combating other viruses with elderberry extract, including HIV, herpes, and Epstein-Barr.

If you take elderberry syrup or extract at the first sign of a cold or flu, chances are excellent that it will work. And if you live in an area where elderberries grow, you may want to consider reviving the tradition of sipping elderberry wine on chilly winter evenings! You can find elderberry remedies at most health food stores. Follow the directions on the label.

20 Ways to Supercharge Your Immune System and Prevent Colds and Flus

1. Stretching helps your lymphatic system do its job of removing toxins from your body. Be sure to stretch your neck muscles and your torso, and to stretch your arms over your head.

2. Get an extra hour of sleep, or go to bed early with a cup of chamomile tea and an uplifting book.

3. Zinc lozenges are powerful weapons in the fight against winter colds. Try the varieties with propolis and vitamin C added.

4. The homeopathic remedy Oscillococcinum will quickly knock out many kinds of flu. The only way to find out if it will work for what you've got is to try it.

5. Reduce the stress in your life through meditation and exercise. Chronic stress depletes your adrenals, which play a vital role in immunity.

6. Stock up on the vitamin C and bioflavonoids. If you feel something coming on, take 1,000 mg of vitamin C and a bioflavonoid such as grapeseed, green tea extract, or quercetin every hour.

7. Drink plenty of clean water, which will help your body keep itself detoxified.

8. Eat plenty of fiber to keep things moving through the digestive system.

9. Eat yogurt once a day for the calcium and beneficial intestinal flora. The friendly bacteria in your intestines are your best weapon against unfriendly bacteria.

10. Skip the candy and soda pop. Try a piece of fruit or some nuts instead.

11. Keep alcohol consumption low. A glass of wine with dinner is fine. More than that and your liver may be diverted from protecting you from illness.

12. Eat your vegetables—fresh and preferably organic.

13. Are you allergic to dairy products? Wheat? Corn? Chronic food allergies can weaken your immune system.

14. Eat more complex carbohydrates and less refined white flour, which causes blood sugar jumps and constipation.

15. Try shiitake or reishi mushrooms with your veggies—the Chinese use them to bolster the immune system.

16. Take one of the cold prevention remedies mentioned in this section preventively when you're under extra stress.

17. If you have a late night or stressful day, balance things out by getting extra rest.

18. If you're going to be traveling on a plane, take plenty of vitamin C and other cold and flu preventives for a few days ahead of time.

19. Seek out the company of loved ones or volunteer for someone less fortunate than you.

20. Exercise keeps everything in the body shipshape, but if you feel weak or tired, don't push it too hard.

Chapter 13

Drugs for Pain Relief and Their Natural Alternatives

Americans love to take pills for pain. We gobble up billions of dollars' worth of pain-reliever pills each year. The large drug companies that sell over-the-counter pain-relieving drugs such as acetaminophen (Tylenol), ibuprofen, and aspirin are always fighting for a share of that huge market. We buy right into their advertising and marketing, believing that the only way to deal with pain is to make it go away with a pill. After all, who doesn't want their pain relieved? And the sooner the better.

The urge to simply suppress pain without addressing the underlying cause can be harmful in the long run. Pain is your body's way of telling you something is wrong. It is a warning signal that has been called the guardian of health, and the sooner you act to heal the source of your pain, the better off you'll be.

If you suffer from some type of chronic pain, you are not alone. Just in the United States, over 100 million people suffer from chronic pain. About 37 million of those suffer from arthritis,

30 million from headaches, and 15 million from the pain caused by cancer. Another 32 million suffer from other types of chronic pain such as back pain, osteoporosis, and nerve pain.

Prescription painkiller abuse is a growing epidemic in the United States. Its consequences can ruin lives and families, and it causes thousands of deaths a year. It's caused primarily by doctors who don't carefully monitor their patients who are on pain drugs, by parents who carelessly make their pain medications accessible to teens, and through thefts of drugs from pharmacies, which are then sold on the street.

On the other hand, nobody should ever suffer unnecessarily from pain out of fear of becoming addicted to a pain drug. If you have acute or temporary severe pain caused by recovery from surgery or a broken bone, for example, it's important to take advantage of the relief that painkilling drugs can give you. That's what they should be used for. The key is to gradually reduce the drug dosage as the pain starts to go away and to stop taking the drugs when they are no longer needed. This may sound obvious, but it may not be when you're taking them. Painkillers are most likely to become addictive when their use isn't closely monitored.

Managing and preventing pain effectively involves much more than just taking a pill to make it go away. It's important to treat the underlying cause of the pain as well. Acute or short-term pain and chronic or long-term pain need to be treated differently. Short-term pain can often be helped by treating both cause and symptom at once, such as ice and some aspirin for a pulled muscle. But chronic pain requires a whole other set of solutions, which will be covered in more depth at the end of the chapter.

In the United States, the terminally ill actually tend to be *undertreated* for pain. If you have severe, intractable, untreatable pain, you should never avoid pain-relief medication out of a sense of guilt or shame, or concern that you will become dependent on it.

If you have chronic pain caused by a disease such as arthritis or fibromyalgia, the waters become a little bit muddier in terms of deciding when and how to take pain medication. Most painkilling drugs don't work for very long or very well for these types of pain. The most important part of managing chronic pain is preventing and eliminating the source of the pain. You'll find solutions that generally work much better than pain-suppressing drugs at the end of this chapter. Please read the chapter on addictive drugs (Chapter 2) if you are dealing with severe pain or think you may be hooked on painkilling drugs.

If you are suffering from severe pain that requires prescription medication, be aware that prescription drugs for pain have the potential to be abused and to cause you harm and even death. All pain medications, without exception, have serious side effects, which become more dangerous as we age. And yet, according to the American Pain Foundation, half of seniors surveyed reported that their doctors didn't tell them about possible harmful interactions between pain drugs and other medications they were taking. Four in 10 seniors reported that their doctors didn't discuss the potential side effects of the pain drugs they prescribed or recommended. We can't repeat this too much: staying safe when you're taking prescription drugs is ultimately up to you. Please take responsibility for your well-being, and if you have a loved one who must take these drugs and can't take care of themselves, please monitor them carefully.

Over-the-Counter Painkillers

Because the over-the-counter painkillers such as aspirin, ibuprofen, and acetaminophen are so common and we can buy them without a prescription, we tend to think they're harmless and that we can take them every day. But they actually have side effects that can range from uncomfortable to deadly. The most commonly reported side effect is gastrointestinal bleeding caused by aspirin and ibuprofen-type drugs, also called NSAIDs (nonsteroidal anti-inflammatory drugs).

Use Caution with NSAIDs

NSAIDs work to decrease inflammation and pain by blocking the production of hormonelike chemicals called prostaglandins. Prostaglandins have other important roles in the body, including the regulation of kidney function. The kidneys maintain fluid and electrolyte (minerals such as sodium and potassium) balance, filtering out excess water and electrolytes and sending them to the bladder to be eliminated in the urine, or retaining them when supplies are low.

NSAIDs (including the new prescription COX-2 inhibitors) can cause the kidneys to hold on to more sodium, potassium, and fluid than they should. What this can translate to is weight gain, swelling of the legs and arms, increased blood pressure, and even heart failure. In heart failure, the heart can no longer pump efficiently, as fluid levels in the body rise and excess fluid passes into the lungs. In a few people who use NSAIDs, the rise in potassium levels has caused irregular and possibly dangerous heart rhythms (arrhythmias).

According to the American Gastroenterological Association, NSAID overuse is one of the leading causes of stomach problems such as bleeding ulcers, and their use leads to more than 100,000 hospitalizations and 16,000 deaths each year in the United States. You may not even know it's coming: four out of five people have no warning signs. When you combine aspirin or ibuprofen-type painkillers with alcohol, you are four times as likely to develop gastrointestinal bleeding.

A study from the University of Massachusetts looked at markers of kidney function in 4,099 patients over the age of 70 and found that the blood tests of regular NSAID users showed early warning signs of kidney failure. Another study found that regular elderly NSAID users have twice the risk of being hospitalized for congestive heart failure (CHF), where the weakened heart muscle loses its ability to pump blood efficiently. There's no evidence to show that the newer "super aspirins"—the COX-2 inhibitors—are less harmful to the heart or kidneys than the older NSAIDs.

Acetaminophen, advertised as a safe alternative to the NSAIDs that cause stomach upset, is not a harmless panacea. Although it is an over-the-counter drug, it can have serious side effects, such as liver and kidney damage. Each year many thousands of people are unknowingly harmed by liver damage caused by acetaminophen. This is especially true of children whose parents carelessly give them liquid acetaminophen at the least sign of discomfort. In 1997, more than 10,000 acetaminophen overdoses were reported. This drug is found in so many over-the-counter cough, cold, fever, and pain preparations—many of which are taken in combination—that it's easy to accidentally take too much.

While aspirin, ibuprofen, and acetaminophen can be very useful for the odd headache or sprain, they are potent drugs with serious side effects that should never be taken for more than a few days in a row or more than a few days a month.

Side Effects of Some Over-the-Counter NSAIDs

NSAID	Action	Side Effects
Acetaminophen (Tylenol)	Relieves pain, reduces fever	Liver and kidney damage, rash, dizziness; do not combine with alcohol or take for a hangover
Aspirin	Reduces fever, relieves pain, reduces inflammation	Allergic reactions, stomach upset, gastrointestinal bleeding, ulcers, ringing ears; should not be used by pregnant women or children
Ibuprofen (Advil)	Reduces fever, relieves pain, effective for menstrual pain, reduces inflammation	Skin rashes, itching, stomach upset, digestive problems
Ketoprofen (Orudis)	Reduces fever, relieves pain, reduces inflammation	Stomach upset, digestive problems, dizziness, itching, skin rashes
Naproxen (Aleve)	Relieves pain, reduces fever, reduces inflammation	Skin rashes, itching, stomach upset, digestive problems, dizziness

What Causes Arthritis Pain

One of the most common types of pain is arthritis pain. Osteoarthritis is the most common form of arthritis and affects more than 27 million Americans. It affects 80 percent of people over the age of 50. Although conventional medicine doesn't have much to offer in the way of relief from arthritis aside from painkilling drugs, we do know a lot about what causes arthritis, and alternative medicine has had great success treating it.

The major risk factors for arthritis are well known. Smoking has been proven over and over again to increase the risk of arthritis. A recent study of twins done in Great Britain compared arthritis in those who smoked and those who didn't, and found that those who smoked had a much higher risk of arthritis.

Obesity may be the single biggest cause of arthritis. According to an article in the *American Journal of Clinical Nutrition*, the single biggest risk factor for osteoarthritis in the hips and hands of people over 60 is being overweight. Reducing the symptoms of this painful disease should be a great inspiration to drop those pounds! Gentle movement and exercise are highly recommended for all types of arthritis.

Naturopathic doctors have discovered that food allergies are often a direct culprit in arthritis pain. Crippling arthritis can clear up simply by elimination of the nightshade family of plants from the diet (tomatoes, potatoes, eggplant).

NSAIDs and Melatonin Don't Mix

Melatonin is a wonderful hormone for treating jet lag, occasional insomnia in younger people, and chronic insomnia in older people. This amazing hormone is secreted in the human brain in response to darkness and is truly important to a good night's sleep.

Some drugs, including NSAIDs, interfere with the brain's production of melatonin. In fact, just one dose of normal aspirin can reduce your melatonin production by as much as 75 percent. If you're taking these drugs, take the last dose after dinner. Other drugs that can interfere with melatonin production in the brain include the benzodiazepines such as Valium and Xanax, caffeine, alcohol, cold medicines, diuretics, beta-blockers, calcium channel blockers, stimulants such as diet pills, and corticosteroids such as prednisone.

If you're in the habit of having a midnight snack, some of the foods that can boost the production of melatonin include oatmeal, corn, barley, bananas, and rice. A hot bath before bed can also raise melatonin levels.

Other common food allergens are citrus fruits, dairy products, wheat, corn, and soy.

In the long term, the NSAIDs and acetaminophen can actually aggravate arthritis because they inhibit collagen synthesis and accelerate the destruction of cartilage. Collagen is the glue that holds tissues together, and any chronic pain relief program should be building collagen, not destroying it.

Track Down the Cause of Your Headache

An estimated 30 million Americans suffer from chronic headaches, and 90 percent of those are thought to be "tension headaches." This doesn't necessarily mean these headaches are caused by emotional tension (though that is often the case); it means they are caused by tension in the muscles of the shoulders, neck, and head, and by constriction or congestion of the blood vessels in the head. Tension headaches have dozens of potential causes and often a combination of causes.

Another 20 to 30 million people suffer from occasional headaches, often called "too much" headaches. This includes "too much" sugar, alcohol, drugs, staying up late, stress, sun, or whatever else it is that gives you a pain in the head. Eyestrain, sinus infection and allergies, ear infection, and fever are also well-known culprits.

Prescription and over-the-counter drugs are probably the single most common cause of headaches in older people. In fact, so many drugs can cause headaches that if you're taking any type of medication, you can assume first that it's the culprit and go from there. If you're taking more than one medication, chances are even better they are the culprit.

Lesser-known causes of tension headaches are constipation, hypothyroidism (low thyroid), high blood pressure, hypoglycemia, caffeine withdrawal, and adrenal exhaustion. Changes in vision or eyestrain can also cause headache, so have your eyes checked if you think this could be part of your problem. Allergies or sensitivities to substances such as perfume, car exhaust, paint fumes, and cigarette smoke can also cause headaches.

Migraine headaches afflict fewer people but make up for that in the intensity of the pain they inflict. The good news is that, in most cases, the causes of migraines are fairly easy to track down once you know how.

For women, hormone imbalance is a common cause of headaches: some 6.1 percent of men compared to 14 percent of women have four or more headaches a month. Three times as many women as men suffer from migraines, and many women's migraines occur premenstrually. (Whenever women are suffering from an ailment twice as much as men, or vice versa, it's a good tip-off that the underlying cause is hormonal.) The culprit in these cases is usually a progesterone deficiency and a resulting excess of estrogen. Synthetic hormone replacement therapy (i.e., Premarin, Provera, Prempro) is probably the most common cause of headaches among menopausal women. Read the book *What Your Doctor May Not Tell You About Menopause* by John R. Lee, M.D., and Virginia Hopkins, or their book *What Your Doctor May Not Tell You About Premenopause* for details on how to balance your hormones naturally.

After stress, food allergies are probably the most common cause of both tension and migraine headaches, especially in children. There have been controlled double-blind studies showing that elimination of allergenic foods cures migraines in a majority of patients. In one study, 83 percent of the patients who eliminated allergenic foods, drugs, or inhalants cured their migraines. The foods that most often cause migraines are dairy products, wheat, citrus, chocolate, coffee, nuts, eggs, the artificial sweetener aspartame, the flavoring monosodium glutamate (MSG), and other artificial additives and preservatives.

Many people who get migraines are sensitive to foods containing large amounts of the amino acid tyramine. These include aged and fermented foods such as aged cheeses, vinegar, beer, wine, and miso; pickled foods including sauerkraut; meats such as sausages and bologna; and avocados.

If you take migraine drugs for pain relief, you should know that the side effects are significant, and some of them are so toxic that they are only prescribed for five days at the maximum.

Back Pain

Acute back pain is among the easiest types of pain to prevent. You do it by lifting properly, keeping your back and stomach muscles strong, and keeping your hamstrings (the muscles that run up the backs of the thighs) flexible. Good alignment is also important; if you aren't properly distributing the stresses on your body, back pain can be the end result. Chronic back pain is an extremely common type of pain, especially in older Americans who are simultaneously putting on weight and suffering from chronic stress. Although back-strengthening exercises have permanently eliminated back pain in many people, there is undeniably an emotional component to the majority of back pain.

If you or someone you love has back pain, read the book *Healing Back Pain* by John Sarno, M.D. (Warner Books, 1991). This book was written by an M.D. who had seen thousands of patients with back pain and had little success in treating them until he began addressing the emotional components of this type of pain. It's an illuminating and useful book, and his suggestions are easy to follow.

Carpal Tunnel Syndrome

Carpal tunnel syndrome is a repetitive motion disorder caused by repeating one movement over and over again with the wrist. Those who work intensively on computers, cashiers, and waitresses are among those who most commonly suffer from carpal tunnel syndrome.

Once you have carpal tunnel syndrome, it can be very difficult to heal, so pay attention to early symptoms and treat them right away by making sure the ergonomics of the repetitive motion are correct. Getting some expert help adjusting the setting in which you perform this motion can do a lot to nip the problem in the bud. If at all possible, take a break from doing the repetitive motion. It's easy to brush off early pain by telling yourself you don't have the time to solve the problem, but if you wait too long, you may solve the problem by being out of a job. You'll get some nutritional pointers for treating carpal tunnel at the end of the chapter.

Drugs for Pain Relief

Examples of Acetaminophen

Acetaminophen (various forms of Tylenol, Children's Feverall, Acephen, Abenol, Apacet, Aceta, Myapap, Maranox, Genapap, Panadol, Neopap, Silapap, Anacin-3, Redutemp, Arthritis Foundation Pain Reliever, Dapa, Ridenol)

Acetaminophen is one of the most overused and abused drugs on the market today because clever advertising and marketing have told us that it is harmless. However, it is potent medicine with great potential to do harm, especially in children. Please use it only when necessary.

Acetaminophen is also used in dozens of prescription and over-the-counter cold, cough, flu, arthritis, and headache remedies in combination with other drugs, including aspirin, caffeine, codeine, hydrocodone, oxycodone, propoxyphene, pseudoephedrine, and various cough and cold medications. Read labels.

What Does It Do in the Body? Relieves pain and reduces fever by increasing the dissipation of body heat. It also relieves pain from inflammation, but does not reduce inflammation.

What Is It Prescribed For? Most commonly it is prescribed for headaches, pain from earaches, teething, toothaches, or menstruation, for the common cold or flu, as well as arthritic and rheumatic conditions. It is also prescribed for people who are allergic to aspirin.

What Are the Possible Side Effects? Acetaminophen is notoriously hard on the liver and for that reason alone should be used with caution. If you have any type of liver disease or dysfunction, or if you are drinking alcohol, you should avoid this drug altogether. Other possible side effects include open sores, fever, jaundice, hypoglycemic coma, low white blood cell count, easy bruising, and excessive bleeding.

CAUTION!

Think Twice About Taking This Drug If . . .

- You have severe allergies.
- You are a chronic alcoholic, drink excessively, or even have one drink a day. The combination of this drug and alcohol can produce significant liver dysfunction.
- You have liver disease or a liver dysfunction.

What Are the Interactions with Food? In general, eating foods while taking this drug decreases or delays the drug's absorption. Eating large amounts of cruciferous vegetables such as cabbage and brussels sprouts; carbohydrates such as crackers, dates, and jellies; and foods high in pectin such as apples increases the effects of acetaminophen.

Examples of Aspirin and Similar Drugs (Salicylates)

Aspirin (Bayer, St. Joseph, Bufferin, Alka-Seltzer)
Choline salicylate (Arthropan)
Diflunisal (Dolobid)
Magnesium salicylate (Bayer Select Maximum Strength Backache)
Salicylate combinations (Tricosal)
Salicylsalicylic acid (Amigesic)
Sodium salicylate
Sodium thiosalicylate (Rexolate)

Aspirin is a near miracle drug, especially if you have a "too much" headache or a minor ache or pain. But it can easily and quickly cause serious gastrointestinal bleeding, it can increase the risk of some eye diseases, and it interacts dangerously with a long list of other drugs, so please use it with caution and don't use it regularly. Aspirin has been loudly and widely touted as a cure-all for heart disease when taken daily in small doses, because of its ability to thin the blood, but it's not worth the risk of gastrointestinal bleeding. See "Should You Be Taking an Aspirin a Day?" in Chapter 10 for more about aspirin and heart disease.

What Do They Do in the Body? Lower elevated body temperatures while also reducing inflammation and pain.

What Are They Prescribed For? Relief from mild to moderate fevers, inflammation, aches, and pains. Aspirin is also prescribed for reducing the risk of heart attacks, although the risk of gastrointestinal bleeding outweighs the benefits for heart disease, especially considering how many other natural supplements can do the same thing without the side effects. Simply taking 300 to 500 mg of magnesium and 400 IU of vitamin E daily will likely do your heart a world more good than aspirin.

Aspirin is prescribed for a variety of inflammatory conditions such as rheumatic fever, rheumatoid arthritis, and osteoarthritis.

What Are the Possible Side Effects? Aspirin is particularly hard on the digestive tract and can cause nausea, upset stomach, massive intestinal bleeding, and peptic ulcers. It can also cause temporary liver dysfunction and skin discomforts such as hives and rashes. Anemia, low white cell blood count, prolonged bleeding, and easy bruising are also possible with this drug, as well as severe allergies, mental confusion, dizziness, headaches, and depression. Ringing in the ears, or tinnitus, is a sign that you have taken too much aspirin.

CAUTION!

Think Twice About Taking These Drugs If . . .

- You are scheduled for surgery in a week or less (to avoid postoperative bleeding).
- You are allergic to any salicylates or NSAIDs.
- Your child or teenager has chicken pox or flu. A physician should check for Reye's syndrome, a rare but serious disease, before giving a child or teenager salicylates.
- You have asthma. Some asthmatics are intolerant of aspirin and can go into shock.
- You have liver damage, poor clot formation, or vitamin K deficiency.
- You have kidney disease or dysfunction. Aspirin may aggravate your condition.
- You have gastric ulcers, mild diabetes, gout, gastritis, or bleeding ulcers.
- You have hemophilia or hemorrhagic states.

- You have advanced kidney dysfunction due to magnesium retention. Do not take magnesium salicylate.

What Are the Interactions with Food? In general, eating food of any kind delays or decreases the absorption of these drugs. Taking one aspirin an hour before drinking can raise alcohol blood levels 26 percent above normal.

What Nutrients Do They Throw out of Balance or Interfere With? Aspirin and similar drugs block vitamin C from getting into the cells and lower levels of iron, folic acid, and potassium.

What Else to Take If You Take These Drugs. Increase your intake of foods high in vitamin C and potassium, and be sure to follow the Six Core Principles for Optimal Health (Chapter 9) to ensure an adequate intake of vitamins and minerals. Be sure you're getting 200 mcg daily of folic acid, especially if there's any possibility of becoming pregnant.

Examples of Ibuprofen and Similar Drugs

Diclofenac (Cataflam, Voltaren)
Etodolac (Lodine, Lodine XL)
Fenoprofen (Nalfon)
Flurbiprofen (Ansaid)
Ibuprofen (Motrin, Advil, Midol IB, Bayer Select Pain Relief, Nuprin, IBU)
Indomethacin (Indocin)
Ketoprofen (Orudis, Oruvail, Actron, Ketoprofen)
Ketorolac (Toradol)
Meclofenamate sodium (Meclomen)
Mefenamic acid (Ponstel)
Meloxicam (Mobic)
Nabumetone (Relafen)
Naproxen (Aleve, Naproxen, Naprosyn, Naprelan)

Oxaprozin (Daypro)
Piroxicam (Feldene)
Sulindac (Clinoril)
Tolmetin sodium (Tolectin)

The ibuprofen-like painkillers are another example of a type of over-the-counter medication that is a potent drug with serious side effects when taken by the wrong person for more than a few days. Ibuprofen is a potent anti-inflammatory drug, so it is often used to treat arthritis pain. As many women are well aware, the ibuprofen-type drugs can bring welcome relief from menstrual cramps. (This is probably a result of reduced prostaglandin synthesis.) What many arthritis sufferers and women with menstrual cramps don't realize is that if you have a sensitive stomach, taking ibuprofen just a few days a month can cause chronic digestive problems all month long. Ibuprofen is closely related to aspirin and can cause diarrhea, constipation, heartburn, gas, gastrointestinal bleeding, and chronic stomach pain and irritation. Taking it with food will help, but it won't eliminate the problem.

Hundreds of thousands of people get stuck on the drug treadmill when they take these types of drugs. Here's the scenario: They take ibuprofen or a similar drug for arthritis pain nearly every day and develop chronic stomach irritation. So their physician recommends Tagamet, which blocks the production of stomach acid. As a result of lower stomach acid, nutrients aren't being properly broken down or absorbed, and the process of low-level malnutrition begins. The irritated digestive tract precipitates food allergies, which aggravate the arthritis, prompting ever-higher doses of pain medication and Tagamet. Pretty soon sleeping pills are prescribed to help get through the night, and the person is groggy during the day. Just a few months of this type of scenario is enough to land an independent elderly person in a nursing home. Please don't underestimate the potency of these drugs.

What Do They Do in the Body? Relieve pain from inflammation and lower elevated body temperatures.

What Are They Prescribed For? Rheumatoid arthritis, osteoarthritis, mild to moderate pain, tendonitis, bursitis, acute gout, fever, sunburn, migraine headaches, menstrual cramps and discomforts, and acne.

What Are the Possible Side Effects? The most common and one of the most dangerous side effects of the ibuprofen-like drugs is damage to the digestive system. They can cause nausea, vomiting, diarrhea, constipation, cramps, and gas, as well as serious bleeding and ulcers, particularly if you are elderly.

These drugs are hard on both the liver and kidneys. They can cause hepatitis, jaundice, and elevated liver enzymes, as well as urinary tract infections, urinary frequency, and a wide variety of kidney problems.

Other side effects include dizziness, headache, drowsiness, fatigue, and nervousness. They can aggravate a wide range of behavioral problems including depression and psychosis. They can also cause muscle weakness or cramps, numbness, changes in blood pressure, vision disturbances and damage, hearing disturbances, shortness of breath, rashes, blood sugar changes, weight gain or loss, mineral imbalances, menstrual problems, impotence and breast enlargement in men, and a wide range of blood disorders, including anemia. Like aspirin, these drugs can prolong bleeding time by as much as three or four minutes.

Piroxicam (Feldene) appears to be particularly likely to cause severe gastrointestinal problems, and the European equivalent of the Food and Drug Administration (FDA) has recommended that it not be a drug of first choice for most types of pain.

CAUTION!

Think Twice About Taking These Drugs If . . .

- You are elderly. Serious side effects are more likely to happen to you if you are over the age of 65.
- You have had an allergic reaction to these or to other similar drugs such as aspirin.
- You have kidney or liver disease or dysfunction.
- You have an ulcer, inflammation, or a history of bleeding in your intestinal tract or rectum.
- You have a history of anemia, excessive bleeding, or poor clotting.
- You are scheduled for surgery in a week or less.
- You have a heart condition or pancreatitis.
- You have eye problems.
- You have an existing controlled infection. These drugs can mask the symptoms of infection.
- You are sensitive to sunlight.

What Are the Interactions with Food? Generally, anytime you eat food and take these types of drugs, the food will delay or decrease the absorption of the drug. Always take these drugs with food to protect your stomach.

What Nutrients Do They Throw out of Balance? Iron levels may be reduced because of blood loss due to gastrointestinal bleeding.

What Else to Take If You Take These Drugs. If you are a premenopausal woman and taking these drugs for more than a few days (which is not recommended), increase your intake of iron.

Examples of COX-2 Inhibitors

Celecoxib (Celebrex)

Both of the COX-2 inhibitors rofecoxib (Vioxx) and valdecoxib (Bextra) were pulled off the market due to safety concerns of an increased risk of cardiovascular events (including heart attack and stroke), but not before Vioxx raked in $2.5 billion in 2003 and was linked to more than 27,000 heart attacks or sudden cardiac deaths in less than four years in the United States alone.

The FDA put a black-box warning on Celebrex that reads as follows:

Celebrex is a NSAID. It may cause an increased risk of serious and sometimes fatal heart and blood vessel problems (e.g., heart attack, stroke). The risk may be greater if you already have heart problems or if you take Celebrex for a long time. Do not use Celebrex right before or after bypass heart surgery.

Celebrex may cause an increased risk of serious and sometimes fatal stomach ulcers and bleeding. Elderly patients may be at greater risk. This may occur without warning signs.

What Do They Do in the Body? They inhibit the production of COX-2 enzymes, which are involved in the production of pain and inflammation.

What Are They Prescribed For? Pain from osteoarthritis and rheumatoid arthritis, dysmenorrhea, and dental procedures or surgery.

What Are the Possible Side Effects? Increased risk of heart attack and stroke, the symptoms of which can include chest pain, weakness, shortness of breath, slurred speech, and problems with vision or balance. In addition to heart attacks and strokes, this drug can cause gastrointestinal bleeding; dizziness; headache; fluid retention (edema); increased likelihood of upper respiratory infection, indigestion, diarrhea, vomiting, abdominal pain, and flatulence; problematic changes in kidney and liver function tests; insomnia; menstrual and female gynecological problems; dermatitis; throat inflammation; runny nose; sinusitis; and accidental injury.

CAUTION!

Think Twice About Taking These Drugs If . . .

- You have kidney or liver disease. They should never be prescribed to people with severe kidney or liver disease.
- You have a history of peptic ulcer disease, especially if you are elderly, alcoholic, a smoker, or use anticoagulant drugs or steroid drugs.
- You are at high risk of heart attack or stroke, or have had a heart attack or stroke.
- You have aspirin-sensitive asthma.
- You are pregnant. These drugs have been shown to cause premature closure of a vital blood vessel in growing fetuses, and this can lead to very dangerous lung problems once the baby is born.

Examples of Nonnarcotic Painkiller Combinations

Nonnarcotic analgesic combinations (Vanquish, Pamprin, Extra Strength Excedrin, Midol, Cope, Anacin, Saleto, Gelpirin, Supac,

Extra Strength Tylenol Headache Plus, Equagesic, Gensan)

Nonnarcotic analgesics with barbiturates (Fiorinal, Esgic, Fioricet, Repan, Amaphen, Butace, Endolor, Femcet, Two-Dyne, Bancap, Triaprin, Lanorinal)

These drugs generally combine acetaminophen or aspirin with a barbiturate, meprobamate, or antihistamine for sedative effects, caffeine to help constrict blood vessels and relieve headaches, belladonna alkaloids to reduce muscle spasms, and pamabrom as a diuretic. They are sold both as prescription and as over-the-counter drugs.

What Do They Do in the Body? These drugs are used as painkillers with specific added effects such as sedation or muscle relaxation.

What Are They Prescribed For? They are prescribed for a wide variety of pain conditions including arthritis, headaches, and muscle pain.

What Are the Possible Side Effects? The side effects can be severe because they are drug combinations and thus more dangerous. Many of these drugs are available without a prescription. If you are going to take them, read the directions!

Examples of Migraine Drugs (Serotonin Receptor Agonists)

Almotriptan malate (Axert)
Eletriptan (Replax)
Frovatriptan succinate (Frova)
Naratriptan (Amerge)
Rizatriptan benzoate (Maxalt)
Sumatriptan succinate (Imitrex)
Topiramate (Topamax)
Zolmitriptan (Zomig)

Other migraine drugs not covered here because they are so rarely used include methy-

sergide maleate (Sansert), ergotamine drugs (Ergomar, Migergot, Cafergot), dihydroergotamine mesylate (D.H.E.45), and the combination drugs Cafatine PB, Cafetrate, Catergot, Ercaf, Midrin, and Wigraine.

In 2007 the FDA pulled 15 ergotamine drugs off the market because they had not been officially approved. Considering the length of time ergotamine drugs have been on the market, and considering that five ergotamine drugs were left alone, this was likely more a political move than an attempt to protect the public interest.

Many other types of pain drugs are used alone or in combination to treat migraines, including acetaminophen, naproxen, SSRI antidepressants, seizure drugs, narcotics, caffeine, and antinausea drugs. None of these combinations are well studied, thus all are risky. The combination of SSRI antidepressants and the "triptan" migraine drugs is proving to be dangerous. Do not combine them without asking your doctor and pharmacist to thoroughly research the possible side effects, as well as reports from the FDA.

What Do They Do in the Body? Serotonin receptor agonists relieve pain from migraine headaches by constricting the blood vessels in the brain.

What Are They Prescribed For? Relieving pain from migraine headaches.

What Are the Possible Side Effects? These drugs have a powerful constricting effect on the heart and blood vessels and as a result have caused fatal heart spasms and possibly fatal strokes. Palpitations, increased blood pressure, heartbeat irregularities, fainting, slow heartbeat, varicose veins, heart murmur, and low blood pressure have been reported. Migraine headaches are unbearable, but they aren't worth dying over. If you have any type of heart disease or are at risk for heart disease or stroke, do not take these drugs. Your physician should fully evaluate your heart disease risk before prescribing these drugs, and the first dose should be given in the physician's office.

Taken regularly, serotonin agonists can cause damage to the eyes.

They often cause a tingling sensation that is not harmful. They can also cause dizziness, a sensation of tightness or heaviness, numbness, coldness or warmth, drowsiness, and a stiff neck.

Other possible side effects include vertigo, aggression, hostility, agitation, hallucinations, panic, hyperactivity, tremors, disorders of thought, sleep disorders, anxiety, depressive disorders, detachment, confusion, sedation, coordination disorders, nerve disorders, suicidal tendencies, diarrhea, unusual thirst, asthma, blood sugar imbalances, weight gain or loss, intestinal bleeding, peptic ulcer, breast tenderness, abortion, speech or voice disturbance, allergy to sunlight, or shock. Dozens of other side effects affecting virtually every body system have been reported.

• **Sumatriptan.** May also cause flushing, nasal discomfort, eye irritation, vision disturbances, weakness, or dry mouth.

• **Naratriptan.** May also cause fatigue; pain or pressure in the neck, throat, or jaw; or nausea.

• **Rizatriptan.** May cause dizziness; sleepiness; headache; pain or pressure in the chest, neck, throat, or jaw; dry mouth; or nausea.

• **Zolmitriptan.** May cause heart palpitations; dizziness; sleepiness; chest, neck, throat, or jaw pressure; weakness; digestive problems (in 11 to 16 percent of users); muscle pain; and sweating.

CAUTION!

Think Twice About Taking These Drugs If . . .

- You have heart disease or have had a stroke, or are at risk for heart disease or stroke.
- Your migraine headache feels different than usual.
- You tend to have hypersensitivity or severe allergic reactions.
- You have kidney or liver disease.
- You have a history of seizures.
- You have eye problems, especially glaucoma.

Central Analgesics

Tramadol (Ultram)

This drug isn't technically classified as an opiate or narcotic, but it has an abuse and addiction profile similar to the opiates. Use with great caution. The only central analgesic commonly used these days is tramadol (Ultram), which will be covered here.

What Does It Do in the Body? It blocks the perception of pain and produces a state of euphoria.

What Is It Prescribed For? Pain management.

What Are the Possible Side Effects? Addiction, seizures, liver and kidney damage, respiratory depression, increased intracranial pressure, dizziness and vertigo, nausea, constipation, headache, sleepiness, vomiting, itching, nervousness and anxiety, weakness, sweating, heartburn, dry mouth, diarrhea, fainting, hypotension (low blood pressure), irregular heartbeat, loss of appetite, gas, stomach pain, rash, vision disturbances, urinary tract disturbances, and menopausal symptoms.

CAUTION!

Think Twice About Taking These Drugs If . . .

You have a history of substance abuse, or kidney or liver damage. In general, please try to avoid this drug if at all possible.

Examples of Narcotic Painkillers

Alfentanil (Alfenta)
Codeine
Combinations (Propacet, Roxicet)
Fentanyl (Sublimaze, Duragesic-25)
Hydrocodone (Lortab, Hydrogesic, Vicodin)
Hydromorphone (Dilaudid)
Levomethadyl (Orlaam)
Levorphanol tartrate (Levo-Dromoran)
Meperidine (Demerol)
Methadone (Dolophine)
Morphine sulphate (Astramorph, Duramorph,
*   MSIR, MS Contin, Roxanol)*
Opium (Pantopon, Opium Tincture, Paregoric)
Oxycodone (Roxicodone)
Oxymorphone (Numorphan)
Propoxyphene (Darvon, Dolene, Darvocet)
Remifentanil (Ultiva)
Sufentanil (Sufenta)

These are addictive, mind-altering drugs that are among the top-selling drugs in the United States. It's likely that tens of thousands of people are addicted to these drugs. The fact that these drugs are such bestsellers tells us that this is an area where both the pharmaceutical industry and the conventional medical industry (physicians, hospitals, insurance companies, HMOs) are profiting from the addictive nature of these drugs. Hydrocodone and codeine are often found in combination painkillers, of which there are dozens, so if it's not on this list, that doesn't mean it's not dangerous and addictive. Don't let your physician become your drug pusher!

Please don't avoid these drugs if you really need them for pain. Nobody should suffer unnecessarily. If you do need to take them for more than a few days, be aware that you will go through a withdrawal reaction.

Please don't take these drugs unless absolutely necessary. If you have a history of drug or alcohol abuse, go off them gradually and under the close supervision of a health care professional.

What Do They Do in the Body? These drugs relieve pain and induce a state of euphoria.

What Are They Prescribed For? The relief of moderate to severe pain, as medication prior to and during surgery, and as cough suppressants.

What Are the Possible Side Effects? The most important side effect of these drugs is that they are addictive. For that reason alone, don't take them unless you must! These drugs alter your perception of pain and reality. Some of their side effects are euphoria, drowsiness, apathy, and mental confusion. They also reduce your respiratory rate and heart rate, which can result in fainting, heart attack, shock, and seizures.

Because they slow down your digestive system, constipation and urine retention can also happen with these drugs, as well as nausea, vomiting, and abdominal pain. These drugs also cause allergic reactions such as skin rashes, water retention, and hypertension. Frequently these drugs cause light-headedness, dizziness, sedation, face flushing, and sweating. Other side effects include palpitations, allergic reactions, and jaundice.

The fentanyl skin patches (Duragesic) are particularly dangerous. The FDA issued a long black-box warning for them, which reads in part:

Duragesic contains a high concentration of a potent Schedule II opioid agonist, fentanyl. Schedule II opioid substances which include fentanyl, hydromorphone, methadone, morphine, oxycodone, and oxymorphone have the highest potential for abuse and associated risk of fatal overdose due to respiratory depression. Fentanyl can be abused and is subject to criminal diversion. The high content of fentanyl in the patches (Duragesic) may be a particular target for abuse and diversion.

Duragesic is indicated for management of persistent, moderate to severe chronic pain that:

- requires continuous, around-the-clock opioid administration for an extended period of time.
- cannot be managed by other means such as nonsteroidal analgesics, opioid combination products, or immediate-release opioids.

It's important to avoid adding heat to a fentanyl patch, because that may cause the patch to release dangerous levels of the drug into the bloodstream. Examples of adding heat would be a heating pad, hot tub, hot shower, heavy exercise, and fever. Do not cut the fentanyl patch, as this could also cause it to release dangerous levels of medication.

CAUTION!

Think Twice About Taking These Drugs If . . .

- You are suicidal or prone to addiction. Drug abuse can and does happen with prolonged use of these drugs. People who are prescribed narcotics for medical purposes over a period of one or two weeks usually

do not develop dependence. But prolonged use of narcotics can lead to psychological and physical dependence and then uncomfortable and difficult withdrawal.
- You are an alcoholic, have bronchial asthma or trouble breathing, have a head injury or brain tumor, have chronic obstructive heart disease, or have liver or kidney dysfunction.
- You are on monoamine oxidase inhibitors (MAOIs) or have been within 14 days. Do not take meperidine.
- You have an acute abdominal condition. These drugs can obscure an accurate diagnosis.
- You have lung or respiratory disease. Be careful—cough reflex is suppressed with these drugs.

The Signs of Withdrawal from Narcotic Drugs

The earliest signs include yawning, sweating, tearing eyes, and runny nose. Later the symptoms can include dilated eyes, flushing, heart palpitations, twitching, shaking, restlessness, irritability, anxiety, and loss of appetite. Signs of severe withdrawal can include muscle spasms, fever, nausea, diarrhea, vomiting, severe backache, abdominal and leg pains and cramping, hot and cold flashes, inability to sleep, repetitive sneezing, and changes in heart rate and breathing rate.

What Are the Interactions with Food? High-fat foods may increase the effects of morphine. Foods that acidify the urine cause a decrease of potency. Foods that alkalinize the urine decrease the ability of the body to excrete morphine.

Examples of Narcotic Agonist-Antagonist Painkillers

Buprenorphine (Buprenex)
Butorphanol (Stadol)
Dezocine (Dalgan)
Nalbuphine (Nubain, Nuban)
Pentazocine (Talwin, Talacen)

What Do They Do in the Body? Relieve pain and induce euphoric mood changes.

What Are They Prescribed For? Relieving pain, particularly for postoperative patients.

What Are the Possible Side Effects? These drugs are potent pain-relieving substances that have a lower abuse potential than pure narcotics, but they can still be addictive—and usually are!

These drugs can cause sweating, chills, flushing, water retention, heart or pulse irregularity, nausea, vomiting, abdominal pain, muscular pain, slowed breathing, rashes, slurred speech, blurred vision, hallucinations, dizziness, urinary frequency, heart attacks, seizures, and skin and muscle damage.

CAUTION!

Think Twice About Taking These Drugs If . . .

- You have an allergic reaction to these drugs.
- You have a drug dependence problem.
- You have liver or kidney dysfunction or disease.
- You have a head injury.
- You have heart disease.
- You must drive or operate machinery (that includes cars).
- You have severe allergic reactions (particularly to sulfur).
- You have acute asthma or other significant respiratory problems.

Drugs for Arthritis Pain

There is an entire class of drugs prescribed specifically for arthritis pain. None of them are well studied, none are widely used, and all are uniquely dangerous. We don't recommend them. Conventional medicine is notoriously unsuccessful at treating arthritis safely and effectively, but there are many alternative approaches that provide great relief and even healing. Please read the later section on arthritis for details.

Natural Remedies for Pain

Most of the pain we suffer we can do something about. We have a pretty good grasp of what causes the pain of headaches, and in alternative medicine we have many effective ways to treat arthritis. Most back pain can be prevented and healed using a combination of physical and emotional healing, and with lifestyle changes alone, the pain of osteoporosis can often be prevented. This means that millions of people can avoid the use of painkilling drugs and their side effects.

If you have an acute pain such as a muscle sprain, you may need to warm up before you exercise in the future. If you have chronic pain such as back pain, you may need to do exercises to strengthen your back muscles. Exercise is the single best cure for chronic back pain and for arthritis. If you have chronic pain such as from arthritis, try an elimination diet to find out whether a food sensitivity is causing inflammation in your joints. Or it could be a side effect of a prescription drug. The anticholinergic drugs can cause muscle stiffness and neck pain, for example. Headache pain is often caused by stress, allergies, or sensitivities to food or chemicals.

The Best Natural Remedies for Occasional Pain Relief

There are many ways to alleviate chronic pain before reaching for pain drugs. Here are a few favorite natural pain relievers. All of the supplements can be found at your health food store.

Hot and Cold Packs. Ice is one of the best and simplest remedies for pain caused by inflammation. The cold very effectively reduces the inflammation. Use a cold pack for 20 minutes every few hours for sprains and strains. For a muscle sprain or strain that's been around for a few days or swelling caused by a bruise, first use a 20-minute cold pack, then a 20-minute hot pack. The cold will reduce the inflammation, and the heat will encourage blood flow into the area and help break up and remove damaged tissue so that healing can take place.

One of the simplest, cheapest, and most effective ways to relieve chronic pain (with the exception of headaches) is with what is known as moist heat. You can apply moist heat by taking a long, hot shower and aiming the showerhead at the area that hurts. You can take a long, hot bath with relaxing herbal oils, or you can use a hot pack or a hot water bottle. If you have access to a Jacuzzi, you can aim the jets of water at the places that are painful.

Digestive Enzymes. If you have pain from a muscle injury or arthritis, try digestive enzymes. Clinical studies show that enzymes help reduce inflammation caused by arthritis and injuries to joints and connective tissues such as muscle sprains, and can even relieve back pain. Enzymes tend to speed up the rate at which many bodily processes work, and injuries are no exception. Enzymes work at the site of an injury to remove damaged tissue, which reduces swelling, and to help the body repair itself. Bromelain, which comes from pineapples, is an enzyme that has anti-inflammatory properties. One of the best combinations is quercetin, an antioxidant, and bromelain.

DL-Phenylalanine (DLPA). This is a combination of L-phenylalanine, an essential amino acid, and D-phenylalanine, a nonnutrient amino acid that helps promote the production of endorphins, natural painkillers made in the brain. DLPA can be very effective in the relief of chronic pain such as arthritis and back pain. While in most studies there have been no side effects at all from DLPA, it has raised blood pressure in a few people. Although this is unlikely to happen, please monitor your blood pressure if it is high and you take DLPA. Don't use DLPA in combination with antidepressant drugs or if you have phenylketonuria (PKU).

Vitamins and Minerals. There are vitamins and minerals that can play a part in reducing inflammation. These include vitamin C, vitamin E, and the B-complex vitamins. Taking a magnesium-calcium supplement can help relieve the pain of muscle spasms and often relieves chronic headaches. A copper deficiency can cause inflammation in the joints, as well as fragile skin and connective tissue. The bioflavonoids, such as grapeseed extract and quercetin, can help reduce inflammation reactions.

Herbs for Pain. White willow bark (*salix* spp.) was used as a pain reliever long before a chemist at the Bayer company in Germany synthesized acetylsalicylic acid, or aspirin, from one of its active ingredients in 1897. Aspirin is a synthetic drug (not found in nature), but various teas, decoctions, tinctures, and poultices of trees of the *salix* species, most commonly known as willow and poplar, have been used to relieve pain for many centuries. White willow bark doesn't cause gastric bleeding or ringing in the ears as aspirin does and can be a very effective pain reliever, especially for headaches and arthritis pain. Traditionally, a tea of the inner bark was used (a small handful of bark to a cup of hot water) to treat headaches. A bath, wash, or poultice was used to treat aches and pains in the joints. You can find white willow bark in capsule or tincture form at your health food store.

Nearly 2,000 years ago, the Roman doctor Dioscorides, one of the first to write a medical textbook, recommended the herb feverfew (*Chrysanthemum parthenium*) for headaches. Feverfew is still the most effective treatment known for migraines. It is the only medicine that will help migraine headaches without side effects. This member of the daisy family is also called bachelor's buttons. Feverfew has undergone much testing and research as a migraine remedy, as pharmaceutical companies are trying to find the active ingredient so they can isolate it and synthesize it. However, the lowly feverfew is not revealing its healing secrets, and the freeze-dried herb in capsules, or a tincture of the fresh leaves, is still the best way to take the plant. Feverfew has also been used successfully to treat arthritis.

Treating Chronic Pain

As scientists research pain, they're finding that a wide variety of techniques that induce relaxation and increase body awareness can be used very effectively to beat the demon of chronic pain. In fact, an expert panel at the National Institutes of Health concluded that there is enough positive research data to now integrate behavioral and relaxation therapies into standard treatment of chronic pain and insomnia. This does not mean it's "all in your head," which implies that somehow it's your fault you're in pain. It means there are techniques you can use to induce deep relaxation and become more aware of stress points in your body and how to relax them.

People in chronic pain tend to tense specific areas of muscle, such as the neck and shoulder areas, creating other areas of pain and skeletal imbalances. This creates a vicious cycle, with a new area of pain leading to increased tension, which creates yet more pain. Pretty soon, pain seems to exist everywhere in the body and the person in pain doesn't want to move at all—the worst thing you can do for most pain!

Emotional factors such as tension, anxiety, depression, loneliness, anger, an inability to communicate, a sense of being a victim, and a sense of being estranged from the world can all contribute to more severe pain by blocking the body's production of natural painkillers called endorphins. People who strive to become more aware of their pain—exactly where it is located, what causes it, what makes it worse, and what makes it better, for example, rather than blocking it with analgesics and narcotics—tend to have a great sense of empowerment and less severe pain. The first tendency for most of us when we're in pain is to try to block it, usually with medication. It's ironic that the reverse approach of becoming more aware and paying more attention can be the key to coping effectively with chronic pain.

Two of the most powerful techniques for both increasing body awareness and inducing relaxation are meditation and the Asian movement disciplines such as yoga, qi gong, and tai chi.

Meditate Your Pain Away. Meditation can bring a greater awareness of what we're doing with our consciousness in any given moment. It may begin simply by paying attention to breathing and progress to a "detached observing" of what is happening with the mind and emotions.

As people learn to separate their physical sensations from their thoughts, pain will often begin to dissipate some. A favorite basic meditation that can be used anytime by anyone for relieving stress or tension is this: Breathe deeply and slowly in through the nose to the slow count of five, hold the breath for the slow count of five, and breathe out to the slow count of five. Repeat at least three times. A few rounds of this elegantly simple technique and you'll be amazed at how relaxed you can feel.

Another simple meditation technique is to repeat one word silently over and over. Many meditation disciplines use the word *om*. You can use any word or phrase you want as long as it has a positive association.

A form of meditation especially designed to induce relaxation is called visualization or guided imagery. In these techniques, you sit or lie down, close your eyes, and take three long, deep breaths. Then you visualize the most relaxing place or situation you can think of and make it your "vacation spot" that you visit whenever you feel tense. Many people like to envision themselves on a tropical beach. As you visualize, engage all of your senses: the sky is deep blue, the water turquoise; you sift the warm, white sand between your fingers and feel the hot sun; you hear the waves breaking and the palm trees rustling; and you smell the salt water and sweet aromas of tropical flowers.

A technique you can use to help you become more aware of your body is to lie on your back in a comfortable place with your eyes closed, perhaps with some soothing music on. Starting at your toes, slowly and in turn, become aware of every part of your body, and as you become aware of it, gently tense the muscles around it for 5 to 15 seconds (keep breathing) and then relax them. For example, feel each toe on your right foot by wiggling it, and then curl all five of them forward. Do the same with your foot and ankle, move to your other foot, and then move up to your calves, your knees, and your thighs, tensing and relaxing each area. By the time you finish with your face, you'll be deeply relaxed.

Exercise Your Pain Away. It is extremely important to exercise in whatever way you can when you're suffering from chronic pain. If you do exercises such as yoga or qi gong, sometimes called "enlightened exercise," you will stretch, tone, and strengthen your muscles; limber up your joints; improve your circulation, coordination, and balance; get your lymph system flowing; bring greater alignment to your musculoskeletal system; improve your posture; increase relaxation; and become more aware of your body. People who do these practices regularly claim that they also speed healing, boost the immune system, improve digestion, increase energy, and improve mood. Studies show they can also reduce blood pressure. If your arthritis pain is severe, work with a physical therapist to create an exercise program or try swimming or water exercise to keep pressure off of tender joints while moving through full ranges of motion.

Much pain, particularly back pain, results from poor posture and improper use of the spine (i.e., lifting something without bending your knees). Greater body awareness will alert you when you're doing something that creates pain and can teach you to move away from habitual patterns of movement and into new, more healing patterns. With any exercise, especially yoga, remember to ease off on whatever you're doing if you experience any pain. Contrary to the "no pain, no gain" philosophy, adopt a new philosophy of "there's no gain in pain." Stretching is an essential part of all the forms of enlightened exercise. You can stretch gently anytime you're starting to feel pain or tension.

Although much pain is caused by the improper use of the muscles and spine, it is also caused by muscles that aren't used and aren't toned. For almost all lower-back pain caused by strained muscles, there are specific exercises you can do that will, in effect, cure the problem. You can get these exercises from almost any physician or physical therapist. Yoga instructors usually have their own set of back exercises, which are equally effective.

Treating Chronic Pain with Herbs. Two of the biggest problems in chronic pain are stress and tension: physical, emotional, and mental. When you hurt all the time, you tend to tense muscles all over your body, creating additional areas of pain. People who suffer from chronic pain often become anxious and fearful, and feel helpless, which is understandable. Waking up and going to bed with pain as a constant companion is a traumatic experience.

For that reason you can try the herb kava with the goal of relieving anxiety and tension, and secondarily to relieve pain. Sometimes a little herbal help in relaxation can help start you on the path to healing.

• **Kava (*Piper methysticum*).** This member of the pepper family grows as a bush in the South Pacific. Kava is a sedative and muscle relaxant. The South Pacific islanders, who use it in much the same way many people in North America use alcohol, describe kava as a calming drink that brings on a feeling of contentment and well-being and encourages socializing.

Kava is also a pain reliever and can often be used in place of the NSAIDs. In a European study, people with anxiety symptoms given a 70 percent kavalactone extract in the amount of 100 mg three times a day were found after four weeks to have a significant reduction in anxiety symptoms such as feelings of nervousness, heart palpitations, chest pains, headaches, dizziness, and indigestion, all with no side effects noted.

For over 100 years, scientists have been trying to figure out exactly what it is in kava that gives it sedative and antidepressant properties. Although they have isolated chemical compounds named kavalactones, which act as sedatives and antidepressants when given alone, an extract of the whole root has always worked better. Kava also has a different action on the brain from any of our other antidepressants or sedatives, possibly working in the limbic brain, the seat of our emotions. Used occasionally in medicinal doses, kava has no known side effects. In very high doses, it can cause sleepiness, and high doses over a long period of time can cause skin irritation and liver damage.

The FDA recently issued a press release cautioning against the use of kava because of "the potential risk of severe liver injury." Virtually all prescription drugs and many over-the-counter drugs have the potential to harm the liver when taken long term in large doses. Acetaminophen (Tylenol) is a perfect example of a widely used over-the-counter drug that quickly becomes toxic to the liver when combined with other drugs or alcohol.

The kavalactones, and lactones in general, are toxic to the liver. However, it turns out that kava also naturally contains glutathione, a substance that protects the liver and is essential to its detoxification processes. The South Pacific islanders, who have used kava for centuries without problems, use the whole root and thus retain the benefit of the glutathione. In Western countries, kava is most commonly sold as a liquid extract of the root: some of the active ingredients are pulled out in a laboratory using alcohol or acetone, leaving concentrated lactones and no glutathione. Some researchers claim that low-alcohol or acetone extracts are safer.

Alternative Medicine Treatments That Work for Chronic Pain

There are dozens of safe, effective alternative medicine techniques for healing pain that don't involve surgery or medication. Here are some that have been proven over time to work for some people:

Acupressure
Acupuncture
Alexander Technique
Biofeedback
Chiropractic
Feldenkrais
Hydrotherapy
Hypnosis
Massage
NLP (neuro-linguistic programming)
Prolotherapy (also known as sclerotherapy or reconstructive therapy)
Rolfing
TENS (transcutaneous electrical nerve stimulation)

One of the truisms of herbal medicine is that the whole plant usually works better than an extract. Kava is a perfect example of this. Kava is useful when used in moderation but can be harmful when overdone or combined with other drugs. It's not a substance to use daily for an extended period of time. It would also be wise to avoid combining kava with alcohol and to avoid the highly concentrated doses offered by some manufacturers.

• **St. John's wort** (*Hypericum perforatum*). This medicinal plant with a beautiful yellow flower has been used by the Chinese, the Greeks, the Europeans, and the American Indians for centuries to treat heart disease, anxiety, insomnia, and depression. In a study of 105 patients who had symptoms of mild to moderate depression, half the patients took 300 mg of St. John's wort extract three times a day for four weeks, and the other half took a placebo. Some 67 percent of the group taking the St. John's wort had positive results, compared to only 28 percent of the placebo group. Another study comparing St. John's wort to two standard antidepressants, amitriptyline (Elavil) and imipramine (Tofranil), showed that St. John's wort had a better positive result. This amazing herb has also been used in studies alongside the antidepressant SSRIs, such as Prozac, and found to be as effective. And you guessed it, those taking the prescription antidepressants suffered from drowsiness, constipation, and dry mouth, while those taking St. John's wort reported no side effects.

Healing Headache Pain Naturally

Headaches are a source of pain that bothers all of us at some time or another, but they can almost always be avoided with a bit of alertness to what might bring them on. Of course, nobody outside of yourself can help you solve the problem of "too much" headaches, as in too much alcohol, sugar, staying up late, TV watching, or Internet use.

How you cure your chronic headaches is a matter of uncovering the cause, and that will take some sleuthing. Once you have a few leads, you can track down the perpetrator and say good-bye to pain. It will be up to you to put together your own personal headache profile, but once you do, avoiding headaches will be a matter of commonsense solutions.

Headaches are an extremely personal matter, in the sense that the cause tends to be a little bit different for everyone. Harry cured his headaches by eliminating certain foods from his diet. Sarah started using natural progesterone cream and tak-

Your Brain Has a Mind of Its Own

The human brain may be the most miraculous creation on earth, aside from life itself. Its inner workings are so complex and instantaneous that it puts even the most sophisticated computer to shame. And computers don't have our rich interplay of thoughts, emotions, creativity, intuitions, and instincts.

An entire field of scientific study, known as psychoneuroimmunology, is devoted just to studying the connection between our emotions, our brains, and our bodies. For example, did you know that serotonin, one of the brain's neurotransmitters that affects mood, is also found abundantly in the small intestine? Have you ever gotten bad news or been about to perform in front of an audience and clutched your stomach because it was suddenly and violently queasy? That's right, your brain lives in your stomach, as well as in your head. In fact, it lives all over the body. The gray matter in your head is just the main terminal.

In his book *Healing Back Pain* (Warner Books, 1991), John Sarno, M.D., an expert who has spent more than 20 years in his field, explains how feelings such as anger, fear, and anxiety that we don't want to be aware of can be the cause of pain almost anywhere in the body. He says we create pain in the body to distract us from these unwelcome feelings. Try reading Sarno's book if your headaches don't respond to the other treatments mentioned here. Everything he says about back pain can also apply to headaches.

Stress factors such as overwork, lack of sleep, anxiety, and depression can all cause or contribute to headaches. Stress causes us to tense muscles we don't even know we have, which deprives them of oxygen and causes pain. Any type of tension that centers in the shoulders, neck, face, or head can affect muscles and blood vessels, causing pain. It is estimated that 50 percent of tension headaches are caused by stress.

---

ing magnesium, and her migraines disappeared. Francine banished her tension headaches by swimming at her local YMCA three or four times a week and taking a yoga class, where she learned some breathing exercises for muscle relaxation.

For most people, headaches are caused by a sequence or combination of triggers. It might be a combination of emotional stress and chocolate; too much time in front of the computer combined with low blood sugar; or a glass of red wine with Chinese food containing MSG. Ultimately, you will be your own best headache detective.

Preventing and Treating Headaches. There are some very simple, basic steps you can take both to prevent and treat headaches. Following the Six Core Principles for Optimal Health is your best bet for a headache-free lifestyle.

• **Exercise.** This is such a simple solution to headaches that it's often overlooked. Moving your body improves circulation and increases oxygen in the blood, improves hormone balance, reduces stress and is relaxing, reduces anxiety and depression, and stimulates our brain's natural mood enhancers and painkillers called endorphins.

• **Magnesium.** If there had to be one magic bullet for both migraine and tension headaches, it would be the mineral magnesium. It's not clear whether magnesium banishes migraines by relieving muscle spasms or changing brain chemistry, but there have been many, many successes curing migraines with this simple solution. If you get migraine headaches, include magnesium in your daily vitamin regimen. You can take 400 mg twice daily (one with breakfast and one before bed), and if you feel a migraine coming on, take 400 mg immediately. In one study done in Germany, 81 migraine sufferers were given 600 mg of magnesium daily or a placebo. After two to three months, those taking the magnesium had 42 percent fewer migraines, while those in the placebo group had only 16 percent fewer migraines.

• **Feverfew.** The herb feverfew is another safe, natural, and effective remedy for both tension and migraine headaches. If you tend to get migraines, it's best to take feverfew daily as a preventive until you've found the underlying cause. You can use it in capsule or tincture form, but since it tastes absolutely terrible, you might want to stick with the capsules! Follow the instructions on the container.

• **Coffee.** If you feel a headache coming on, a cup or two of coffee can constrict your blood vessels enough to prevent it. On the other hand, too much coffee can cause a headache, as can coffee withdrawal. Coffee is a stimulating drug and should be treated as such.

• **Relaxation.** Almost anything that helps you relax will help prevent and treat headaches. That includes massage, breathing exercises, visualization techniques, and meditation. Soothing herbal teas such as chamomile, skullcap, and passionflower can be helpful, and when necessary, you can use the more powerful antianxiety and antidepressant herbs St. John's wort or kava.

Treating Arthritis Pain Naturally

Sometimes you can take care of arthritis naturally, covering all your bases with nutrition and exercise, and still get a painful flare-up that leaves permanent damage to joints. Mary is a good example. A couple of years ago, Mary's pain and stiffness had been increasing in her hands and her hips, and the aspirin she had been taking to keep it under control was causing stomach pain. She started taking glucosamine and EFAs (essential fatty acids) and started easing off the aspirin gradually, over a period of two weeks. She also tried an elimination diet. Within a few months her arthritis was virtually gone.

But a few months after that, Mary experienced a painful flare-up of her arthritis that left her with a permanent knob on the knuckle of one of her hands. After closely examining her lifestyle changes during the flare-up, Mary realized that during the summer months she had been eating fresh tomatoes at least once a day, sometimes twice. Tomatoes belong to the nightshade family (along with potatoes, eggplant, bell peppers, hot peppers, and tobacco) and are renowned for aggravating arthritis in some people. As soon as Mary stopped eating the tomatoes, her arthritis symptoms eased up entirely.

To avoid permanent damage caused by a severe flare-up of arthritis, it's important to treat the symptoms immediately, as well as look for the underlying cause and eliminate it as soon as possible. For immediate treatment of symptoms, you can keep a cortisone cream on hand and rub it on the affected area every few hours until the pain begins to subside. (Cortisone creams are easily available at your pharmacy. They are not for long-term use, but are very effective in reducing inflammation for the short term.) For minor flare-ups, you can also use a cream containing capsaicin (cayenne).

In addition to the cortisone cream, you can take the supplements listed at the end of this section. Most important is to play detective and make a list of everything you've done differently in the week preceding the flare-up, to track down the culprit.

Other factors besides dietary allergens that may cause an arthritis flare-up are primarily related to inflammation. These can include exposure to environmental toxins such as pesticides, excessive estrogen caused by hormone replacement therapy (HRT), a leaky gut caused by taking NSAIDs (e.g., aspirin and ibuprofen), overdoing it with exercise or some other type of physical exertion, or a sudden onset of stress such as can happen when traveling and visiting family.

If the culprit is stress, resist the temptation to blame the stress on the outer cause (e.g., travel, family, illness of a loved one) and work on your inner response to the stress. You can't control your outer environment much of the time, but you can always control your inner environment, and that is one of the great secrets to serenity.

Delayed Food Allergies Are the Biggest Culprits. Alternative health care professionals are finding that nearly all of their patients with arthritis can be helped at least some by eliminating food allergens from the diet, and some patients can be cured this way. You can find out how to accomplish elimination of food allergies in detail in Chapter 11. According to a Scandinavian study, delayed food allergy tests (such as the ELISA) do not seem to be good predictors of foods that cause arthritis. This means that the very best course of action at this time is an elimination diet. This is one step that everyone with arthritis should take.

Glucosamine. A natural treatment for arthritis in clinical studies relieved the symptoms of osteoarthritis and in some cases reversed the disease. This substance is glucosamine, a naturally occurring compound in the body that can help keep cartilage strong and flexible, and can also play a role in repairing damaged cartilage.

Like bones, the cartilage found in tendons, ligaments, and other connective tissue is very much alive. When it becomes damaged in a healthy person, it is slowly but surely replaced by new cartilage. As we grow older, our bodies become less efficient at repairing cartilage.

Glucosamine is a key substance in the cartilage rebuilding process. It provides basic cartilage building blocks and stimulates the growth of cartilage. Animal studies have also shown that through a presently unknown mechanism, glucosamine reduces inflammation.

There have been at least five excellent studies done comparing the effects of glucosamine versus NSAID drugs such as acetaminophen, ibuprofen, and aspirin. In each study, the NSAIDs group improved faster during the first two weeks, but after a month the effectiveness began to wear off and side effects such as stomach and digestive problems began to appear. In contrast, after four to eight weeks, the glucosamine group showed a high degree of relief from pain, joint tenderness, and swelling. A study that did before-and-after electron micrographs of cartilage taken from both a placebo and a glucosamine group showed continuing arthritis in the placebo group and nearly healthy cartilage in the glucosamine group. In one recent study that compared the effects of glucosamine sulfate and a placebo on the progression of knee osteoarthritis, it was found that three years of treatment with 1,500 mg a day of glucosamine sulfate halted the progression of cartilage deterioration and joint space narrowing. Those who took the placebo showed progressive joint space narrowing, to the tune of 0.19 mm over three years. Symptoms improved 20 to 25 percent with glucosamine sulfate and only modestly with the placebo. Other studies have shown glucosamine therapy to be as effective at relieving arthritis pain as the NSAID ibuprofen. None of the glucosamine groups reported any significant side effects.

If you are suffering from osteoarthritis, bursitis, joint pain, swelling, or tenderness, you might want to try glucosamine. Take one 500-mg capsule three times a day for eight weeks, and then taper it down to one 500-mg capsule daily for maintenance.

Fish Oil Continues to Be a Winner. Research continues to indicate that omega-3 fatty acids found in fish oil can reduce arthritis pain considerably. A study from the Fred Hutchinson Cancer Research Center in Seattle that looked at diet and arthritis found that people who ate baked or broiled fish more than twice a week had less risk of rheumatoid arthritis. Other kinds of fish, such as fried fish, didn't have an effect. You can take fish-oil capsules, but watch for rancid oil, which will do you more harm than good. (Refer to Chapter 9 for guidelines on choosing the best fish-oil supplement.) Whether or not you supplement, make a point of eating cold-water fish two or three times a week.

You can also get omega-3 fatty acids from flax oil, but it's not recommended in high doses for the long term, as it can suppress both "good" and "bad" prostaglandins, the hormonelike substances that create or subdue inflammation. Flax oil is also notoriously unstable, meaning that it goes rancid almost immediately, which is counterproductive. If you would like to add flax to your diet, take it in the form of whole flax-seeds ground to a powder with a coffee grinder just before you add it to your food. Try it in smoothies, in yogurt, on cereal, sprinkled over salad, or mixed with nut butters.

DHEA May Be Good for Arthritis, Too. A researcher from the National Institutes of Health was the author of an article in the *Journal of Rheumatology* stating that men and women with rheumatoid arthritis tend to have lower than normal levels of DHEA (dehydroepiandrosterone), and men have low testosterone levels. For many of the chronic problems of aging, including arthritis, you can try taking a DHEA supplement of 5 to 10 mg daily or every other day for women and 25 mg daily for men.

Vitamin C Saves Joint Tissues. A study from a researcher at Boston Medical Center in the journal *Arthritis and Rheumatism* reported that people with rheumatoid arthritis who had higher levels of vitamin C had significantly less progression of the disease and less knee pain, due to a reduction in the loss of cartilage. Cartilage is made from collagen, and vitamin C is a key component of collagen. You can take up to 3,000 mg daily in divided doses to prevent and treat arthritis.

Other Supplements to Reduce Inflammation. One of the first steps in cooling down an arthritis flare-up is reducing inflammation, which should be done as quickly as possible. Following are some herbs, vitamins, and other nutrients that reduce inflammation. As a preventive measure, you can take them in one of the many arthritis formulas that contain combinations of these supplements. For flare-ups, increase the dose of the formulas or take them separately.

To prevent both chronic arthritis and flare-ups, it's extremely important to follow the Six Core Principles for Optimal Health, taking the vitamins, drinking plenty of water, and getting some exercise. Keeping muscles strong will support joints better, and movement helps move toxins out of the joints.

• **Pregnenolone**, a steroid hormone, can be very helpful in treating arthritis. Most of the studies were done decades ago, but interest in it as an arthritis treatment was dropped because it can't be patented. It has no known side effects and often improves memory as well. You can take 100 mg two to three times daily.

• **Bromelain** (from pineapple) is an enzyme that helps heal tissues and speed up the removal of inflammatory waste products from the joint. Other digestive enzymes such as papain (from papaya) can also be helpful.

• **Turmeric** or **curcumin** (curcumin is the active ingredient of turmeric), which you mainly know as a spice, is a powerful anti-inflammatory that works as well as cortisone for some people during arthritis flare-ups. For a flare-up, you need to take 300 to 600 mg of curcumin, three times a day in capsules. (If you take turmeric, you may need as much as 50 grams a day, which is overdoing it!)

• **Cat's claw** or **una de gato** (*Uncaria tomentosa*) is a South American tree. Its inner bark is used to treat arthritis. You can take it as a tea (the way the natives take it), in capsules, or in tincture form. Take 1 to 6 grams for a flare-up, or drink a cup or two of the tea a week as a preventive measure.

• **Ginger** is one of the best healing herbs that is effective in reducing inflammation of all kinds. Experiment with adding fresh ginger to foods. Ginger tea is delicious with a touch of honey and is great for relieving nasal, sinus, and chest congestion.

• **Vitamin D** is essential for healthy joints. Recent research has shown that low levels of vitamin D can contribute to the progression of osteoarthritis. Be sure you're getting out in the sunlight for at least 15 minutes a week, summer and winter, and if you live in a cloudy climate, you may want to include 1,000 to 2,000 IU of vitamin D in your daily vitamin intake during the winter months.

Treating Carpal Tunnel Syndrome Naturally

Although the general wisdom is that carpal tunnel syndrome is caused by repetitive movement, our great-great grandparents did plenty of repetitive movement—just think of plowing, spinning, sewing, and churning butter, to name a few—and yet carpal tunnel syndrome was relatively unknown until the past few decades. Repetitive motion may just be the final insult to already aggravated wrist nerves.

It's very likely that there are nutritional and hormonal factors associated with carpal tunnel syndrome that are important to pay attention to. It's clear that a vitamin B_6 deficiency is involved in carpal tunnel syndrome, and a B_6 deficiency may have even more to do with carpal tunnel syndrome than repetitive motion. Pyridoxal-5'-phosphate, the active form of vitamin B_6, is a cocatalyst for a large number of enzymes. It reduces inflammatory reactions in connective tissue and promotes collagen repair. Vitamin B_6 is also essential to the production of progesterone, a hormone that balances excessive estrogen.

Women get carpal tunnel syndrome more than men do, some women get it when they're pregnant, and both sexes get it around middle age, leading us to suspect that hormonal imbalance may aggravate or precipitate carpal tunnel syndrome. We also know that low thyroid and birth control pills are associated with carpal tunnel syndrome.

When estrogen is present in excess, it can cause salt and fluid retention, interfere with thyroid hormone, reduce the level of oxygen in all cells, and reduce vascular tone. All of these conditions aggravate carpal tunnel syndrome. We're living in a sea of xenoestrogens (environmental estrogens) from pesticides, plastics, and even soaps, not to mention exposure through hormone-treated meat, so that even men are exposed to excessive amounts of estrogen.

A woman named Beth who uses a computer for a living began to have wrist pain and stopped using her computer immediately. The pain persisted, so she tried taking vitamin B_6 and that helped some, but she had to take large doses to get relief. Then Beth realized she was eating a snack food every day that contained yellow dye no. 5 (tartrazine), which depletes vitamin B_6.

Within days of avoiding yellow dye, her wrist pain began to go away.

Once carpal tunnel gets established in the nerves of the wrist, it is very difficult to treat. It's important to pay attention to any type of pain in the wrist that doesn't go away after a few days and to stop doing the aggravating motion immediately.

To aid in healing carpal tunnel, in addition to 50 to 100 mg of vitamin B_6 daily you can take ginkgo biloba to improve blood supply to the affected area. Since ginkgo improves circulation to the extremities, it seems a logical choice for carpal tunnel syndrome.

Chapter 14

Antibiotics, Antifungals, and Their Natural Alternatives

A*nti-infectives* is the general term to describe the drugs we take to fight all kinds of infections such as bacteria, fungi, parasites, and viruses. The types of anti-infectives covered in this chapter are antibiotics, antivirals, and antifungals.

Kill the germ with an antibiotic, and your infection problem—sinus congestion, carache, urinary tract infection, cough—is solved. Right? Well, for the past 50 years, this is how conventional medicine has been treating patients. But 98 percent of those infections would have become better with some very basic care, like rest and fluids. Antibiotics do nothing to get rid of a virus when you have a cold or the flu.

Your life may depend on avoiding antibiotics until you really need them. The notion that the neat solution to every infection is to find the right antibiotic is not only incorrect but also has led us into big trouble. We are addicted to antibiotics. We think they'll cure everything from cholera to a hangnail. If you think this is an exaggeration, check out these numbers: about 145 million courses of antibiotics are prescribed each year in doctors' offices and emergency rooms across the United States. Add to this the 190 million doses handed out in American hospitals each year, and you've got a good idea of the rampant overuse of these drugs. Data from the National Center for Health Statistics indicates that antibiotics have been given to millions of patients who had viral infections that antibiotics are useless against. And if you think antibiotic abuse isn't about money, think about the billions of dollars those millions of prescriptions represent.

Alexander Fleming, discoverer of penicillin, warned us nearly a century ago that the overuse of antibiotics would create resistant bacteria. Even Louis Pasteur, the father of germ warfare using antibiotics, is said to have admitted on his deathbed, "The germ is nothing, the terrain is everything." This was his way of saying that a healthy body and a healthy immune system will fight off most infections, and an unhealthy body and immune system will be susceptible to infection.

In fact, antibiotics are a major cause of recurrent infections, and our overuse of them is breeding highly resistant strains of "superbugs" that are immune to all known types of antibiotics. To add insult to injury, we have lost the war on infectious diseases, even with all these antibiotics and better hygiene. According to a recent press conference held by the American Medical Association, infectious diseases have reemerged as a serious health threat. Just in the past decade, death from infectious diseases has risen a stunning 58 percent worldwide. Even after subtracting the deaths caused by the HIV virus, it's still up by 22 percent. Most of these deaths are caused by infections in the lungs and the blood that are resistant to antibiotics.

By using antibiotics as a cure-all, the magic bullet has come back to hit us. Every time we take antibiotics, we give harmful bacteria a new opportunity to become resistant. The consequence is that many antibiotics are useless. An increasingly common scenario in American hospitals is a hospitalized patient who gets a hospital-based staph infection or pneumonia that is totally resistant to antibiotics. People with antibiotic-resistant diseases often die.

According to the U.S. Centers for Disease Control and Prevention, each year nearly 2 million patients in the United States get an infection in a hospital. *Of those patients, about 90,000 die as a result of their infection.* More than 70 percent of the bacteria that cause hospital-acquired infections are resistant to at least one of the drugs most commonly used to treat them. The cost to treat these people with hospital-acquired infections is $1.2 billion each year in the United States.

Tuberculosis is making a comeback because it is now resistant to most antibiotics, along with highly resistant strains of pneumonia. Think twice and question your physician very closely before using an antibiotic.

Superbugs are just one of the downsides of these drugs. According to Canadian researchers, children who receive antibiotics before the age of 1 are more likely to have childhood asthma. Researchers in British Columbia combined the results of seven studies involving about 12,000 children. They found that when a child receives a course of antibiotics before his or her first birthday, that child is twice as likely to develop asthma than a child who receives no antibiotics during that time. Multiple courses in early childhood were found to bump risk higher, with an increase in risk of 16 percent with each course of antibiotics taken before the age of 1.

Antibiotics kill our beneficial gut bacteria, which provide a frontline defense system against harmful bacteria, viruses, and other environmental irritants such as allergens, and toxins such as pesticides. Antibiotics also weaken the immune system, promote the growth of harmful candida, create a friendly environment for parasites, and cause excessive loss of vitamins and minerals through digestive problems. They cause diarrhea and create a susceptibility to food allergies by destroying the protective bacteria that line the gut.

Clearly we need to find other ways to fight infections and to support our immune systems when we get sick. Antibiotics should only be used as a final resort in fighting a potentially life-threatening infection. Before he or she prescribes an antibiotic, your physician should do a culture to find out (1) if bacteria are present, and if so, (2) what strain of bacteria is present and thus what type of antibiotic to give you. Avoid wide-spectrum antibiotics whenever possible.

An Overview of Antibiotics

Antibiotics are anti-infective drugs that destroy specific types of bacteria. Penicillin, cephalosporins, tetracycline, macrolides, and aminoglycosides are some of the more common types of antibiotics. There are many different types of penicillin drugs, but by far the most prescribed penicillins are amoxicillin and the combination amoxicillin and potassium clavulanate (another antibiotic). Some of the brand names of amoxicillin are Amoxil, Trimox, and Augmentin, which you will probably recognize if you have been a parent in the past few decades.

• **Penicillins** stress the kidneys significantly and are particularly hard on children's kidneys. If your child has been prescribed a penicillin

for more than a week, make sure your physician monitors his or her kidney and liver function.

• **Cephalosporins** are broad-spectrum antibiotics. The most prescribed of these drugs are Cefaclor, Cephalexin, Duricef, Lorabid, Cefzil, Ceftin, and Suprax.

• **Fluoroquinolones** are synthetic broad-spectrum bacterial agents. The most common brand name of this drug is Cipro, the antibiotic made famous during the anthrax scares that occurred in the aftermath of 9/11. Side effects can be very serious with this drug, including allergic reactions to sunlight. It also interacts badly with any food that contains caffeine and can produce insomnia, the jitters, and heart palpitations. It can also cause ruptured tendons.

• **Tetracycline** used to be prescribed much more often than it is today. The most common tetracycline prescribed today is doxycycline. It is prescribed for acne as well as some dangerous infections such as Rocky Mountain spotted fever. This drug is so hard on your liver and kidneys that your physician should monitor the function of these organs periodically to avoid kidney and liver damage.

• **Macrolide antibiotics** are also tough on your body. They are effective for limiting the growth of a variety of infections, but their serious side effects could stay with you permanently. Some patients who had severe reactions to this drug—such as hearing loss, hallucinations, and abdominal pain—had a recurrence of these allergic reactions even after they stopped taking the drug. So don't take macrolides unless you absolutely have to!

• **Neomycin sulfate** is the most frequently prescribed aminoglycoside antibiotic. This drug suppresses intestinal bacteria and also has potentially dangerous side effects that necessitate monitoring of both kidney and nerve function during the course of therapy. In fact, the side effects are so common that 8 to 28 percent of patients who take this drug develop impairment of their kidney function. This is another anti-infective to stay away from unless you really need it.

• **Antifungal agents**, of course, fight fungal infections, and fluconazole is the most popular drug in this class. A single dose of this drug can bring on unpleasant side effects such as nausea and vomiting. Several doses can cause severe reactions, including liver dysfunction and seizures.

Because antibiotics are limited in the types of infections they can effectively fight, physicians are supposed to—but rarely do—determine exactly what kind of infection a patient has before prescribing an antibiotic. Not only does testing tell the physician if the infection is bacterial or viral in nature, but also exactly what kind of virus or bacteria it is. Again, antibiotics only destroy specific kinds of bacteria. If you have an infection that is caused by bacteria or a virus other than the type your prescribed drug kills, then taking that drug will prolong your illness, waste your money, and subject you to unnecessary side effects.

Antibiotics can be very effective in combating bacterial infections. However, many people are allergic to antibiotics and experience severe allergic reactions—even fatal ones. You can experience many varied reactions, but they usually begin with skin rashes, followed by one or more of the following: itching, hives, severe diarrhea, shortness of breath, wheezing, sore throat, nausea, vomiting, fever, swollen joints, and unusual bleeding or bruising. If any of these symptoms occur after you take an antibiotic, contact your physician immediately.

If You're Taking Antibiotics, Don't Reach for an Antacid

Antibiotics can play havoc on your digestive system, bringing on unpleasant symptoms such as gas, diarrhea, abdominal cramping, and indigestion. It would be natural to rifle through your medicine cabinet for Tums, Pepto-Bismol, or another brand of antacid to relieve yourself of these discomforts. But don't. If you take an antacid with most antibiotics (particularly tetracycline or quinolone antibiotics), you'll be reducing their effectiveness by 50 to 90 percent. When taking an antibiotic, hold yourself back from taking an antacid or you'll undermine the antibiotic's ability to fight your infection.

Antacids That Interfere with Antibiotics

Aluminum hydroxide gel	Mylanta II
Amitone	Phillips' Milk of
Calcium carbonate	Magnesia
Chooz	Riopan
Dicarbosil	Riopan Plus
Di-Gel Advanced	Rolaids
Formula	Rolaids Calcium
Gas-X	Rich/Sodium Free
Gaviscon	Rulox
Gaviscon Cool	Rulox Plus
Mint Flavor	Simaal 2 Gel
Gaviscon ESR	Titralac
Gaviscon-2	Titralac Plus
Gelusil	Tums
Kudrox	Tums Anti-Gas
Maalox HRF	Tums E-X Extra
Milk of magnesia	Strength
Mylanta Double	WinGel
Strength	

Antibiotics May Reduce the Effectiveness of Birth Control Pills

In the digestive tract, antibiotics kill bacteria that are key players in maintaining blood levels of contraceptive hormones. Studies have shown that unintended pregnancies have occurred from a birth control pill and antibiotic interaction. (The same reaction may be true for antifungal medications, too.) Even the most vocal critics of this theory recommend that women receiving broad spectrum antibiotics with oral contraceptives should use alternative means to protect themselves from unplanned pregnancies.

Kinds of Antibiotics

Examples of Penicillins

Amoxicillin (Amoxil, Trimox, Augmentin, Biomox, Polymox, Wymox)

Ampicillin (Polycillin-N, Amicillin, Omnipen, Totacillin, Principen, D-Amp)

Ampicillin with probenecid (Probampacin)

Ampicillin and sulbactam (Unasyn)

Bacampicillin HCl (Spectrobid)

Carbenicillin indanyl (Geocillin)

Cloxacillin (Tegopen, Cloxapen)

Dicloxacillin (Pathocil, Dynapen, Dycill)

Methicillin (Staphcillin)

Mezlocillin (Mezlin)

Nafcillin (Unipen, Nafcil, Nallpen)

Oxacillin (Bactocill, Prostaphlin)

Penicillin G (Pfizerpen, Pentids, Wycillin, Permapen, Bicillin)

Penicillin V (Veetids, V-Cillin, Beepen, Betapen, Robicillin)

Piperacillin (Pipracil)

Piperacillin and tazobactam (Zosyn)

Ticarcillin (Ticar)

Ticarcillin and clavulanate (Timentin)

Antibiotics That May Affect Oral Contraceptives

Achromycin V	Ala-Tet
Amcill	Amoxil
Augmentin	Azlin
Bactocill	Beepen-VK
Betapen-VK	Bikomox
Biomox	Cloxapen
Coactin	Declomycin
Doryx	Doxy-Caps
Doxychel	Dycill
Dynacin	Dynapen
Geocillin	Geopen
Ledercillin	Minocin
Monodox	Nallpen
Omnipen	Panmycin
Pathocil	Pentids
Pen-V	Pen-Vee K
Polycillin	Polymox
Principen	Prostaphlin
Robicillin VK	Robitet
Spectrobid	Staphcillin
Sumycin	Tegopen
Terramycin	Tetracap
Tetracyn	Tetralan
Totacillin	Trimox
Unipen	Uri-Tet
V-Cillin K	Veetids
Vibramycin	Vibra-Tabs
Wymox	

What Do They Do in the Body? Halt bacterial infections.

What Are They Used For? Treating mild to moderately severe penicillin-sensitive bacterial infections, including pneumonia, some respiratory tract infections, ear infections, some sexually transmitted diseases, and meningitis.

What Are the Possible Side Effects? Mild to serious and occasionally fatal immediate allergic reactions. These reactions can include skin rashes, fever, problems with breathing, wheezing, abnormality of the tongue, sore throat, swollen joints, chills, water retention, breathing problems, and death.

Penicillins also can create distress in the digestive and eliminative systems such as cramping, abdominal pain, gas, vomiting, bloody diarrhea, rectal bleeding, upset stomach, taste abnormalities, and kidney inflammation.

Possible side effects also include imbalance of blood chemistry, including suppression of the immune system and anemia. These drugs can also produce lethargy, dizziness, convulsions, anxiety, depression, combativeness, insomnia, seizures, and hyperactivity.

These drugs are particularly hard on young kidneys. Your child's physician should be monitoring your child's organ system function closely when your child is taking this type of drug.

If you are receiving this drug through an IV drip, you should know that potassium or sodium is added to the solution and can cause an imbalance of those minerals in your body.

CAUTION!

Think Twice About Taking These Drugs If . . .

- You have an allergic reaction to any type of penicillin.
- You have asthma, hay fever, or other allergies. If you take penicillin or any other antibiotic, your allergic reactions to it could be immediate and severe.
- You bleed or bruise easily or have any kind of kidney dysfunction.

What Are the Interactions with Food? Taking food with most penicillins reduces their effec-

tiveness. (Amoxil, Augmentin, and Trimox are exceptions. They can be taken without regard to food.)

Having an alcoholic drink while taking these drugs can produce uncomfortable symptoms such as headaches, stomach cramping, and vomiting.

Acidic fruit juices, sodas, wines, carbonated drinks, syrups, and other acidic beverages decrease the effectiveness of penicillins. Don't take penicillins with acidic food or drink.

What Nutrients Do They Throw out of Balance or Interact With? Vitamin K, amino acids, calcium, folic acid, magnesium, potassium, and vitamins B_6 and B_{12} are all depleted.

What Else to Take If You Take These Drugs. Supplements of the preceding nutrients. Take them two hours after a meal. Also be sure to take probiotics during and after a course of antibiotics. See the section on natural alternatives at the end of the chapter.

Examples of Cephalosporins

Cefaclor (Raniclor, Ceclor)
Cefadroxil (Duricef)
Cefamandole (Mandol)
Cefazolin (Ancef, Kefzol, Zolicef)
Cefepime (Maxipime, Kefurox, Zinacef)
Cefixime (Suprax)
Cefmetazole (Zefazone)
Cefonicid (Monocid)
Cefoperazone (Cefobid)
Cefotaxime (Claforan)
Cefotetan (Cefotan)
Cefoxitin (Mefoxin)
Cefpodoxime Proxetil (Vantin)
Cefprozil (Cefzil)
Ceftazidime (Fortaz, Tazidime, Ceptaz, Tazicef)
Ceftibuten (Cedax)

Ceftizoxime (Cefizox)
Ceftriaxone (Rocephin)
Cefuroxime (Ceftin)
Cephalexin (Keflex, Keftab, Biocef)
Cephalothin (Keflin)
Cephapirin (Cefadyl)
Cephradine (Velosef)
Loracarbef (Lorabid)

What Do They Do in the Body? They are related to penicillins and destroy specific bacterial infections.

What Are They Used For? Halting bacterial infections.

What Are the Possible Side Effects? Allergic reactions, particularly for people who have a history of allergy, asthma, or hay fever. These reactions include rashes, open sores, breathing difficulties, vaginal infections, dizziness, drowsiness, nervousness, insomnia, confusion, and anemia.

Intestinal problems are common when using these drugs. They can cause nausea, vomiting, diarrhea, stomach and abdominal cramping, gas, and heartburn. A more serious side effect is colitis, or inflammation of the colon. This problem results in colicky-like cramps and either diarrhea or constipation, and is caused by a depletion of vitamin K as well as an imbalance of the friendly and unfriendly bacteria in the intestinal tract.

These drugs are also particularly hard on kidney and liver function and have caused liver dysfunction, jaundice, and kidney failure. Because of this, your physician should monitor you closely if you are elderly or debilitated. Children should also be watched closely for any indications of kidney or liver system dysfunction. These drugs can cause seizures in people with kidney problems.

Like penicillin, these drugs also create changes in blood chemistry that suppress the immune system and can cause abnormal and heavy bleeding and mineral imbalances such as anemia.

CAUTION!

Think Twice About Taking These Drugs If . . .

- You have or have had asthma, hay fever, or an allergic reaction to this type of antibiotics.
- You have kidney dysfunction or kidney disease.
- You have a problem with excessive bleeding.
- You have liver dysfunction or liver disease.
- You have colitis or any other problem with your digestive tract.

What Are the Interactions with Food? Do not take these drugs with food. Food delays or reduces the absorption of these drugs into your system. (Cephalexin, Duricef, and Ceftin are exceptions.)

What Nutrients Do They Throw out of Balance or Interact With? Vitamin K, copper, sodium, vitamins B_6 and B_{12}, zinc, amino acids, calcium, folic acid, magnesium, and potassium may all be depleted by antibiotics.

What Else to Take If You Take These Drugs. Take supplements of the preceding nutrients and be sure to use probiotics. See the section on natural alternatives at the end of the chapter.

Examples of Fluoroquinolones

Ciprofloxacin (Cipro)
Enoxacin (Penetrex)
Gatifloxacin (Tequin)
Lomefloxacin (Maxaquin)
Norfloxacin (Noroxin)

Ofloxacin (Floxin)
Sparfloxacin (Zagam)

What Do They Do in the Body? These drugs are synthetic antibacterial agents with specific components not present in antibiotics that enhance their ability to efficiently destroy some infections.

What Are They Used For? Patients over 14 years old who have cystic fibrosis and who experience exacerbated lung problems from infection, with malignant external ear infections, or with tuberculosis.

Patients over 18 years old who have lower respiratory infections, skin infections, bone and joint infections, urinary tract infections, infectious diarrhea, typhoid, and gonorrhea.

Cipro is the first-line treatment for inhalation or skin anthrax infection.

What Are the Possible Side Effects? Allergic reactions—particularly to light of any kind. The reactions include skin burning sensation, redness, swelling, blisters, rash, or itching. Other allergic reactions can range from serious to fatal. They include loss of consciousness, tingling, water retention in the face, dizziness, drowsiness, and itching. There have also been reports of cataract development.

Numbness and pain in the hands and feet, convulsions, tremors, confusion, and hallucinations have occurred with these drugs.

Colon inflammation and diarrhea that can occur from these drugs ranges from mild to life threatening in severity and can result in chronic diarrhea or constipation. These drugs are hard on the eliminative systems and can cause kidney damage and kidney failure as well as jaundice and hepatitis.

These drugs can also cause respiratory problems, heart attacks, vaginal infections, intestinal bleeding, and stomach disturbances.

These drugs also caused lameness in immature dogs from permanent cartilage lesions and joint destruction. People who take these drugs have a very real risk of ruptured tendons, even for some time after the drugs have been discontinued. If you must take these drugs, you should be extremely cautious about exercise, and inform your physician if you experience any type of pain or swelling after taking the drugs.

Canadian health officials report serious swings in blood sugar in people taking Tequin.

CAUTION!

Think Twice About Taking These Drugs If . . .

- You are allergic to these drugs or other antibacterial agents such as cinoxacin and nalidixic acid.
- You have eye problems such as cataracts or are sensitive to sunlight or to light from sunlamps.
- You have pressure from fluids or growths under the skull.
- You have or suspect any brain disorder such as severe cerebral arteriosclerosis, epilepsy, or other factors that make you susceptible to seizures.
- You have diarrhea or colitis.
- You have kidney disease or kidney problems of any kind.

What Are the Interactions with Food? Food in general delays the absorption of these drugs. Take them two hours after a meal. (Cipro is an exception. It is absorbed better without food but may be taken with food to avoid stomach upset.)

These drugs interact poorly with mineral supplements of any kind. Take them two hours after taking a mineral supplement.

Avoid coffee or tea while taking these drugs. Fluoroquinolones intensify the caffeine effect and can give you jitters, insomnia, and heart palpitations. Check labels for products that contain caffeine that you may not be aware of.

What Nutrients Do They Throw out of Balance or Interact With? Acid/alkaline balance is often upset. Vitamin K, amino acids, calcium, folic acid, magnesium, potassium, and vitamins B_6 and B_{12} can all be depleted.

What Else to Take If You Take These Drugs. Plenty of water! Take supplements of the preceding nutrients. Take two hours after ingesting these drugs. Also, be sure to use probiotics during and after taking them. See the section on natural alternatives at the end of the chapter.

Other Tips on These Drugs. If you are taking these drugs for a prolonged amount of time, your physician should periodically assess your kidney and liver function as well as your blood chemistry.

Do not take antacids within four hours before or two hours after taking these drugs.

These drugs require sufficient fluids to ensure that you maintain the correct amount of water in your system and enough urine to eliminate required amounts of these drugs from your system.

Since these drugs can cause dizziness or light-headedness, do not drive or perform tasks that require alertness or coordination.

Examples of Tetracyclines

Demeclocycline (Declomycin)
Doxycycline (Doxychel, Vibramycin, Monodox, Doxy Caps, Doryx)
Methacycline (Rondomycin)
Minocycline (Dynacin, Minocin)
Oxytetracycline (Uri-Tet, Terramycin)
Tetracycline (Achromycin, Arestin, Sumycin, Spectracef, Tetralan, Panmycin, Robitet, Teline, Tetracyn)

What Do They Do in the Body? Tetracyclines inhibit the multiplication and the growth of bacteria but do not kill the bacteria.

What Are They Used For? Severe acne, infections in the excretory and reproductive systems, a type of conjunctivitis, different kinds of infections related to gonorrhea and Rocky Mountain spotted fever. Sometimes tetracyclines are used to prevent diarrhea from occurring while one is traveling in foreign countries. They are also prescribed for early stages of Lyme disease. However, their efficacy has been questioned.

What Are the Possible Side Effects? Allergic reactions—particularly to sunlight and sun lamps, weakness, shortness of breath, heart abnormalities, headaches, dizziness, open sores, and rashes.

These drugs are very hard on both the kidneys and liver and can impair the function of both of these vital organs. Because of this, you may experience kidney impairment or liver poisoning, hepatitis, or an increase in liver enzymes. In fact, they are so hard on these organs that your physician should monitor your liver and kidney functions periodically. In addition, physicians are warned that prescribing an additional drug that is also hard on your liver could be dangerous to you.

Headaches and blurred vision are possible with these drugs. These drugs can also cause nausea, vomiting, diarrhea, indigestion, sore throat, abnormalities of the tongue, colitis, hernias, discoloration of teeth and nails, and ulcers in the esophagus. It has also been reported that they can discolor the thyroid gland to a brown-black color.

There are increasing reports that minocycline, commonly prescribed for acne in young people, can cause a lupuslike reaction that can last for more than a year after going off the drug. It's not worth it.

Prescription and Over-the-Counter Medicines That Contain Caffeine

AAC tablets

Acetaminophen pain relief tablets super strength

Added strength headache relief capsules/
    tablets

Added strength pain reliever

Adult analgesic tablets

Adult strength pain reliever tablets

Alagesic

Alertness Aid Tablets/Alertness Tablets Extra
    Strength

Amaphen

Americet

Anacin Analgesic Adult Strength Tablets

Anodynos Dhc

Anodynos Forte

Anolor 300

Anoquan

APAP/butalbital/caffeine

Aqua-Ban Plus

Arcet

Arthritis Strength BC Powder

Bayer Select Maximum Headache Capsules

BC Headache Powders/BC Tablets

Belcomp-PB

Buffets II

Butalbicet

Butal Compound

Cafacit

Cafatine

Cafatine PB

Cafergot

Cafetrate

Caffedrine

Caffeine Sodium Benzoate

Cope

Cotanal 65

Darvon Compound 65

DeWitts Pills

Dexatrim Natural (Green Tea Formula)

DHC Plus

Diurex Long-Acting Water Capsules/
    Diurex Water Pills

Dolmar

E-Caff PB

Endolor

Energy Formula Advanced

Enerjets

Ercaf

Ercatab

Ergo-Caff PB

Ergotamine, pendoparbital, belladonna,
    caffeine (rectal)

Esgic

Esgic Plus

Equate Chocolate-Flavored Laxative

Equate Extra Strength Pain Relief

Equate Stay Awake

Excedrin Extra-Strength/Excedrin Aspirin
    Free/Excedrin Migraine

Ex-Lax Chocolate

Exolise Capsules

Extra Strength Pain Relief

Ezol

Farbital

Fembutal

Ferncet

Fioricet

Fioricet/Codeine

Fiorinal

Fiorinal #3

Fiormor

Fiorpap

Fiortal

Flexible Dose Pep Back

Fortabs

Gelprin

Gensan Tablets

Geone

Goody's Extra Strength Tablets/Goody's
    Headache Powders

Gotu Kola with Guarana

Guarana Tablets

Headache Formula

Herbal Energy Capsules

Hi Ener G Tablets

Hyomine Compound

Ide-Cet

Invagesic

Invagesic Forte

Isocet

Laniroif

Lanorinal

Laxative Chocolate Flavored

Laxative Natural Senna Chocolate

Luden's Natural Herbal Throat Drops/Luden's
    Natural Orange Throat Drops

Margesic

Maximum Strength Arthriten

Maximum Strength Menstrual Formula
    Caplets

Maximum Strength PMS Caplets

Medigelsic

Medigesic

Metabalite

Metabolife 356

Metabolift

Metabolize and $ave

Micomp PB

Midol Maximum Strength/Midol
    Maximum Strength Multisymptom
    Menstrual

Mikarcet

Minotal

NoDoz

Norgesic

Norgesic Forte

Orphengesic

Orphengesic Forte

Pacaps

Pain Reliever Tablets

PC-Caps

Pep-Back

Pharmagesic

Phenaphen with Codeine #3

Propoxyphene compound 65, propoxyphene
    HCl, ASA, caffeine

Quick Pep

Repan

Revco Adult Strength Pain Reliever

Saleto/Saleto D

Scot-Tussin Original 5 Action Cold Formula/
    Scot-Tussin Original 5 Action Liquid

Senokot Liquid, Chocolate

Stay Awake

Summit Extra Strength

Supac

Synalgos CD

Tenake

Tencet

Tirend

Triad

Tussirex Sugar Free

Tussirex Syrup

Ultra Pep-Back

Vanquish Caplets/Vanquish Extra Strength

Viactiv Milk Chocolate

Vivarin

Walgreens Added Strength Pain Relief Tablets/
    Walgreens Aspirin Plus/Walgreens Awake
    Tablets/Walgreens Stay Awake

Wigraine

XS Hangover Relief Caplets

Your Life Complete Spectra
    Multivitamin/Herb Tablets

CAUTION!

Think Twice About Taking These Drugs If . . .

You are allergic to sulfites. Allergic reactions can be life threatening and can create severe asthmatic episodes.

What Are Their Interactions with Food? Eating food with these drugs decreases their absorption. (Doxycycline is an exception. Take with food.) Take these drugs with a full glass of water. Avoid eating dairy products within two hours of taking them.

Iron, calcium, magnesium, riboflavin, vitamin C, zinc, or any mineral supplements taken at the same time as tetracyclines can reduce their absorption as well as reduce absorption of these nutrients. Take these supplements two hours before or after taking tetracyclines.

Also avoid antacids, laxatives, or iron- or magnesium-containing products. If you must take an antacid, take it at least two hours before or after tetracyclines.

Caffeine enhances the effects of tetracyclines.

What Nutrients Do They Throw out of Balance or Interact With? Vitamin K, riboflavin, vitamin C, amino acids, copper, folic acid, potassium, zinc, calcium, and vitamins B_2, B_6, and B_{12} can all be depleted by antibiotics. These drugs can cause severe headaches when taken with high doses of vitamin A.

What Else to Take If You Take These Drugs. Take supplements of the preceding nutrients. Be sure to take probiotics during and after a course of antibiotics. See the section on natural alternatives at the end of the chapter.

Other Tips on These Drugs. Children under the age of 8 should not be given these drugs.

During long-term therapy, your physician should periodically monitor your organ systems, including kidney and liver functions and blood chemistry.

Examples of Macrolide Antibiotics

Azithromycin (Zithromax)
Clarithromycin (Biaxin, Biaxin XL)
Dirithromycin (Dynabac)
Erythromycin (Ery-Tab, E-Mycin, Robimycin,
    E-Base, Eryc, Ilosone, Eramycin, EryPed)
Troleandomycin (Tao)

What Do They Do in the Body? These drugs either kill or stop multiplication and growth of specific bacteria.

What Are They Used For? Tonsillitis, sinus infections, chronic bronchitis, pneumonia, skin infections, ear infections, and acne; or for the prevention or destruction of bacteria and fungal infections in advanced HIV patients.

Azithromycin is prescribed for all of the preceding conditions as well as bacterial infections of patients with chronic obstructive pulmonary disease (COPD) or community-acquired pneumonia.

Erythromycin is prescribed for moderately severe upper and lower respiratory infections, whooping cough, diphtheria, conjunctivitis of newborn, pneumonia of the infant, genital infections during pregnancy, syphilis, Legionnaires' disease, rheumatic fever, prolonged diarrhea, and early Lyme disease.

What Are the Possible Side Effects? The most frequently reported side effects are related to the digestive system. They include diarrhea, nausea, abnormal taste, upset stomach, abdominal cramping, headache, and vaginal infections. In children, side effects can include diarrhea, vomiting, abdominal pain, rash, and headache.

Allergic reactions can range from life threatening to mild. These can include loss of hearing, rashes, behavioral disorders, disorientation, dizziness, hallucinations, insomnia, nightmares, vertigo, palpitations, chest pain, liver dysfunction, abnormal heartbeats, and death. Allergic reactions have reoccurred in patients using azithromycin and erythromycin even after they stopped taking the drugs.

Erythromycin can cause life-threatening disturbances in heart rhythms.

Erythromycin (e.g., E-Mycin) and clarithromycin interact dangerously with many common drugs. For example, erythromycin interacts with some calcium channel blockers and the cholesterol-lowering drug lovastatin (e.g., Mevacor), as well as some not-so-common drugs such as vinblastine (e.g., Velban), a chemotherapy drug. These drugs should be used with extreme caution or not at all. They raise levels of many other drugs due to their blocking action on certain enzymes in the liver responsible for metabolizing the drugs. This means they could affect hundreds of other drugs that simply haven't been studied yet and even substances such as coffee and alcohol. Your best bet is to stay away from these drugs unless you are in a life-threatening situation.

Azithromycin appears to be the safest of the macrolide antibiotics.

CAUTION!

Think Twice About Taking These Drugs If . . .

- You have heart problems of any kind, particularly those involving irregular heartbeats—please ask your doctor to reconsider prescribing this drug.
- You have colitis, inflammation of the intestinal tract, severe diarrhea, or constipation.
- You have liver or kidney disease or dysfunction—particularly if you are elderly.

What Are the Interactions with Food? Food delays the absorption of these drugs. Take one hour before or two hours after a meal. Acidic fruits or juices, carbonated drinks, sodas, wines, and syrups decrease the effectiveness of these drugs. Alkaline foods such as milk, dairy products, and vegetables also decrease the effectiveness of these drugs.

What Nutrients Do They Throw out of Balance or Interact With? Amino acids, calcium, vitamins B_6 and B_{12}, folic acid, potassium, and vitamin K may be depleted.

What Else to Take If You Take These Drugs. Take supplements of the preceding nutrients. Take two hours after taking macrolides. Be sure to take probiotics during and after a course of antibiotics. See the section on natural alternatives at the end of the chapter.

Examples of Ketolide Antibiotics

Telithromycin (Ketek)

The FDA approved this new type of antibiotic in 2004, so it is a relatively new and untested drug. By 2008 enough people had taken it to let us now know it can cause severe liver damage leading to liver failure and death.

What Do They Do in the Body? These drugs either kill or stop multiplication and growth of specific bacteria.

What Are They Used For? This drug is approved for the treatment of community-acquired pneumonia (of mild to moderate severity) due to *Streptococcus pneumoniae, Haemophilus influenzae, Moraxella catarrhalis, Chlamydophila pneumoniae,* or *Mycoplasma pneumoniae,* for patients 18 years old and older.

What Are the Possible Side Effects? The most common side effects are nausea and diarrhea. It can also cause headache, dizziness, vomiting, and distortions in the sense of taste.

Other less common side effects can include a wide variety of gastrointestinal problems including abdominal distension, abdominal pain, dyspepsia, gas, constipation, and pancreatitis; a variety of liver dysfunctions, including hepatitis and fatal liver toxicity; and a variety of heart problems, including hypotension, atrial arrhythmias, and palpitations. Also, swelling of the face, oral candidiasis, glossitis, inflammation of the mucous membranes in the mouth, dry mouth, fainting, fatigue, sleepiness, loss of consciousness, insomnia, vertigo, increased sweating, anxiety, blurred vision, vaginal candida and fungal infections, various skin rashes and disorders, increased platelet count, bradycardia, elevated blood bilirubin, flushing, increased blood alkaline phosphatase, increased eosinophil count, paresthesia, and muscle cramps.

People with myasthenia gravis should not take this drug, as it can cause respiratory failure.

This drug interacts dangerously with many other drugs. Please read the prescribing information sheet carefully and talk with your pharmacist about any other drugs you're taking before taking this drug.

CAUTION!

There doesn't seem to be any good reason to take this drug unless you have a life-threatening infection that is resistant to all other antibiotics.

What Else to Take If You Take These Drugs. Be sure to take probiotics during and after a course of antibiotics.

Examples of Aminoglycosides

Amikacin (Amikin)
Gentamicin (Garamycin, Jenamicin)
Kanamycin (Kantrex)
Neomycin (Neo-Tabs, Mycifradin, Neo-Fradin)
Netilmicin

Paromomycin (Humatin)
Streptomycin
Tobramycin (Nebcin)

What Do They Do in the Body? They block proliferation of intestinal bacteria.

What Are They Used For? Suppression of intestinal bacteria. Because of the high potential for toxicity from these drugs, they are only prescribed for periods shorter than two weeks.

What Are the Possible Side Effects? The side effects of these drugs are serious. Therefore, monitoring of kidney and nerve function is critical. Eight to 28 percent of patients who took these drugs for several days or more developed renal (kidney) impairment. Toxicity is so prevalent that physicians are warned against prescribing additional drugs that are at all hard on the kidneys or the liver.

Hearing loss, fainting, ringing in the ears, skin tingling, muscle twitching, and convulsions. Hearing loss that occurs with these drugs may be irreversible.

These drugs also cause problems in the digestive tract and inhibit absorption of nutrients. This can produce nausea, vomiting, diarrhea, and colitis, not to mention malnutrition.

CAUTION!

Think Twice About Taking These Drugs If . . .

- You have muscular disorders such as Parkinson's disease. These drugs can worsen muscle weakness.
- You have open sores in your intestinal tract or have digestive problems.
- You have kidney or liver problems of any kind.
- You have hearing problems.
- You have an electrolyte imbalance.

What Are the Interactions with Food? Acidic foods taken with these drugs can increase the effects and length of effectiveness of the drug. Alkaline foods can decrease the effectiveness of these drugs.

What Nutrients Do They Throw out of Balance or Interact With? Magnesium, calcium, potassium, vitamin A, carbohydrates, and vitamin K.

What Else to Take If You Take These Drugs. Take supplements of the preceding nutrients several hours apart from taking an aminoglycoside, and be sure to use probiotics during and after a course of antibiotics. See the section on natural alternatives at the end of the chapter.

Examples of Antifungal Agents

Amphotericin B (Abelcet, Amphotec, Fungizone)
Fluconazole (Diflucan)
Flucytosine (Ancobon)
Griseofulvin (Fulvicin, Grifulvin, Grisactin)
Itraconazole (Sporanox)
Ketoconazole (Nizoral)
Miconazole (Monistat)
Nystatin (Mycostatin, Nilstat)
Terbinafine (Lamisil)
Voriconazole (Vfend)

Most of the antifungal drugs have very nasty side effects and dangerous interactions with a long list of other drugs. Be extremely cautious with their use. It has become something of a fad in alternative medicine to prescribe antifungal drugs for intestinal candida infections that are diagnosed by symptoms. The long-term effect of this treatment is often that the candida returns, worse than ever, within a year. You are better off treating candida infections, both vaginal and intestinal, with one of the suggested alternatives

at the end of this chapter that supports your good bacteria.

Antifungals are also notoriously ineffective for treating toenail fungus. Again, chances are it will come back worse than ever, even after a long course of the drugs.

What Do They Do in the Body? They inhibit fungal growth.

What Are They Used For? Fungal infections. Most commonly, vaginal infections from candida, the prevention of fungal infections during surgery, and meningitis.

What Are the Possible Side Effects? These drugs can be prescribed for women with yeast infections, but they have 10 percent more side effects than intravaginal agents that accomplish the same thing. See the section on natural alternatives.

Side effects can include headache, nausea, abdominal pain, diarrhea, dizziness, and drowsiness. Patients receiving multiple doses may experience all of the preceding side effects plus seizures, skin disorders, and serious liver reactions. Australian drug authorities report numerous cases of abnormal red and white blood cell counts in people taking Lamisil.

Injury to your liver is possible. Toxicity is rare but has ranged from mild to fatal.

Allergic reactions can occur, such as rashes, shortness of breath, and dizziness. Some people have had serious skin disorders from these drugs, which have produced open sores.

CAUTION!

Think Twice About Taking These Drugs If . . .

- You have malignant cancer or AIDS.
- You have any dysfunction of the liver or liver disease.

- You have kidney dysfunction or kidney disease.
- You have a serious skin disorder.

Antiviral Drugs

Antiviral drugs are targeted for very specific viruses. We now have antivirals for HIV, herpes, hepatitis B and C, and influenza (flu) A and B.

Antiviral drugs for the flu weren't routinely used until the bird flu (H5N1) scare of 2005, when oseltamivir (Tamiflu) was widely marketed as the only medication available to treat humans with bird flu. This created a flood of sales and worldwide stockpiling of the drug. The truth is, however, that the drug had never been tested in humans with bird flu. According to an article at worldnetdaily.com, a Vietnamese doctor from the Center for Tropical Diseases in Hanoi who used the drug for 41 bird flu patients concluded that the drug is "useless." The World Health Organization (WHO) agrees that the drug has not been very useful in treating bird flu. Those defending the drug claim that it was not started soon enough to help.

These drugs are said to shorten the duration and severity of the flu, but the human research showing this to be a consistent effect is limited.

Examples of Neuraminidase Inhibitor and Amantadine Derivative Antivirals for Flu

Neuraminidase inhibitor antivirals for flu: oseltamivir (Tamiflu), zanamivir, inhaled (Relenza)

Amantadine derivative antivirals for flu: amantadine hydrochloride (Symmetrel), rimantadine hydrochloride (Flumadine)

What Do They Do in the Body? If taken early enough, these drugs can help block the spread of a viral infection and reduce the duration of flu symptoms by about one and a half days.

What Are They Used For? The neuraminidase inhibitor antivirals are approved for preventing and treating influenza virus A and B. To be most effective, treatment must be started within 48 hours of when symptoms begin. The amantadine derivatives are approved for treating influenza A infection.

These drugs are most often prescribed to so-called high-risk people, including the elderly—especially in nursing homes, those with lung or heart disease, those with compromised immune systems (e.g., HIV), and those who serve the public and may be exposed to large numbers of people with the flu, such as hospital workers and police.

All of these drugs can cause viruses to become resistant, a good reason to be cautious about taking them.

What Are the Possible Side Effects? The most common side effects of the flu antivirals are gastrointestinal and can include abdominal pain, nausea, vomiting, loss of appetite, diarrhea, and heartburn. They can also affect the nervous system, in bizarre and contradictory ways (read on for specifics). Geriatric patients are much more susceptible to these side effects.

- **Flumadine.** Can cause insomnia, sleepiness, depression, dizziness, nervousness, agitation, and foggy thinking.

- **Symmetrel.** Causes an increase in dopamine release in the animal brain, and considering the wide range of nervous system side effects possible with this drug, it may be safe to assume that it does the same in the human brain. Side effects can include confusion, hallucinations, nightmares, nervousness, anxiety, irritability, hyperkinesia (increase in body movements), impaired concentration, amnesia, difficulty in coordination, slurred speech, mental depression, decreased libido, weakness, euphoria, seizures, severe mood or mental changes, thoughts of suicide, or attempts at suicide. Other Symmetrel side effects can include fainting, high blood pressure, blurred vision, irritation or swelling of the eye, difficult urination, edema (water retention), congestive heart failure, shortness of breath, fever, chills, sore throat, and rash. As little as a 1 gram overdose of Symmetrel has caused death.

• **Tamiflu.** Has caused serious skin reactions, including toxic epidermal necrolysis, Stevens-Johnson syndrome, and erythema multiforme. These can be fatal side effects of this drug. Tamiflu is much more widely used in Japan than in the United States. Doctors there have reported that in children and teens, the drug is associated with delirium and abnormal behaviors (such as jumping out of buildings) that have resulted in injury and death. Tamiflu side effects may include bronchitis, dizziness, headache, insomnia, vertigo, fatigue, abnormal liver tests, irregular heartbeat, gastrointestinal bleeding, colitis, seizure, aggravation of diabetes. Side effects specific to children can include middle ear infection or inflammation, nosebleed, asthma, pneumonia, eye infection, and swollen lymph glands.

• **Relenza.** Side effects are similar to Tamiflu. Although Relenza is less convenient and more expensive because it is inhaled, it appears to have fewer side effects, and less severe side effects than the other antivirals.

CAUTION!

- Do not use these drugs if you are pregnant or nursing.
- Do not use these drugs if you have a seizure disorder.

- These drugs may interact dangerously with antidepressants.
- There are reports that amantadine can interfere with male fertility.
- Do not use Relenza if you have asthma or any other chronic lung problem, as it could cause serious spasms in the lungs.
- Considering the extreme nature of Symmetrel side effects, it does not appear sensible to take this drug.
- Please monitor children and teens very carefully for nervous system side effects when taking these drugs.

Natural Alternatives to Antibiotics

When penicillin was discovered, we thought we had discovered a magic bullet that would kill any and all infections. Physicians tend to prescribe it for anything from a cut to a cold, knowing all the while that it doesn't kill the viruses that cause colds—it only kills bacteria. We Americans have become hooked on antibiotics. If our physician doesn't write us out a prescription for them, we go to another physician.

The bacteria in our bodies that antibiotics are supposed to kill have an intelligence all their own when it comes to building resistance to these drugs. Every time we take antibiotics or get them in dairy products or meat, we are giving bacteria a new opportunity to become resistant. The consequence of this is that many antibiotics have become useless—a wide variety of bacteria that are the cause of many serious illnesses are resistant to them. Clearly we need to find other ways to fight infections and to support our immune systems when we get sick.

Use Probiotics When You Take Antibiotics

One of the most serious side effects of taking antibiotics is killing the "good" bacteria that live in your large intestine. The colon, in contrast to the germ-free stomach and small intestine, is lavishly populated with bacteria, which are normal intestinal flora that keep the "bad" bacteria under control. These bacteria, also called probiotics, are also found in the mouth, the urinary tract, and the vagina. There are about 100 trillion of these bacteria living in our bodies and over 400 species. The three most common friendly bacteria are called *Lactobacillus acidophilus*, *Lactobacillus bulgaricus*, and *Bifidobacterium bifidum*.

Probiotics are intimately tied into how our immune system works. They manufacture the B vitamins, help us digest our food, reduce cholesterol, and help keep hormones in balance. If you take an antibiotic and kill them off, it can seriously compromise your health. Steroids such as prednisone, poor digestion, nutritional deficiencies, and stress can also kill off these good bacteria, leaving an overgrowth of the bad guys, most of whom are a fungal yeast called *Candida albicans*. An overgrowth of yeast in the intestines can cause fatigue, bloating, gas, diarrhea, constipation, skin problems, and a long list of secondary symptoms such as headaches, mental fogginess, achy joints, and pollen allergies.

If you must take antibiotics for some reason, be sure to take probiotics both during and after the course of antibiotics. Take them at least two hours before or after you take the antibiotic, and keep taking them for at least two weeks after you finish the antibiotics.

Probiotic supplements are "alive" and have a relatively short shelf life of a few months. If you use probiotic supplements, please stick to the refrigerated brands. A good probiotic supplement will contain fructooligosaccharides (FOS), which promote the growth of good bacteria. Bananas are a plentiful source of FOS; they're a good food to have around during and after a course of antibiotics.

There is much disagreement among health professionals and probiotic manufacturers about which types of probiotic supplements are best. Most people do just fine with a mixture of lactobacillus, bifidus, and acidophilus. The loose powder is the ideal way to get a concentrated dose of probiotics, but if this is going to be too much trouble, take it in capsules. When we're talking about billions of bacteria, the loss of a few million won't hurt too much! You need to keep the capsules refrigerated when you get them home. Since stomach acid rises when you eat, you'll get more of them into your digestive system by taking them between meals.

You can get probiotics in your diet by eating yogurt with live cultures (this is listed on the label). Many supermarkets and health food stores also sell acidophilus milk, which contains live cultures.

Natural Remedies for Resisting Infections

The best way you can create hostile terrain for "bad" bacteria is to follow the Six Core Principles for Optimal Health and make them a way of life. They will give your body a solid foundation from which to fend off bacteria and viruses. It's important to be aware that we are always being exposed to billions of potentially infectious germs, and our bodies naturally fend them off. When your immune system is weakened through poor nutrition, high stress levels, not enough sleep, and the rigors of travel, the germs have the opportunity to get a foothold in your body.

One of the keys to resisting an infection is to begin helping your body fight it as soon as you are aware it's there. We all know the symptoms: fatigue, achiness, sore throat, swollen glands, runny nose, cough, and fever. If you have a sore throat and ignore it, stay up late, and eat a bowl of ice cream, it's bound to get worse. If you gargle with salt water, go to bed early with a cup of chamomile tea, and avoid sugary foods, chances are it will be gone by morning.

Here are some simple, specific steps you can take to stay free of infections:

• **Wash your hands.** If you have been around people with colds or the flu, keep your hands away from your face and wash your hands before eating. Don't, however, be fooled into thinking that all of those antibacterial household cleansers and soaps are going to protect you. It has been found that the bacteria-busting chemicals they contain create an ideal environment for the formation of resistant bacteria. Soap and water works just fine for the hands, and vinegar (dilute and put in a spray bottle) is the perfect kitchen cleaner.

• **Gargle.** If you're coming down with a sore throat, one of the simplest and most effective solutions is to gargle with a germ-killing mouthwash (make sure the gargle reaches your throat) or a simple salt water solution (1 teaspoon of salt to 1 cup of water). A sore throat is often caused by mucus from the sinuses dripping down the back of the throat, so giving that area an antibacterial bath can work wonders. There are some herbal throat sprays on the market that are excellent for banishing throat infections.

• **Sinus rinse.** A great remedy for an encroaching sinus infection is to rinse the sinuses with a saltwater solution (1 teaspoon of salt and a pinch of baking soda per 1 cup of water). This remedy takes some discipline and focus, and it's not recommended for most children. The best tool for the job is called a neti pot, which looks like a little teapot with a spout that is made for rinsing the sinuses. You can buy a traditional ceramic neti pot or get the plastic version at the drugstore. Mix the solution of salt and baking soda in the neti pot. Tip your head sideways, and insert the spout gently into one of your nostrils. If you hold the spout at the right angle, the water will flow in one nostril and out the other. The real experts allow the water to flow in one nostril and out the mouth, but this can cause gagging if you swallow some of the water. This technique can work wonders for a stubborn sinus infection.

• **Avoid sugar and alcohol.** As your body fights infection, it helps to eat wholesome, healthy foods. Sugar and alcohol suppress the immune system and can make it harder for your body to do its job.

• **Extra vitamin C** can help fight infections and viruses. If you take 1,000 to 2,000 mg every three to four hours as soon as you feel a cold coming on, drink plenty of water, and avoid sugar, you can often knock the cold out before it ever gets started. Vitamin C will work even better if you combine it with bioflavonoids.

• **Vitamin A** is a powerful infection-fighter is an immune stimulant that boosts thymus gland function and helps maintain healthy cells in your mucus membranes. You can take 10,000 to 30,000 IU daily for a week to help fight off an infection. (If you're pregnant, don't take more than 10,000 IU daily.)

• **Zinc and selenium** are your two most important infection-fighting minerals. A wide variety of lozenges are available at your health food store that contain zinc, selenium, and vitamin C. Pass on those with a lot of sugar.

• **Vitamin D** is essential for a healthy immune system. People who don't get out in the sun or who have long, gray winters should take at least 2,000 IU of vitamin D3 daily.

• **Allow a fever to run its course.** Bacteria are adverse to high temperatures, which is why we sometimes get a fever when we get infections. This is why it's important to not bring down a fever unless it's dangerously high. The fever is the very thing that will kill the bacteria or virus that's making you sick. In children in particular, a fever is part of the body's mechanism for training the immune system to recognize hostile bacteria and viruses and forming antibodies that will recognize them in the future. If you suppress the fever with acetaminophen (Tylenol), your child could be more likely to get sick again the next time the bug comes to visit. Talk to your doctor about exactly how high to allow a fever to go with your child. You can help yourself or your child through a fever with a few commonsense measures:

1. Remain warmly dressed in soft, natural-fiber clothing. If it's a cold day, cover your head and wrap your neck, and keep feet in warm socks. This will help speed the passage of the fever.
2. Stay hydrated, but don't eat a lot, and stay away from heavy foods. Stick with light soups, cooked vegetables, or whole-grain crackers. Eating less cranks up your immune system a notch.
3. Stay where things are quiet and peaceful. The less stimulation you have, the more your body can focus on getting well.
4. If the discomfort becomes too much, the arms and legs can be sponged off with water, but try not to undress completely or bathe until the fever has broken.

• **Grapefruit seed extract** is a product you can use if you feel an infection coming on. It is a grapefruit bioflavonoid concentrate that works well to help knock out a cold. You can take one 100 mg tablet every four to five hours or a few drops of the liquid. There are anecdotal reports from women that grapefruit seed extract will effectively cure urinary tract infections.

• **The herb echinacea**, sometimes combined with goldenseal in formulas, is an effective immune stimulant but works best when used early on in an infection. Some people are allergic to it, so if you take a dose and feel worse, stop taking it!

• **Oscillococcinum** is a homeopathic remedy for preventing and relieving the symptoms of the flu. This is a great remedy to travel with and to keep in the medicine cabinet, as it can quickly knock out a flu.

• **Yin Chiao** is a Chinese herbal remedy for preventing colds and flus. It can actually prevent a full-blown cold if taken soon enough. When using Chinese medicines, it's important to use reputable brands.

• **EpiCor** is a fermented yeast product that enhances natural killer cell activity and helps modulate and strengthen the immune system. It contains a unique blend of vitamins, minerals, amino acids, and antioxidants that research has shown to be very effective in warding off colds and flus. This is a supplement that can be taken daily during cold and flu season as a preventive. There are excellent human clinical studies on EpiCor, which you can read about in detail at embriahealth.com.

• **Russian Choice Immune** is a probiotic that originated as a fermented milk product in

Eastern Europe. Technically speaking, it's "a preparation of cell-wall fragments made from a specific strain of *Lactobacillus rhamnosus*. . . . Such probiotic bacteria are known to stimulate both the innate and adaptive immune systems. . . ." The bottom line is that it supports the immune system and the gastrointestinal system.

• **Olive leaves** have been used medicinally for centuries to treat fever, malaria, colds, and fungal infections. Modern research shows that a bitter constituent of olive leaves called oleuropein has antibacterial, antiviral, and antiprotozoal effects. Research at the pharmaceutical company Upjohn found that elenolic acid, another chemical found in olive leaves, stopped certain cold viruses dead in their tracks. The best way to take olive leaf as a supplement is as an extract in capsule or liquid form.

• **Elderberries** have a long history of use by American Indians, who used it primarily for the treatment of infections. Elderberries contain anti inflammatory bioflavonoids that have been shown in test tube studies to inhibit viral growth. Specifically, elderberry flavonoids can stifle the activity of a protein needed by the flu virus to multiply and spread. It's no surprise that elderberry is especially effective against viral infections such as the flu and the common cold. In one study, a patented elderberry extract was given to flu patients. They showed significant improvement in symptoms, including muscle aches, respiratory symptoms, and fever, in the space of only 24 hours.

Bladder Infections. For bladder or urinary tract infections, drink 4 ounces of unsweetened cranberry juice or take 1 capsule of cranberry concentrate three times a day along with grapefruit seed extract.

Ear Infections. For recurrent ear infections:

• Eliminate sugar.
• Identify and eliminate food allergens.
• Take vitamin C to tolerance.
• Take vitamin A, 10,000 to 15,000 IU a day for up to two weeks.
• Chew xylitol gum.

Recent studies have found that antibiotics make little to no difference in the course that children's ear infections take. Many children have had multiple courses of antibiotics for recurrent ear infections before they've passed through toddlerhood, and this just sets children up for weakened immunity and more infections. Watchful waiting and allowing the infection to resolve naturally—along with children's echinacea, a multivitamin, vitamin C, and a no-sugar, no-refined-carbohydrate diet—may stop the cycle of repeat infections in children.

A study published in the *British Medical Journal* looked at the effects of a course of probiotic therapy for the prevention of recurrent ear infections. The researchers recruited 130 children from ages 6 months to 6 years, all of whom were suffering from ear infections and had a history of recurrent otitis media. They gave all the children 10 days' worth of antibiotics. Once the antibiotic therapy was over, half the kids got a probiotic nasal spray for 10 days, while the other half got a placebo. A second course of probiotics and placebos was given two months later. Over the three months of the study, 42 percent of the probiotic group avoided getting another ear infection, while only 22 percent of the placebo group avoided another ear infection.

In Great Britain and Europe, the sweetener xylitol is being used with great success to treat ear infections, often in the form of chewing gum. Xylitol has antibacterial properties that work specifically against the pathogens that cause ear infections.

Internal Fungal Infections. Candida is a common fungus that grows out of control in many people, thanks to too many antibiotics and too much sugar. Your best strategy for fighting a fungal infection is to boost your body's natural resources as much as possible, so that your own "good" bacteria can fight off the candida.

It's extremely important to eliminate sugar from your diet if you're fighting a candida infection, and it helps to eliminate or cut back on fermented foods such as beer, wine, vinegar, aged cheeses, and anything made with yeast.

If you suspect you have a serious candida overgrowth in your intestines, read the book *Optimal Wellness* by Ralph Golan, M.D. (Ballantine Books, 1995). He covers the subject in detail and gives an excellent protocol to follow for bringing candida under control.

Grapefruit seed extract, garlic oil, and oregano oil are all very effective antifungals. It's certainly worth giving them a try before taking a potent antifungal drug. Be sure to take probiotics to enhance your body's production of its own "good" bacteria.

Vaginal Yeast Infections. Vaginal yeast infections are an overgrowth of candida, usually caused by taking antibiotics. They cause itching and redness and a white discharge from the vagina. Yeast infections can also be caused when the pH of the vagina is altered, creating a favorable environment for candida growth. The pH of the vagina can be altered by frequent sex, because semen creates a more alkaline environment in the vagina. It can also be altered by the use of commercial douches, which in general cause a lot more unpleasant odors than they cover up.

Fortunately, vaginal yeast infections are usually easy to treat, especially when caught early. The first thing you can try is douching at least twice a day with a vinegar and water solution, ¼ cup white or apple cider vinegar to 1 quart of water. You can also use a yogurt douche for the probiotics in it, although it's probably easier and less messy just to insert a probiotic gelatin capsule into the vagina.

To avoid future yeast infections, use a vinegar douche once a day if you are having frequent sex, and avoid using commercial douches. If you are taking antibiotics and you have a tendency to get yeast infections, take your probiotics orally *and* vaginally!

A recent study found that a significant proportion of the women who buy over-the-counter yeast infection remedies have misdiagnosed themselves with vaginal yeast infections when the problem is a bacterial infection such as trichomoniasis or bacterial vaginosis. Some women are right about the yeast infections but have bacterial infections in addition. Vaginal discharge that smells fishy or "off," or a discharge that is greenish or yellowish, could indicate infection. Left untended, these types of infections can cause pregnancy complications or even infertility due to pelvic inflammatory disease (PID). Reestablishing the proper balance of good bacteria in the vagina will go a long way toward preventing and controlling these types of infections, as will promoting good immune function with vitamin C, zinc, and a high-potency multivitamin. Visit your ob-gyn if you are concerned about a vaginal infection.

Toenail Fungus. Toenail fungus is unsightly and uncomfortable and can cause the loss of toenails. It's extremely difficult to get rid of, and conventional drugs used to treat it are ineffective or dangerous. The imidazole antifungal drugs can cause headaches, dizziness, rashes, digestive problems, and photosensitivity, and they interact dangerously with a long list of other drugs, including antihistamines, any drug that puts extra stress on the liver, and alcohol. Drugs that suppress stomach acid can reduce the effectiveness of antifungals. Birth control pills can be made ineffective by antifungal drugs. Many of the antifungal drugs, but especially ketoconazole (Nizoral), can cause acute liver toxicity.

The worst part is that toenail fungus often comes back after the drugs are discontinued. There must be another way, right? Well, you can beat toenail fungus naturally, but you need to be rigorous about it for months and sometimes more than a year. Going barefoot in clean areas can help, because your feet stay dry and aired out, but avoid going barefoot in gyms and other public areas. You must keep your feet clean and dry as much as possible and not wear shoes that cause your feet to sweat.

To avoid reinfecting yourself, you'll need to douse your shoes with an over-the-counter antifungal powder to kill any lingering fungus there, and be sure to wash your socks in hot water and detergent. Also wipe down the bathroom, shower, and any other place you go barefoot with a mixture of soap and tea tree oil to kill fungus there.

Tea tree oil, garlic, and vinegar are effective antifungals. Here's a natural strategy for banishing toenail fungus: Every night before bed, soak your feet in a vinegar-and-water solution (1 cup per ½ gallon of water) for 10 minutes. Then soak them in a mixture of tea tree oil, and if you can stand the smell, garlic oil (6 to 8 drops of each) and warm water for half an hour. After that, thoroughly dry your feet, apply tea tree oil directly to the nails, and wear white cotton socks to bed. You will have to do this for at least three months to get rid of the fungus.

Just as with an internal fungus infection, it's important to support your body by avoiding sugar and taking probiotics.

Chapter 15

Drugs for Insomnia, Anxiety, and Depression and Their Natural Alternatives

In 2005, newer sleep drugs such as Ambien, Lunesta, and Rozerem were prescribed some 45 million times in the United States. It's amazing that so many Americans are having so much trouble falling asleep and staying asleep, but let's put that aside for now and look at rare side effects that are causing concern and conversation: sleepwalking, binge eating while asleep, and even sleep-driving.

Rosalind Cartwright, a 60-something college professor, took Ambien a few hours following some over-the-counter cold medicine. She headed to bed. At 3:30 A.M., she found herself on the floor hurting but too sleepy to do much about it, so she crawled back into her bed and fell asleep again. Cartwright had no history of sleepwalking. When she awoke in serious pain and bleeding, a trip to the ER revealed bleeding on the brain, four pelvic fractures, three broken ribs, and a fractured left wrist. What had she done in her sleep to be injured so severely?

This side effect of new sleep drugs combined with other medicines first gained notoriety in 2006, when Rhode Island representative Patrick Kennedy crashed into a barrier near Capitol Hill and blamed it on Ambien and another medication he had used with it. Others have reported similar examples of strange activities while under the drug's influence; over a dozen reports of sleep-driving have been made to the Food and Drug Administration (FDA). Laura J. Liddicoat, a forensic scientist who works at a lab in Wisconsin, reported in the *New York Times* that Ambien had been detected in the blood work of 53 drivers who exhibited erratic driving behavior. In Washington in 2005, Ambien played a role in 78 impaired-driver arrests. In some of these cases, drivers are doing more than weaving or running red lights: they're driving the wrong way or slamming into other cars and objects head-on. In many instances, they don't recognize or communicate with the officers who arrest them. One air traveler was arrested for tearing off his shirt and threatening other passengers—he remembered nothing between having taken Ambien, downing two of those airplane-sized bottles of wine, and waking up in a jail cell.

Many of the instances where Ambien and related sleep drugs cause problems have to do with its combination with alcohol or other medications. If you do decide you need to take sleep medications, don't go near alcohol, cold medicines, tranquilizers, or any other drugs that have potential hypnotic or sedative effects. And don't

make the mistake described in several reports of Ambien-related driving mishaps: the user took the drug on the way home so that it would "kick in" by the time he or she arrived.

One woman who took a single Ambien at bedtime woke up after having had a car accident and urinating in the middle of the street. She found a half-drunk bottle of wine on her kitchen counter after returning home and did not remember having consumed it. She had done so and then gotten behind the wheel, all while mostly asleep.

Although these side effects are rare, it just doesn't seem worth it to turn to sleep drugs when insomnia strikes. In this chapter you'll find many effective, natural, safe ways to encourage healthy and rejuvenating sleep without medications that can be addicting or dangerous.

Popping sleeping pills can be a tactic we use to avoid dealing with the issues that are causing us to lie awake tossing and turning at night. If emotions such as worry, frustration, stress, or anger are keeping you up, do the needed spiritual, practical, or interpersonal work to help you manage and put them aside when it's time to rest. Humans will never be free of worry—but we can learn to set it aside when we choose to do so.

Lack of sleep is one of the most common causes of daytime fatigue. Whether it's not being able to get to sleep, or waking several times each night, or never feeling as though you've gotten a good night's sleep, insomnia can take a huge toll on your quality of life. Fortunately for most people, it's relatively easy to remedy restless nights. The most obvious sleep robbers are the most common ones: stress, lack of exercise, caffeine, and prescription drugs. Having to get up at night repeatedly to urinate can disturb sleeping patterns enough to cause problems, as any man coping with an enlarged prostate gland can tell you. For women, menopause may bring on hot flashes and night sweats that disturb sleep.

Often when people are under stress and feel helpless to do anything about it, they lie awake at night tossing and turning with repetitive "tapes" going through their heads, or they wake up very early in the morning and can't get back to sleep. Big decisions, the illness or troubles of a loved one, major life changes, financial difficulties, and any number of the other lumps and bumps life hands out can all cause sleeplessness. Depression and anxiety will often cause sleeplessness, which creates a vicious circle of more depression and more sleeplessness.

Depression and Anxiety: Part of Being Human

Depression and related disorders are very common, with some 17 million Americans having the experience of depression each year. In the United States, depression is the most common cause of disability. According to predictions from the World Health Organization, it will be the most common cause of disability worldwide by the year 2020. Anxiety disorders include panic disorder, obsessive-compulsive disorder (OCD), post-traumatic stress disorder (PTSD), social phobia, other specific phobias, and generalized anxiety disorders. They are believed to affect even more people than depression: the National Institute of Mental Health estimates that 40 million Americans ages 18 and up have at least one of these anxiety disorders, and it states that most people with anxiety problems also have issues with depression.

In 2006, more antidepressants were sold than any other class of drug, with pharmaceutical companies raking in $20.6 billion. In 2007, there were more FDA warnings about the dan-

gers of antidepressants than any other class of drug. Most of the warnings were related to suicidal thoughts in adolescents who take these drugs. How many of those prescriptions were written to treat a clear case of severe depression or anxiety, and how many were written to people who were just feeling a bit blue or a bit stressed and thought that a little dose of this or that would save them the pain of experiencing and processing difficult, uncomfortable emotions and situations? How many saw an ad for one of these drugs and decided to heed its exhortations to "just ask your doctor"?

Prescribing data aren't specific enough to answer these questions with certainty. The most important question here is whether the drugs so widely used to medicate unhappiness are safe enough to hand out so freely, or whether they are, in fact, much less safe and effective than most people believe them to be.

Many respected experts agree that depression and anxiety are overdiagnosed and overmedicated. Although many who end up on drugs may not have really needed them, let's make one thing clear: *those of us who have never experienced a major depression or intense anxiety can never understand the experience of people who have.* Any person who has ever been severely depressed or anxious has been told at some point by a well-meaning loved one or friend, "Just snap out of it!" or "Get on with your life and you'll feel better!" or "Just relax!" or "Smile!" Depression and anxiety are both real problems for millions of people, and telling them they don't really have a problem or that it's something they should be able to shake off and "get over" does little good. These kinds of comments only make the person who is suffering feel more alone.

Of course, the question remains: where should the line be drawn between feeling down-

and-out or worrying too much, and the existence of a mental disorder that merits the use of medication? The psychiatric community has put a lot of time and effort into creating diagnostic criteria for depressive disorders and anxiety disorders, but making a diagnosis is far more subjective than some people might think. The diagnostic criteria for mental illnesses, all codified in the *Diagnostic and Statistical Manual of Mental Disorders* (DSM), have been created by committees of psychiatrists and other scientists, based on symptoms commonly seen. The DSM criteria are constantly changing; new diagnoses appear often.

No clinical test of brain chemicals exists to definitively answer the question of whether a person "has" a mental disorder or not. When we say someone has depression or anxiety, we're insinuating that the line between sick and not-sick is solid—but it isn't when it comes to these very common complaints. It's really just an educated guess. That fuzzy line has led to the prescription of brain neurotransmitter-tweaking medications to millions of people who might have been able to work through their issues with natural remedies and therapy.

A person who is clinically depressed is in pain—psychological pain with feelings of inadequacy, hopelessness, and sadness that often lead to suicidal ideation and, in some cases, suicide attempts, and sometimes, physical pain. The world begins to look sinister and ugly to a depressed person, and the things that once gave that person joy now do nothing to raise him or her up out of the quagmire. A depressed person might be unable to get out of bed, speak coherently, or engage in work, play, or relationships. In today's fear-drenched world, anxiety is a fact of life for most of us; the difference for a person with an anxiety disorder is that he or she is so fearful that normal functioning becomes extremely difficult or impossible. An anxious person is very often in a state of fight-or-flight, with all the physical manifestations of a creature in danger—danger that never seems to go away. Anxiety disrupts sleep and brings on distinctly physical symptoms. The diagnosis of anxiety disorder is often first considered when a patient goes to a doctor for physical symptoms like chest pain, dizziness, or shortness of breath. People who have panic attacks often report they feel like they are dying during the attacks.

Back in the 1950s, scientists doing studies on the old-school antidepressants reserpine and isoniazid found that these drugs changed neurotransmitter activity—and that in the majority of patients, they eased symptoms of depression. This led to a theory that a biochemical imbalance—specifically, an imbalance of neurotransmitters—was responsible for depression. This neat, tidy theory created an absolutely massive market for drugs designed to manipulate neurotransmitter levels. The theory lasted for half a century, and the huge market for drugs that affect the reuptake of serotonin and other neurotransmitters promises to long outlive it. But as the saying goes, the most beautiful theories are often slain by facts, and this theory was no exception. The truth, according to psychiatrist and director of the North Wales School of Psychological Medicine, David Healy, M.D., is that "no abnormality of serotonin in depression has ever been demonstrated."

In the world of psychiatry and psychiatric research, no one is talking about these chemical imbalances anymore. The real death-knell of this theory is the fact that the newest antidepressants, Cymbalta, Serzone, and Effexor, inhibit the reuptake not only of serotonin, but also of another neurotransmitter, norepinephrine. The drugs belong to a new class, the serotonin-norepinephrine reuptake inhibitors (SNRIs). Everything old is new again, including the idea that the best antidepressants are not highly specific magic bullets designed to correct an "imbalance" in a single neurotransmitter, but are those that have broader effects. (Natural therapies for depression and anxiety have broad effects as well.)

Neurotransmitter levels are responsive to your emotional state. If anyone ever does establish physical differences in neurotransmitter activity between depressed or anxious people and healthy people, they'll then face another daunting challenge: unraveling whether any changes in neurotransmitter levels or other kinds of brain activity that are found in depressed people are a cause or an effect of depression or anxiety. Neurotransmitters are active throughout our bodies in many, many ways, and when we alter their activity with drugs, we're entering territory that is far from completely mapped. John Horgan, in his book *The Undiscovered Mind*, writes, "Given the ubiquity of a neurotransmitter such as serotonin and the multiplicity of its functions, it is almost as meaningless to implicate it in depression as it is to implicate blood."

The risks of popular antidepressants make headlines often, with shocking revelations that drug companies have actively sought to suppress the public's knowledge of side effects (including suicidality, loss of libido and sexual function, severe withdrawal effects that convince the patient that he or she has to get back on the medications, and akathisia, a restlessness that can be severe enough to make the patient violent or suicidal).

Akathisia, which involves extreme restlessness, jitteriness, anxiety, and inability to sit still, is a major issue with all SSRIs. Prozac, the original, has been found to induce akathisia in between 9.7 and 25 percent of patients (this according to a review performed at Har-

vard University). In its labeling for Paxil, GlaxoSmithKline intentionally avoided the use of this term, choosing instead to describe the symptoms of akathisia as various other side effects — spreading the incidence out to reduce the appearance of akathisia as a significant issue with this drug. This would have enabled them to market their product as less likely to cause anxiety and jitteriness than other SSRIs. Akathisia can swoop in very quickly on a patient in the first three days of taking SSRIs, even at the lowest dose. Antidepressants now have to carry black-box warnings of increased risk of suicidal and violent behavior in those who use them. If you take antidepressants or have a loved one who makes this choice, please know that they all can increase risk of suicidal thinking or suicide attempts. This is more true in people under the age of 24.

The black-box warnings for these drugs state that "[a]ll patients being treated with antidepressants for any indication should be monitored appropriately and observed closely for clinical worsening, suicidality, and unusual changes in behavior, especially during the initial few months of a course of drug therapy, or at times of dose changes, either increases or decreases." Antidepressant information sheets for prescribing doctors also warn that

> . . . anxiety, agitation, panic attacks, insomnia, irritability, hostility, aggressiveness, impulsivity, akathisia, hypomania, and mania, have been reported in adult and pediatric patients being treated with antidepressants for major depressive disorder as well as for other indications, both psychiatric and nonpsychiatric. Although a causal link between the emergence of such symptoms and either the worsening of depression and/or the emergence of suicidal impulses has not been established, there is

concern that such symptoms may represent precursors to emerging suicidality.

Not only are antidepressants less safe than people are led to believe; they are also less effective than most people know. A team that used the Freedom of Information Act to access both published and unpublished studies on SSRI effectiveness found that these drugs were only barely more effective than placebo. A study published in the January 17, 2008, issue of the *New England Journal of Medicine* reinforces this question mark. The study's authors found that while 94 percent of antidepressant studies published in medical journals had positive results (i.e., the drug had more beneficial effects than placebo pills on people with depression), only 51 percent of studies on antidepressants in the FDA's registry had positive results. In other words, the studies published in medical journals have not given an accurate picture of the effectiveness of antidepressant drugs. If you do try an antidepressant, don't be surprised if it doesn't work or if you try two or three different versions before you find one with the desired effect. If you take the drugs for a long time, don't be surprised if they become ineffective. At that point, you may find yourself being prescribed ever-higher doses of medication or even having drugs added to the mix. This is not a scientific practice, folks. In doing this kind of trial-and-error prescribing, psychiatry is conducting a massive, uncontrolled experiment on millions of people's brains. Don't go there unless absolutely necessary.

Today, anxiety is often treated with the same kinds of drugs used to treat depression. The benzodiazepines (such as Ativan, Xanax, Halcion) and other tranquilizers that once were commonly prescribed for anxiety are addictive and produce too many side effects for long-term use, including drowsiness, memory impairment, and poor coordination. Withdrawal from these drugs can cause psychosis, insomnia, even seizures. In some cases, these antianxiety drugs become the *cause* of anxiety that just happens to manifest in a person who is using them to treat depression. Anxiety is a known side effect of antianxiety drugs, just as depression is a known side effect of the antidepressants.

In the short term, if a person is in great distress and needs fast help, these prescription drugs may be the lesser evils—even though they are not always effective and may make things worse. But they are not long-term solutions, and for many people who are not in extreme states of anxiety or depression, they may not be necessary at all. So if we are to turn away from the pharmaceutical fix-it for depression and anxiety, what do we turn *to*? This is the question we would like to begin to answer in the latter half of this chapter.

First, let's look at the most-prescribed sleeping pills, antidepressants, and antianxiety drugs. If you do choose to take them, please educate yourself well about side effects, potential for abuse, and potential for addiction. Please remember they are not lightweight drugs. None has been proven safe for long-term use (more than two years), and many have been essentially banned for use by children 12 and under.

Of particular concern is the effect of antianxiety drugs and sleep-inducing drugs on drivers. According to an organization called Citizens Against Drug-Impaired Drivers (CANDID), prescription and over-the-counter medications that cause drowsiness contribute to more than 100,000 car crashes a year. If your drug insert warns against driving while under the influence of the drug, please take that warning seriously!

Examples of Prescription Drugs for Sleep

Zolpidem tartrate (Ambien, Ambien CR)

What Does It Do in the Body? This drug has a hypnotic, sedative, muscle relaxant effect, which it achieves by altering neurotransmitter channels in the brain. *CR* stands for "controlled release," a version of the drug that has longer-lasting effects.

What Is It Used For? To aid sleep.

What Are the Potential Side Effects? In clinical trials of this drug, 4 to 6 percent of subjects stopped taking Ambien because they were so bothered by side effects. The most common is headache. Others include drowsiness, dizziness, lethargy, a "drugged" feeling, light-headedness, depression, abnormal dreams, amnesia, anxiety, nervousness, sleep disorder, allergy, back pain, flulike symptoms, chest pain, fatigue, nausea, stomach upset, diarrhea, abdominal pain, constipation, loss of appetite, vomiting, muscle pain, upper respiratory infection, sinus and throat inflammation, runny nose, rash, urinary tract infection, palpitations, and dry mouth. Dozens of other side effects may occur, but they are more rare.

CAUTION!

Ambien should be used only for 7 to 10 days at a time. Insomnia may at its root be caused by an underlying physical or psychiatric disorder, and if you need to use drugs to get to sleep for more than a week to 10 days, you should look deeper and try to solve the problem. Other important tips:

- Be sure to use the smallest effective dose of this drug.
- If you have breathing problems such as asthma or emphysema, use sedatives with caution, as they can depress the body's instinctual drive to breathe.
- If you have been addicted to any drug, you should know that zolpidem tartrate can be addictive.

- Any sedative or hypnotic drug can cause abnormal thinking and behavioral changes much like those caused by alcohol. Decreased inhibition and increased aggression, bizarre behavior, hallucinations, feelings of unreality, and amnesia could be attributed to taking this drug.
- If you are suffering from depression, this drug may make it worse and even precipitate suicidal thinking.
- Abrupt discontinuation of Ambien can lead to withdrawal symptoms ranging from a mild downshift in mood and insomnia to abdominal or muscle cramps, vomiting, sweating, tremors, and convulsions.
- This drug has a very rapid onset of action, so only take it right before going to bed. It may affect your ability to drive or operate machinery, even the following day, so use caution.
- Those with impaired liver function should use this drug with caution if at all.
- If you are elderly or debilitated, you may have heightened sensitivity to this drug, and you should be monitored carefully.

Be Aware. Do not combine Ambien with alcohol or narcotics.

Zaleplon (Sonata)

What Does It Do in the Body? It affects neurotransmitter channels in the brain, bringing on sleepiness and relaxation, and relieving anxiety. Its mechanism of action is similar to that of Ambien, but it is a faster-acting drug.

What Is It Used For? A sleep aid.

What Are the Potential Side Effects? Three-and-a-half percent of subjects who took Sonata in clinical trials discontinued the drug because of adverse effects. The most common included migraine, depression, nervousness, difficulty

Sleep Aids Associated with Strange Sleep Behaviors

In 2007, the FDA released a warning about the danger of sleepwalking, sleep-eating, sleep-driving, and other complex behaviors occurring in people under the influence of the following sleep drugs:

Ambien/Ambien CR
Lunesta
Rozerem
Sonata
Butisol sodium
Carbrital
Seconal (barbiturates; rarely prescribed)
Dalmane
Doral
Halcion
Prosom
Restoril (benzodiazepines)
Placidyl (a highly addictive and rarely prescribed sleep medicine)

These behaviors are more likely in people who use other medications or drink alcohol after taking the sleep drug. The FDA also warns that the drugs in this list have significant risk of causing a severe allergic reaction.

CAUTION!

Insomnia should not be treated with Sonata for more than 7 to 10 days. This drug can cause changes in thinking and behavior, including uncharacteristic aggression, extroversion, agitation, and hallucinations. Sudden stopping of the drug can cause symptoms of withdrawal; talk to your doctor about tapering off if you must use this drug. Take Sonata only right before bed, and be aware that it could affect your coordination and alertness in the morning.

Be Aware. Never mix zaleplon with alcohol or narcotics. If taken with a heavy, high-fat meal, concentrating, rash, itching, constipation, dry mouth, exacerbation of arthritis symptoms, bronchitis, conjunctivitis, back pain, and chest pain. Higher doses were more likely to bring about adverse effects.

Sleep Problems Can Be a Result of Other Conditions

All of the hypnotic sleep drugs carry a warning in their prescribing information about the possibility that difficulty sleeping could be a symptom of some other health problem that needs to be addressed. Doctors are directed to thoroughly evaluate patients with sleep problems before prescribing these drugs, to make sure that no other physical or psychological issue needs to be addressed to heal the insomnia. Some people who were enrolled as subjects in studies of these kinds of drugs had worsening insomnia or other thought or behavior abnormalities emerge during drug treatment.

Keep in mind, however, that the use of a consciousness-altering medication could easily be the cause of these seemingly new abnormalities. This is a common issue with psychiatric drugs: the patient goes to the doctor with a psychiatric complaint, gets on a medication, and then has some other "previously masked" psychiatric complaint "emerge" while on the drug. No one really knows whether the drug is unmasking these previously masked conditions—or causing them.

the drug's absorption may be delayed. The drug rifampin can decrease zaleplon's effectiveness, and cimetidine increases it.

Eszopiclone (Lunesta)

What Does It Do in the Body? No one is quite sure how eszopiclone works to bring on sleep. It is believed to work via effects on receptors for the relaxant neurotransmitter GABA.

What Is It Used For? A sleep aid.

What Are the Potential Side Effects? The most common complaint with this drug is an unpleasant taste in the mouth, which affected about one-third of those taking the highest dose and about one-fourth of those taking the lower dose in preapproval studies. Other side effects are memory impairment, sleepiness, headache, infection, dry mouth, upset stomach, vomiting, anxiety, confusion, depression, dizziness, hallucinations, decreased libido, nervousness, and rash.

CAUTION!

Insomnia should not be treated with Lunesta for more than 7 to 10 days. This drug can cause changes in thinking and behavior, including uncharacteristic aggression, extroversion, agitation, a feeling of detachment, amnesia, and worsening of pre-existing depression or suicidal thinking. There have been reports of withdrawal symptoms after several weeks of use, leading to symptoms such as anxiety, abnormal dreams, intense sensitivity to stimuli, or neurosis. Talk to your doctor about tapering off if you must use this drug. Only take Lunesta right before bed, and be aware that it could affect your coordination and alertness in the morning.

Be Aware. Never mix eszopiclone with alcohol or narcotics. If taken with a heavy, high-fat meal, the drug's absorption may be delayed. The drug olanzapine can interact to increase cognitive impairment when taken with eszopiclone, and rifampin can decrease its effectiveness.

Ramelteon (Rozerem)

What Does It Do in the Body? It affects receptors for the hormone melatonin, which is produced in the brain and brings on sleep.

What Is It Used For? To aid sleep in people with insomnia characterized by difficulty falling asleep (as opposed to difficulty staying asleep). Unlike other sleep drugs, Rozerem has not been found to have risks of rebound insomnia, addiction, or withdrawal symptoms.

What Are the Potential Side Effects? Sleepiness, fatigue, dizziness, nausea, worsening insomnia, upper respiratory tract infection, muscle pain, depression, distortion of sense of taste, joint pain, flu, increased blood cortisol levels.

Galactorrhea (milk production) in nonnursing women, cessation of menstrual periods, decreased libido, or reduced fertility can indicate an effect of ramelteon on levels of the hormones prolactin and testosterone.

CAUTION!

Think Twice About Taking This Drug If . . .

- You have been diagnosed with sleep apnea or chronic obstructive pulmonary disease (COPD).
- You are depressed or have had suicidal thoughts. Ramelteon has been associated with worsening of both depression and suicidal thinking.
- You have kidney impairment.

Be Aware. Ramelteon should not be taken with fluvoxamine (Luvox). Taking ramelteon with or just after a high-fat meal may reduce the drug's effectiveness.

Examples of Nonprescription Antihistamine Sleep Aids

Diphenhydramine (Benadryl, Dormin Caplets, Miles Nervine Caplets, Nytol, Sleep-Eze 3, Sleepwell 2-nite, Sominex 2, Extra Strength Tylenol PM, Aspirin Free Anacin P.M. Caplets, Bayer Select Maximum Strength Night Time Pain Relief Caplets, Sominex Pain Relief, Bufferin AF Nite Time Caplets, Excedrin P.M., Unisom with Pain Relief, Compoz Nighttime Sleep Aid, Sominex Caplets, Twilite, Compoz Gel Caps, Dormin, Maximum Strength Sleepinal Capsules and Soft Gels, Maximum Strength Unisom SleepGels, Nighttime Pamprin)
Doxylamine (Unisom Nighttime)

What Do They Do in the Body? These drugs contain antihistamines, which cause sleepiness. Some contain pain relievers to help those in pain to sleep.

What Are They Used For? Relief of insomnia and pain. More than 30 percent of adults use nonprescription drugs to help them sleep.

What Are the Potential Side Effects? Dry mouth and throat, constipation, ringing in the ears, and blurred vision may occur. In older men, prostate enlargement and difficult urination can be side effects of these drugs. Elderly people are prone to other side effects such as delirium, excitement, nervousness, and agitation.

CAUTION!

Think Twice About Taking These Drugs If . . .

- You have asthma, chronic lung disease, glaucoma, or prostate gland enlargement.
- You still need them after two weeks. (Look for the underlying cause.)

Never use over-the-counter sleep aids for more than two weeks at a time.

Avoid driving or other hazardous tasks requiring coordination or dexterity while using these medications.

Be Aware. Any sedating drug will add to the depressant effects of sleeping pills. Avoid using prescription sedatives and alcohol with doxylamine or diphenhydramine.

Antianxiety Drugs

The "benzos" are divided into two subclasses: the hypnotics (sleep-inducing) and the anxiolytics (anxiety-reducing). Hypnotics are shorter-acting than anxiolytics—their effect is more intense and lasts for less time—and are usually the choice for treating insomnia. Withdrawal symptoms between doses and cravings for the next dose are more likely with short-acting versions. All benzodiazepine generic names end in *-pam* or *-lam*.

Examples of Hypnotic and Anxiolytic Benzodiazepines

Hypnotic benzodiazepines: brotizolam (Lendormin), estazolam (ProSom), flunitrazepam (Rohypnol, Hypnodorm), flurazepam (Dalmane), loprazolam (Dormonoct), lormetazepam (Loramet), midazolam (Versed, Dormicum), nimetazepam (Ermin), nitrazepam (Alodorm, Mogadon), temazepam (Normison, Restoril), triazolam (Halcion)

Anxiolytic benzodiazepines: alprazolam (Xanax), bromazepam (Lexotan, Lexotanil), chlordiazepoxide (Librium), clonazepam (Klonopin, Rivotril), clorazepate (Tranxene), diazepam (Valium), lorazepam (Ativan, Tavor, Temesta), oxazepam (Serax, Serepax), prazepam (Centrax, Lysanxia)

What Do They Do in the Body? We don't have an in-depth understanding of how these drugs work, but we do know that they affect the action of neurotransmitters in the brain, bringing about relaxation and decreased anxiety.

What Are They Used For? Small doses quell anxiety. Often, they are prescribed in tandem with antidepressants to reduce the anxiety that the antidepressant drugs may cause. In higher doses, benzodiazepines are prescribed as sleep aids. Benzodiazepines are also used as antiseizure and antiepileptic drugs, and as muscle relaxants. They may be given right before an unpleasant medical procedure or as a preparation for more intense anesthesia before surgery. These drugs are also prescribed for irritable bowel syndrome, restless legs syndrome, nausea and vomiting caused by chemotherapy, panic attacks, depression, and premenstrual syndrome (Xanax), acute withdrawal from alcohol addiction, and chronic insomnia. They do not heal any of these health problems; they only temporarily relieve symptoms.

What Are the Potential Side Effects? Transient mild drowsiness in the first few days of use is common. This side effect may be more pronounced in the elderly or debilitated, who are more likely to experience loss of muscular coordination and confusion when starting out on a course of benzodiazepines.

Other possible side effects include sedation, depression, lethargy, apathy, fatigue, decreased activity, light-headedness, memory impairment, disorientation, amnesia, restlessness, confusion, crying, delirium, headache, slurred speech, loss of voice, stupor, seizures, coma, fainting, rigidity, tremor, abnormal muscle tone, vertigo, dizziness, euphoria, nervousness, irritability, difficulty concentrating, agitation, inability to perform complex mental functions, paralysis of half the body, unsteadiness, loss of coordination, strange dreams, glassy-eyed appearance, paradoxical reactions (increased anxiety or hyperactivity), behavior problems, hysteria, psychosis, suicidal tendencies, constipation, diarrhea, dry mouth, coated tongue, sore gums, nausea, changes in appetite, vomiting, difficulty swallowing, increased salivation, stomach inflammation, incontinence, changes in libido, urinary and menstrual problems, heart rhythm and blood pressure changes, cardiovascular collapse, retention of fluid in the face and ankles, palpitations, vision disturbances, twitching of the eyeballs, decreased hearing, nasal congestion, auditory disturbances, rashes, itching, hair loss or growth, hiccups, fever, sweating, tingling of the extremities, muscular disturbances, growth of breasts in males, milk production in the breasts of females, respiratory disturbances, increased levels of enzymes in the bloodstream indicating tissue damage, hepatitis or jaundice (both very rarely), changes in blood cell counts, decrease in body weight, swelling of lymph nodes, and joint pain.

CAUTION!

- Don't take these drugs if you have a psychological disorder that doesn't have anxiety as a prominent feature and is mainly manifested as depression.
- The long-term effectiveness (four months or more of treatment) of these drugs has not been assessed. Please don't use these drugs long term.

- These drugs may cause drowsiness, so avoid driving or other tasks that require alertness.
- Dependency can occur in as little as two weeks. Withdrawal symptoms may include anxiety, sensory disturbances, sleeping too much, flulike symptoms, difficulty concentrating, fatigue, restlessness, loss of appetite, dizziness, sweating, vomiting, insomnia, irritability, nausea, headache, muscle tension or cramping, tremor, vocal changes, confusion, abnormal perception, depersonalization, muscle twitches, psychosis, paranoid delusions, hallucinations, memory impairment, and grand mal seizures. If you have been using benzodiazepines regularly for a couple of weeks or more, decrease the dosage gradually and carefully.
- Rarely, people have what are known as paradoxical reactions to benzodiazepines: instead of becoming calmer, less anxious, or more sleepy, they may become manic, angry, impulsive, anxious, or suicidal, or even display symptoms of schizophrenia. If symptoms like these emerge during benzodiazepine therapy, your medical team may want to see it as the emergence of a previously masked mental illness—but it may be simply a drug side effect.
- Alcoholics may be put at extra risk if they take benzodiazepines. A study published in the journal *Behavioral Pharmacology* found that when people who tend toward alcoholism take even low doses of a benzodiazepine, they tend to consume more alcohol.
- Use caution if you have liver problems or if you are elderly or debilitated; you may need a lower dose.

Be Aware. Benzodizepines can interact dangerously with many other drugs. Do not add a new drug without consulting a pharmacist or reading the drug information sheet.

Reportedly, the herb kava-kava can potentiate (increase) the intensity of a benzodiazepine's effects—severely enough to lead to coma.

What Are the Interactions with Food? Don't drink alcohol while using these drugs. Avoid charcoal-broiled foods, as they increase the rate at which this drug is emptied from your system. You can take benzodiazepines with water or food if stomach upset occurs, but this may slow down the absorption of the drug.

Antidepressant Drugs

Examples of Tricyclic Antidepressants

Nortriptyline (Pamelor)
Amitriptyline (Elavil)
Imipramine (Tofranil)
Clomipramine (Anafranil)

What Do They Do in the Body? They affect levels of the neurotransmitters serotonin, norepinephrine, and dopamine in the synapses between nerve cells.

What Are They Used For? Tricyclics are older drugs, first developed to treat depression. They can help relieve symptoms of anxiety disorders, including panic disorder and obsessive-compulsive disorder. They may also be used to treat attention-deficit/hyperactivity disorder (ADHD), chronic headache pain, diabetic neuropathy, cancer pain, and bed-wetting, and are sometimes prescribed for migraine prevention.

What Are the Potential Side Effects? Tricyclics have a long, long list of adverse effects, which is one reason they have been almost completely replaced for treatment of depression and anxiety with newer SSRI and SNRI drugs. These effects may include sedation; dry mouth; blurred vision; problems focusing; increased intraocular pressure that can lead to glaucoma; dilation of the pupils; constipation; dysfunction of parts of the small intestine; urinary problems; drastic dips in blood pressure when going from lying to sitting or from sitting to standing; high blood pressure; heart rhythm abnormalities; congestive heart failure (CHF); stroke; electrocardiogram changes (indicating damage to heart tissue); confusion (especially in the elderly); disturbed concentration; hallucinations; disorientation; impaired memory; feelings of unreality; delusions; anxiety; nervousness; restlessness; agitation; panic; insomnia; nightmares; mania; worsening of psychotic symptoms; drowsiness; dizziness; weakness; fatigue; headache; depression; excessive tension in the muscles or artery walls; sleep disorders; psychosomatic disorders; yawning; abnormal dreaming; migraines; depersonalization; irritability and mood swings; numbness; tingling; hyperactivity; lack of coordination; tremors; peripheral neuropathy; seizures; twitching; partial paralysis; allergic reactions, including rash, itching, and swelling; changes in blood cell counts; nausea; vomiting; loss of appetite; diarrhea; flatulence; trouble swallowing; strange taste in the mouth; increased salivation; abdominal cramps; inflammation of the stomach, throat, or esophagus; black tongue; indigestion; breast development in males; testicular swelling; breast enlargement; spontaneous flow of milk; vaginitis and menstrual difficulties in women; changes in libido; painful ejaculation; voiding of urine during the night; cystitis; urinary tract infection; changes in blood glucose levels; increased secretion of the hormones prolactin and vasopressin (antidiuretic hormone); pharyngitis; laryngitis;

sinusitis; coughing; spasm of the airways; nosebleed; shortness of breath; problems speaking; ringing of the ears; excessive tearing of the eyes; conjunctivitis; difference in the size of the pupils; inner ear inflammation; eye allergy symptoms; nasal congestion; excessive appetite; body weight changes; increased sweating; high body temperature; flushing; chills; hair loss; dental problems; abnormal skin odor; chest pain; fever; bad breath; thirst; back pain; and joint aches. In some people, tricyclic antidepressants cause increased sensitivity to the sun.

CAUTION!

Think Twice About Taking These Drugs If . . .

- You have recently had a heart attack. If you have any other heart problems, use extreme caution.
- You are taking an MAOI.
- You have any of the following health problems: seizure disorders, difficulty urinating, spasm of the urethra or ureter, angle-closure glaucoma (even the average dose can cause an attack of glaucoma and permanent loss of vision), high intraocular pressure, or high levels of thyroid hormone (hyperthyroidism), or if you are taking any kind of drug to regulate thyroid hormone levels, or kidney or liver disease. You should be closely monitored while taking tricyclics.
- You are taking anticholinergic drugs such as those prescribed for Parkinson's disease. You may not react well to tricyclics, so use caution.

Your ability to drive and perform hazardous tasks may be impaired while using tricyclics. The symptoms of both manic depression and schizophrenia may be worsened by tricyclic antidepressants.

You should stop taking tricyclics for as long as possible before having elective surgery. Work with your doctor on this, though; don't stop cold on your own.

If you develop a fever or sore throat while taking this medication, it may be an indication of a serious drug-related side effect.

Be Aware. When combined with cimetidine, methylphenidate (Ritalin), antipsychotic drugs, or calcium channel blockers, levels of tricyclic antidepressants in the bloodstream can rise to dangerous levels.

Drugs given to regulate heartbeat can interact dangerously with tricyclics, leading to potentially fatal changes in heart rhythm. So can antipsychotics and the antihistamines astemizole and terfenadine. Never mix tricyclics with alcohol, benzodiazepines, or barbiturates, as they will have additive effects.

Stopping these drugs suddenly can cause symptoms like nausea, dizziness, headache, lethargy, and flulike symptoms.

Suicidal thoughts or depression may get worse while you are taking tricyclics.

Examples of Monoamine Oxidase Inhibitors (MAOIs)

Phenelzine (Nardil)
Tranylcypromine (Parnate)
Isocarboxazid (Marplan)

What Do They Do in the Body? These drugs, which belong to the oldest existing class of antidepressant medicines, block an enzyme that breaks down the neurotransmitters serotonin, norepinephrine, and dopamine in the brain.

What Are They Used For? Treatment of panic disorder, social phobia, and depression.

What Are the Potential Side Effects? Because they cause a long list of potentially serious adverse effects, these drugs are not used unless others prove ineffective or inappropriate. They include drowsiness, constipation, nausea, diarrhea, stomach upset, fatigue, dry mouth, dizziness, low blood pressure, light-headedness, reduced urine output, reduced sexual function, sleep disturbances, muscle twitching, increased appetite, weight gain, blurred vision, headache, restlessness, shakiness, trembling, weakness, and sweating.

What Are the Interactions With Other Drugs? The MAOIs interact dangerously with a very long list of other medications. These interactions usually involve a spike in blood pressure or a spike in levels of serotonin great enough to cause a life-threatening "serotonin storm." A partial list of medications that can have either or both of these effects when combined with MAOIs: desipramine, clomipramine, bupropion, SSRIs, trazodone, nefazodone, mirtazapine, venlafaxine, bronchodilating asthma inhalers, theophylline, terfenadine, dextromethorphan, oxymetazoline, phenylephrine, pseudoephedrine, dopamine, isoproterenol, metaraminol, carbamazepine, lithium, L-tryptophan, and methyldopa. Overall, any person taking an MAOI should never add a drug or herbal supplement without clearance from his or her psychiatrist and pharmacist.

When MAOIs are combined with insulin or hypoglycemic drugs, blood sugar may drop too fast.

Some blood-pressure-lowering drugs may cause pressure to fall too low when combined with MAOIs; others may cause it to rise too high.

When combined with alcohol, barbiturates, buspirone, or tranquilizers, MAOIs can have additive effects, causing extreme sleepiness.

What Are the Interactions with Food? MAOIs can be deadly when combined with foods that contain the amino acid tyramine. It interacts with MAOIs to cause a rapid, extreme spike in blood pressure, leading to severe headache, sweating, palpitations, and even heart arrhythmia, heart failure, or brain hemorrhage. Any person on MAOIs is best off avoiding alcoholic beverages entirely, as well as nonalcoholic beers and wines. Fava beans, cheeses (except for cream and cottage cheese), tofu, miso, aged meat, smoked fish, fermented fish, pickled fish, and other fermented soy products must also be avoided. Also not allowed are ginseng, meat extracts (as might be found in a seasoning packet), protein powders, avocado, soy sauce, sausage, bologna, pepperoni, salami, sauerkraut, shrimp paste, soups, and yeast. If you end up taking MAOIs, your doctor will give you a comprehensive list of foods to avoid.

Buspirone (BuSpar)

What Does It Do in the Body? It is not known exactly how buspirone works.

What Is It Used For? Treatment of anxiety.

What Are the Potential Side Effects? Buspirone may cause temporary or permanent damage to the nervous system. It can also cause drug dependence, sedation, and withdrawal reactions. Adverse reactions have included dizziness, drowsiness, restlessness, nervousness, insomnia, light-headedness, nausea, numbness, headache, fatigue, dream disturbances, tinnitus, sore throat, and nasal congestion. There are dozens and dozens of individualized side effects possible with

this drug, most having to do with interference with or damage to the nervous system.

CAUTION!

Please think twice about taking this drug, period. There are too many other safer alternatives.

Examples of Selective Serotonin Reuptake Inhibitors (SSRIs)

Citalopram (Celexa)
Escitalopram (Lexapro)
Fluoxetine (Prozac, Sarafem)
Fluvoxamine (Luvox)
Paroxetine (Paxil)
Sertraline (Zoloft)

What Do They Do in the Body? Neurons use a neurotransmitter substance called serotonin to relay messages through the nervous system. Researchers found that some people who suffer from depression have low levels of serotonin in their synapses. SSRIs inhibit the reuptake of serotonin and so allow more of it to remain in the synapses for a longer period. SSRIs also weakly inhibit the neuronal uptake of norepinephrine and dopamine, which also play a role in mood.

What Are They Used For? Depression (fluoxetine, paroxetine, sertraline, citalopram, escitalopram), generalized anxiety disorder (paroxetine, escitalopram), obsessive-compulsive disorder (fluvoxamine, fluoxetine, paroxetine, sertraline), bulimia nervosa (fluoxetine), panic disorder (sertraline, paroxetine), and premenstrual syndrome (fluoxetine, paroxetine, sertraline).

These drugs are also prescribed off-label for just about any ailment you can think of, for periods of time that extend far beyond what is known to be safe. According to a 2005 report published by the Medical Expenditure Panel of the Agency for Healthcare Research and Quality (AHRQ), 11 percent of noninstitutionalized women and 5 percent of noninstitutionalized men in the United States are taking an antidepressant.

While it's true that a small number of people with serious psychological problems can benefit from the short-term use of these drugs, in the majority of instances they are used to treat people who are only mildly depressed, going through a tough time in their lives, or think their personality or feelings are somehow wrong and are improved on medication. General practitioners and ob-gyn physicians untrained in psychiatry are passing out prescriptions for these drugs without a second thought. Taking antidepressants for these reasons is the ultimate symptom of thinking we all should behave alike and be happy all the time.

SSRIs create a false sense of emotional detachment, allowing those who use them to disengage from their problems rather than solve them.

What Are the Potential Side Effects? According to a report in *New Scientist*, researchers at the Weill Cornell Medical Center found that men who take SSRI antidepressants have more sperm with damaged DNA, which is not viable for fertilizing an egg. This could be significant to couples who are trying to get pregnant.

Multiple new studies suggest that SSRIs can substantially increase the risk for bleeding ulcers and other gastrointestinal upset, especially when combined with NSAIDs such as aspirin and ibuprofen.

In clinical trials, 15 percent of those on Prozac, 20 percent of those on Paxil, 10 to 15 percent of those on Zoloft, 22 percent of those on Luvox, and 16 percent of those on Celexa stopped using the drugs because of adverse effects.

Nervousness, insomnia (especially with Zoloft), drowsiness (especially with Paxil), fatigue, weakness, tremor, increased sweating, dizziness, anxiety, irritability, headache (especially with Paxil), dry mouth (with Zoloft and Paxil), loss of appetite, nausea (seen most with Luvox, but experienced by more than 20 percent of subjects for all the SSRIs), diarrhea, stomach discomfort (Prozac and Zoloft), altered appetite and weight, and constipation (Paxil). Because SSRIs reduce testosterone levels, there is substantial risk of sexual dysfunction and loss of libido in both men and women who take them.

Rash, fever, joint pain, abnormal changes in blood cell counts, swelling, excessive excretion of protein in the urine indicating liver or kidney damage, and elevated enzymes in the bloodstream (also indicating tissue damage) have occurred in some people who use Prozac. If you experience any of these symptoms, you probably are sensitive to it and should stop taking it. People who continue to use it after developing these symptoms may end up having a life-threatening anaphylactic reaction.

For the prescribing physician, figuring out which antidepressant to prescribe involves far more guesswork and trial-and-error than you might imagine. Only half of the time does the first antidepressant prescribed work well without negative side effects that make the person want to go off of the drug. Switching to new drugs and adding drugs to try to balance out side effects is standard practice. In recent years, genetic testing has been studied as a way to circumvent this process of trial and error; with a blood test, the action of specific detoxification enzymes in the body can be "typed" in a way that helps predict which antidepressants will cause the most side effects. This type of testing measures how fast your body processes antidepressants, which also helps the doctor rule out the antidepressants least likely to be effective at improving your mood and to prescribe a dose level that is least likely to bring on side effects. Unfortunately, the test can't be used to measure the effects of all antidepressants — only of a few SSRIs (fluoxetine, paroxetine, venlafaxine) and a few of the tricyclics (imipramine, desipramine, nortriptyline, clomipramine).

SSRIs can interact with other drugs to cause potentially fatal "serotonin syndrome." Synapses become so flooded with serotonin that hallucinations, agitation, confusion, fluctuating blood pressure, seizures, fever, stiffness, and irregular heartbeat result. SSRIs can also bring about abnormal (excessive) bleeding when used along with aspirin, warfarin, or NSAIDs.

Significant withdrawal syndromes are often experienced when discontinuing the SSRIs, especially with the short-acting SSRIs such as Paxil, Zoloft, and Luvox. The effects of withdrawal can include dizziness, nausea, headache, fatigue, poor concentration, electric shocklike sensations, visual hallucinations, mental fogginess, and moodiness. If you're withdrawing from SSRIs, do it gradually, over a period of one to two weeks, and if you need to, use the natural alternatives given at the end of this chapter under the supervision of a health care professional who is familiar with their use.

CAUTION!

- Clinical trials of most of these drugs have lasted only for 5 to 16 weeks. Studies of Prozac have lasted for up to a year. In other words, the long-term effects of these drugs have not been systematically studied.
- Because of the risk of serotonin storm, which can be fatal, none of the SSRIs should be taken with any MAOI, additional SSRI, SNRI, or tricyclic antidepres-

sant. The weight-loss drug sibutramine (Meridia) works on serotonin-reuptake channels and should also not be added to SSRIs. Don't take SSRIs with MAOIs or within 14 days of stopping MAOIs. The antibiotic drug linezolid, which can have effects on monoamine oxidase similar to those of MAOIs, should also be avoided with SSRIs. For the same reasons, avoid using other serotonin-raising substances in combination with these drugs, including amphetamines, buspirone, amantadine, bromocriptine, St. John's wort, the amino acid tryptophan, and 5-HTP.

- Please avoid these drugs if you have impaired liver function.
- If you tend to be manic, SSRIs may make you more so. In an article published in 2006, psychiatrist Peter Breggin, M.D., wrote about a phenomenon he called medication spellbinding. Those who develop this rare but dangerous side effect while on SSRIs enter a manic state where committing crimes or harming others does not seem wrong. In one case related by Dr. Breggin, a man with no criminal record robbed banks while under the influence of SSRIs and didn't even seem perturbed when sent to prison — until the drugs wore off. In other more tragic cases, people on these medications harm themselves or others without realizing that what they are doing is wrong. Psychiatrists sometimes point the finger at a pre-existing psychosis that is somehow "activated" or "unmasked" by the SSRIs — an explanation that seems to go against the medical school dictum, "When you hear hoofbeats, think horses, not zebras." In other words, when you give someone a drug and the person drops into psychosis, doesn't

the source of the problem seem plenty obvious? Dr. Breggin, the world's best-known expert on the harmful effects of SSRIs and other psychiatric drugs, thinks so.

- Use caution when taking this drug if you have a history of seizures.
- If you are using diuretics to lower blood pressure, Prozac and Paxil can make it more likely that you will have electrolyte imbalances. These imbalances can cause heart rhythm disturbances.
- If you are diabetic, you should know that Prozac can make low blood sugar more likely, and high blood sugar can hit when the drug is stopped. Dosages of insulin and sulfonylurea drugs may require adjustment when taken with this drug.
- If depression has made you feel suicidal, be aware that SSRIs could increase the likelihood that you'll follow through on thoughts of suicide or violent behavior.
- SSRIs can cause drowsiness or dizziness. Use caution while driving, performing tasks requiring alertness, or operating machinery.

Be Aware. Fluvoxamine inhibits enzymes that metabolize warfarin, theophylline, propanolol, and alprazolam. This could cause an increase in levels of these drugs.

What Are the Interactions with Food? You can take SSRIs with or without food. Avoid alcohol while taking SSRIs.

Other Antidepressants

Bupropion (Wellbutrin, Zyban)

What Does It Do in the Body? This drug is a tetracyclic antidepressant. It weakly inhibits the reuptake of serotonin and dopamine, neurotrans-

mitters that play important roles in determining your mood. This drug doesn't fit into any of the categories most antidepressants do, and no one knows just exactly how it works.

What Is It Used For? Treatment of depression, nicotine withdrawal.

What Are the Potential Side Effects? Ten percent of the people who took this drug in clinical trials stopped because of problems with side effects. The most common were rashes; psychological disturbances such as agitation and mental status changes; neurological disturbances such as seizures, headache, and sleep disturbances; and gastrointestinal disturbances such as nausea and vomiting.

Other side effects may include constipation, weight loss (may be up to 5 pounds), increased appetite, stomach discomfort, menstrual problems, dry mouth, excessive sweating, tremor, insomnia, auditory disturbances, blurred vision, taste disturbances, dizziness, cardiac arrhythmias, high blood pressure, palpitations, fainting, agitation, confusion, hostility, decreased libido, anxiety, euphoria, fever, and chills.

CAUTION!

Think Twice About Taking This Drug If . . .

- You have a seizure disorder; it increases your risk of seizures.
- You have or have had bulimia or anorexia.
- You are switching from MAOIs to Wellbutrin. At least 14 days should elapse between your last dose of MAOIs to the first of Wellbutrin. Don't take this drug with MAOIs.
- You have recently had a heart attack or any other kind of unstable heart disease. Bupropion should be used with care.

- You are taking other antidepressants or antipsychotic drugs. If you have had head trauma or have any history of seizures, you are much more likely to experience seizures as a side effect of this drug. High doses or sudden changes in dosage of this drug can cause seizures.
- You have manic-depressive (bipolar) disorder. This drug may trigger manic episodes. Use with caution.

Your ability to drive or to perform other tasks requiring judgment or motor skills may be impaired. Wait a few days before operating a car or machinery to be sure the dose you're taking isn't too sedating.

Bupropion has been shown in animal studies to be toxic to the liver in large doses. If you already have liver or kidney impairment, you should avoid this drug altogether or start at a low dose.

If you start to feel extremely restless, agitated, or anxious, or can't sleep when you start taking Wellbutrin, you may need to discontinue it. You may be sensitive to it and prone to delusions, hallucinations, psychosis, confusion, or paranoia with continued use.

Take Wellbutrin in equally divided doses, three to four times a day, in order to minimize risk of seizure.

Be Aware. MAOIs such as phenelzine increase levels of bupropion in the body, possibly resulting in deadly toxicity.

Don't take this drug with alcohol, as this combination can cause seizures.

Mirtazapine (Remeron)

What Does It Do in the Body? Mirtazapine, a tetracyclic antidepressant like bupropion, increases the activity of mood-elevating neuro-transmitters in the brain. Unlike many other antidepressants, mirtazapine has strong sedative effects.

What Is It Used For? Treatment of depression.

What Are the Potential Side Effects? About 16 percent of subjects who participated in trials of this drug dropped out because of side effects. Side effects reported included increased appetite with weight gain (nearly 8 percent increased their body weight by 7 percent or more during the studies), low blood pressure, heart pains, heart attack, slow or otherwise irregular heartbeats, dizziness, migraine, apathy, depression, listlessness, vertigo, twitching, amnesia, restlessness, numbness, acne, dermatitis, dry skin, loss of appetite, urinary tract infection, abnormal thirst, aches and pains, cough, sinusitis, eye or ear pain, malaise, and abdominal pain.

There is no reason to use a drug this dangerous when so many safer alternatives are available.

CAUTION!

- If you experience sore throat, fever, or other signs of infection soon after you begin using mirtazapine, you may be developing a rare blood disorder called agranulocytosis that can be caused by this drug. Call your doctor.
- If you have glaucoma or problems with urinary retention, this drug should be avoided. It can increase intraocular pressure and worsen urinary retention.
- If you have heart disease or a history of irregular heartbeats, avoid this drug. It can aggravate both of these problems.
- If you tend to get dizzy when standing up from a prone position, be aware that mir-

tazapine can increase this effect, increasing your risk of falls.

Venlafaxine (Effexor)

What Does It Do in the Body? Alters neurotransmitter activity in the brain. It is an SNRI, which means it is a weak inhibitor of the reuptake of the neurotransmitters serotonin and norepinephrine. Inhibiting reuptake of these neurotransmitters leaves more of them active in the synapses. Effexor also affects reuptake of dopamine.

What Is It Used For? Treatment of depression.

What Are the Potential Side Effects? In clinical studies of Effexor, 19 percent of patients stopped taking it because of side effects. Nausea, sleepiness, insomnia, dizziness, abnormal ejaculation, headache, nervousness, dry mouth, anxiety, weakness, and excessive sweating were the adverse effects most often experienced with this drug.

While venlafaxine may help alleviate depression, it can increase feelings of anxiety or cause insomnia. If you are often anxious, this may not be the right drug for you. Loss of appetite and body weight, mania, seizures, and elevated heart rate are other side effects to look out for.

CAUTION!

- Don't combine this drug with MAOIs. High body temperature, sudden rapid muscular twitches, extreme agitation, delirium, and even coma and death have resulted from this deadly mix of drugs. Allow a minimum of 14 days between stopping MAOIs and starting venlafaxine, and a minimum of 7 days between stopping venlafaxine and starting MAOIs.

- If you have hypertension, you should know that venlafaxine may cause a sustained increase in blood pressure. The higher the dose, the greater the increase.
- If you have kidney or liver impairment, use this drug with caution.
- Use of this drug for longer than four to six weeks has not been evaluated with clinical trials. Work with your physician to be sure that the drug is continuing to have benefit for you.
- If you have another illness that affects your blood pressure or metabolism, use caution when taking Effexor.

Duloxetine (Cymbalta)

What Does It Do in the Body? Alters neurotransmitter activity in the brain. Like venlafaxine, duloxetine is an SNRI, which means it inhibits the reuptake of the neurotransmitters serotonin and norepinephrine. Inhibiting reuptake of these neurotransmitters leaves more of them active in the synapses.

What Is It Used For? Treating depression, generalized anxiety disorder (GAD), and pain caused by diabetic nerve damage.

What Are the Potential Side Effects? Nausea, dry mouth, diarrhea, dizziness, insomnia, fatigue, sleepiness, constipation, reduced appetite, increased sweating, and sexual dysfunction. These drugs can also cause difficulty with urinating or emptying the bladder completely during urination.

CAUTION!

Think Twice About Taking This Drug If . . .

- You have liver or kidney disease.
- You have narrow-angle glaucoma.

- You are diabetic. Duloxetine can affect glycemic control; you may need to adjust your insulin or other medications.
- You have an alcohol problem. In a few cases, duloxetine users have turned up with liver failure because they drank heavily while on this SNRI. Alcohol is best avoided with any SSRI or SNRI.
- You have any tendency to become manic. This is one medication that has been known to "activate" a so-called latent mania, precipitating a slide into bipolar disorder. This is not a good medication for bipolar disorder treatment.

Be Aware. As with any drug that affects serotonin, combining duloxetine with other drugs in its class or related classes can lead to serotonin syndrome. This includes SSRIs, tricyclics, MAOIs, and even 5-hydroxytriptan drugs for migraine, which work through a mechanism affecting serotonin levels.

Natural Alternatives for Insomnia, Anxiety, Depression, and Stress

We have become accustomed to running to the medicine cabinet for a drug when we're suffering from insomnia, anxiety, or depression, but 90 percent of the time the cause of these problems is something that can be remedied without taking medication.

Sugar, alcohol, and coffee are our legal American drugs, and it's a good bet that these drugs plus food allergies contribute to the vast majority of insomnia, anxiety, and minor depression. Both sugar and alcohol (which is high in sugar) can cause depression. Sometimes fatigue caused by sugar or alcohol is mistaken for depression. If you have a sugar habit (and if you have

one, you know it), it's likely that fatigue is always dogging your tracks. Sugar stimulates your adrenal glands, and taken in excess it will wear them out. When your adrenals are tired, the rest of the body follows, and then when you're stressed, you'll get irritable and depressed. If you think your depression might be fatigue, try cutting out all sugar for three weeks and see what happens. And yes, alcohol counts as sugar. Artificial sweeteners such as NutraSweet (aspartame) found in diet sodas are also not allowed, as they are brain stimulants and may even give the adrenals the same signals that sugar does.

Is Your Medication Making You Depressed?

One of the most common causes of depression is prescription drugs. Here is a list of some of the most common prescription drugs that can cause depression.

Amphetamines (including antihistamines)
Antibiotics
Anticonvulsants
Antidepressants (!)
Barbiturates
High-blood-pressure drugs (beta-blockers, diuretics)
Hormones (estrogen, including Premarin, and synthetic progestins such as Provera)
Narcotics
Painkillers
Sleeping pills
Systemic corticosteroids (prednisone, cortisone, etc.)
Tagamet and Zantac
Tranquilizers (Halcion, Librium, Restoril, Xanax, etc.)

Some research has shown that in depressed people the balance of essential fatty acids is off. Supplementation with high-quality fish oil, as well as eating plenty of fish, walnuts, pumpkin seeds, and dark leafy greens (all sources of omega-3s), can help return the body to balance and give some relief. Harvard professor Andrew L. Stoll, M.D., has discovered that high-dose fish oil—in the neighborhood of 1.5 to 12 grams of eicosapentaenoic acid (EPA) per day—has had powerful healing effects on study subjects who suffer from bipolar disorder, depression, and postpartum depression. His findings are detailed in his book, *The Omega-3 Connection* (Simon & Schuster, 2001).

If you're taking drugs to lower your cholesterol levels (e.g., statins) and are feeling a bit down in the dumps, you should know that drug-induced low cholesterol has been linked with symptoms of depression. Quitting a smoking habit can also bring on depression. Both cholesterol-lowering drugs and smoking cessation affect serotonin levels.

Do you need to be told that coffee can cause anxiety? Coffee is a drug and should be treated as such. Among other things, it stimulates the production of adrenaline, one of the hormones secreted by the adrenal glands to help us in extreme emergency situations. Our adrenals evolved to give our early ancestors the extra strength and alertness needed to escape a saber tooth tiger attack, but we don't often need that much adrenaline these days. Like sugar, coffee constantly stimulates the production of adrenaline, putting excessive wear and tear on the adrenal glands. And let's not forget that green tea and black tea contain caffeine, and even decaf still contains some caffeine. If you're sensitive to caffeine, it can keep you awake at night even if you haven't had any since noon. For those suffering from insomnia, nonstimulating herbal teas such as chamomile or mint are

your best bet in the evening. If you need a boost in the afternoon, try a cup of ginseng tea.

More than a couple of alcoholic drinks a day can cause enough ongoing stress to all systems of the body to bring on depression. Then you have a couple more drinks to banish the depression, and you're in a vicious cycle. Like most things, alcohol in small amounts can be beneficial and in large amounts detrimental. You may escape temporarily from your problems, but excess alcohol is more likely to keep you up at night than put you to sleep. Alcohol also robs your body of many nutrients.

Researchers are discovering that what you eat has a lot to do with how you feel. In a study of 275 people suffering from many different conditions, including fatigue, insomnia, and depression, elimination of allergenic foods resulted in significant improvement, with relief of nearly all symptoms. This is another reason to be moderate about your consumption of refined sugars, white flour, caffeine, and chocolate.

Exercise Is Your Cure-All

Exercise is one of the best sleep aids around. Does this mean you need to get up in the middle of the night and run around the block? Not at all. The point is that if you've taken a brisk walk or have had some other kind of exercise during the day, you'll sleep better and wake up more refreshed.

When we are depressed, we tend to want to stop moving. When we are anxious, we tend to move unproductively, fidgeting or pacing. If you've slowed down to a crawl and can't seem to get your engines started, or if you can't sit still or can't sleep, try some exercise. Several studies have demonstrated that a moderately intense workout, enough to get your heart pounding and your body hot and sweaty, has as strong an antidepressant effect as an SSRI.

Cognitive-Behavioral Therapy: Change the Way You Think to Heal from Anxiety and Depression

Research has demonstrated that brain chemistry can actually be altered by a kind of therapy called cognitive-behavioral therapy (CBT). CBT is based on the understanding that in an otherwise healthy brain, thought patterns create and perpetuate states of anxiety and depression. These thought patterns can change brain biochemistry in negative ways, and changing those patterns can change it for the better.

CBT is based on the idea that our thoughts, not external events, are what create our feelings and behaviors. One person can handle the worst adversity and maintain his or her optimism and zest for life, while another person can be devastated by the smallest problem—or as is the case for many depressed or anxious people, can *make up* problems, and then let those problems sink them like the *Titanic.* These two people think differently. CBT helps the latter person think more like the former.

A CBT therapist can effect big changes in a person's life in only a few months—on average, the length of therapy is 16 sessions. Rather than the traditional "talk therapy" relationship, CBT resembles a teacher-student relationship, complete with homework!

For more information, go to the website of the National Association of Cognitive-Behavioral Therapists, nacbt.org/whatiscbt.htm. This site is for psychologists, but it has a lot of great information that is easy to understand.

Let the Sun Shine In

Depressed people are often depleted of vitamin D, the "sunshine vitamin." Lack of vitamin D is linked to seasonal depression, where people get down in the dumps during the dark, short days of winter. Simply getting out into some direct sun (without sunscreen) for 15 to 30 minutes leads to a boost in vitamin D levels.

If you tend to get down in the dumps every winter and feel better in the spring, you may have seasonal affective disorder (SAD), and you may want to try light therapy, where you spend two hours a day in a room lit at 80 times the brightness of indoor lighting. This can help adjust your hormonal rhythms in a way that boosts mood. You can gain very quick relief with light therapy if you have SAD. If you think this might be for you, check your local health food store for a source of full-spectrum lighting. That being said, the ideal solution is still to get outside and get some sunshine every day.

Track Down Your Sleep Robber

Many over-the-counter painkillers, cold and allergy remedies, and appetite suppressants contain caffeine and other substances that can cause insomnia. Some examples of drugs that contain caffeine are Anacin, Extra Strength Excedrin, Bayer Select Maximum, Midol, and Vanquish. Herbal products with zippy names and energy-boosting claims may be nothing more than concentrated caffeine or guarana, a South American herb that contains high levels of caffeine.

Allergy and cold medicines may contain synthetic variations of ephedrine, such as pseudoephedrine (Sudafed), which can keep you awake. The over-the-counter asthma drugs, Bronkaid and Primatene for example, that contain stimulants such as ephedrine and epinephrine can make sleeping difficult.

The cortisones, such as prednisone, can also cause sleeplessness. The heart drugs propranolol, furosemide, and lovastatin may cause insomnia, as can too high a dose of thyroid medication such as Synthroid. Ironically, many of the antidepressants cause insomnia, which can cause depression due to lack of sleep!

Unfortunately, if one of these medications is keeping you awake at night, your physician is most likely to write you a prescription for a sleeping pill. In nearly all cases, that is the worst possible thing you can do for insomnia. Sleeping pills cause either dependence or outright addiction very quickly, tend to lose their effectiveness over time, and have a rebound effect if you stop, causing worse insomnia than ever. They also tend to suppress your dream or REM sleep, sometimes resulting in severe mental disturbances and psychoses if used over a long period of time. If someone hands you a prescription for a sleeping pill, think twice before using it.

If you're having trouble sleeping and you are taking any type of medication, including over-the-counter drugs, read the label or package insert to find out if it can cause insomnia, restlessness, or irritability.

Don't drink a lot of fluids before bed. If prostate problems are keeping you up with repeated bathroom trips, try the herb saw palmetto.

If you like to watch TV at night before you go to sleep, choose nonviolent, upbeat shows. When you're sleepy, your unconscious is particularly susceptible to suggestion. Violence and mayhem can show up in disturbing dreams that leave you feeling less rested in the morning. If you need a non-TV bedtime ritual, try reading (again, nothing too upsetting or violent) or a warm bath (not hot—that can be stimulating).

When you know that the next day is going to be busy or you have something coming up that you are tense about, make sure you are prepared. Sit down and make a list of things you need to remember, look at your schedule, and organize the day on paper. If you are going to an important meeting, you can visualize it coming out well (you don't need to visualize the whole thing, just the happy ending). That way you won't be worrying about it as you're trying to sleep.

Should you eat right before you go to sleep? Some people say it gives them nightmares, and others say it helps them sleep better. This is very individual and depends on your blood sugar, your digestion, and your metabolism. However, if you do eat before bed, stick to simple, complex-carbohydrate-rich foods like a piece of toast, a bowl of cereal (without added sugar), fruit (bananas work well), or crackers (low salt). Avoid white sugar, spicy foods, and foods high in protein and fat—they can keep you awake, and fat is harder to digest.

Things That Go Bump in the Night

For those of us who travel a lot, live in a noisy neighborhood, have neighbors with a barking dog, or have a spouse who snores, noise can be a real sleep inhibitor. Some primitive part of us is on guard at night, ready to wake us up if something is wrong. Unfortunately, this guard isn't always discriminating about what noises it deems important enough to wake up for.

Here's a sleeping tip that can work wonders: if there's a sound that's been waking you up at night, such as a barking dog, sirens, or garbage trucks, have a little conversation with the "part" of you that's waking up. Thank it for being attentive enough to wake you up, and explain that this particular sound is not a sign of danger. Tell it that it doesn't need to wake you up for this specific sound and that it's perfectly safe to keep on sleeping. It may seem strange, but try it—it works!

When all else fails, earplugs can be a real gift. Get the soft foam type at your local drugstore. White-noise machines that make pleasant, repetitive sounds such as the babbling of a brook or the crashing of ocean waves can help drown out more intrusive sounds. Sleep masks are also available to remove sleep disturbances caused by light.

Melatonin

The hormone melatonin is secreted in tiny amounts from the pineal gland at the base of the brain. As each day draws to an end and darkness falls, melatonin gives us the hormonal signal that it's time to rest for the night. Because we live in a culture that stays up long into the night, with lights blazing, our pineal glands can get a little confused. Night-shift work, newborn babies, and crazy schedules also disrupt our natural circadian rhythms, and quality of sleep suffers.

Melatonin production in the brain is important to a good night's sleep. As we age, our pineal gland secretes less melatonin, and we tend to have more trouble going to sleep and sleeping through the night. Fortunately, thanks to the miracles of modern science, you can buy supplemental melatonin to help you get back into a pattern of deep, rejuvenating sleep.

It's best to take melatonin at least eight hours before you want to wake up, or you may experience some mild grogginess in the morning. Other than that, melatonin has repeatedly been shown to be completely free of side effects when used as directed and is nonaddictive.

Since it regulates sleep-wake cycles, melatonin can also be very useful for banishing jet lag by adjusting circadian rhythms to match your geographic location. You do this simply by taking melatonin about an hour before you want to sleep in your new location. It will give your brain the message that it's time to sleep, regardless of what time zone you're in. One or two nights of melatonin should put you back on the right track.

As for the claims that melatonin is an anti-aging drug, we need to be cautious in making the leap from extending lifespan in a particular strain of mice to extending lifespan in humans. In some studies, mice that were given melatonin lived 20 percent longer, but other strains of mice in other studies died sooner. Some younger mice given melatonin developed cancer. Melatonin in high doses suppresses sex hormones. And how much can we presume about supplemental melatonin based on studies of nocturnal rodents?

Melatonin can also work very well for older people who are having trouble sleeping, but be aware that we simply don't know the long-term effects of using melatonin every night. Anytime we take a hormone in higher doses than the body would naturally produce, we're asking for an imbalance.

If you are over the age of 65 and your melatonin levels have dropped so far that you can't sleep at night, and you have eliminated other possible causes of your insomnia, taking 0.5 to 2 mg at night is tantamount to correcting a deficiency. It is also perfectly safe to take melatonin for an occasional bout of insomnia. Melatonin is a natural hormone, so when it is used occasionally, your body should have no trouble excreting any excess. If you need melatonin, it only takes a very small dose to help you sleep better. If low melatonin levels aren't your problem, even a big dose won't make any difference.

The melatonin sold in health food stores is manufactured but has the exact same molecular structure as the melatonin made by the body. Sublingual forms of melatonin are more expensive but act more quickly. Look for a reputable brand that states on the label that it is pharmaceutical grade melatonin. Take melatonin tablets about one hour before you want to go to sleep, and the sublingual tablets half an hour before you want to go to sleep.

Some drugs, including NSAIDs (e.g., aspirin, ibuprofen, acetaminophen), interfere with the brain's production of melatonin. In fact, just one dose of normal aspirin can cut your melatonin production by as much as 75 percent. If you're taking these drugs, take the last dose after dinner.

Other drugs that can interfere with melatonin production in the brain include the benzodiazepines such as Valium and Xanax, caffeine, alcohol, cold medicines, diuretics, beta-blockers, calcium channel blockers, stimulants such as diet pills, and corticosteroids such as prednisone.

Even the smallest amount of light at night can inhibit the production of melatonin. After sundown, keep artificial lighting gentle. Once it's time to sleep, be sure your bedroom is completely dark, with drapes or blinds drawn to block out streetlights and passing headlights if necessary. Even light as dim as the glowing display of a digital clock has been *found* to adversely affect melatonin production, so turn your clock away or cover it with a cloth.

Valerian

Sometimes at the end of a long day, we're "tired but wired." The body is telling us it's time to sleep, but the mind is keeping us awake. When that happens, you can try taking a dropperful of valerian tincture in water, which should send you to dreamland within 30 minutes. Valerian (*Valeriana officinalis* L.) is a plant that has been used for thousands of years as a folk remedy for "nervous stomach" and as a sedative. Valerian has few, if any, side effects and is not habit-forming. Valerian can be taken as a tincture (a

fluid extract of the herb suspended in alcohol or glycerine) or in capsule form. If you can, get the fresh root tincture. Valerian can make some people weepy when taken for more than a few nights in a row. This is a rare side effect, but well-known among herbalists.

Natural Remedies for Stress

There are many, many positive ways to cope with stress. One of them is to try a form of meditation that focuses on becoming aware of the mind and of your "self-talk" as well as on breathing and chanting techniques that can help focus the mind. If you are unconsciously saying negative things to yourself all day long, it can be more than enough to keep you up at night! Many forms of meditation will assist you in replacing that destructive self-talk with something more positive.

Another way to cope with stress is to talk to a trained therapist. Just talking out loud about a problem to another human who is willing to listen attentively can be enough to begin the emotional healing process. Often, when we talk about our problems out loud, resolutions begin to appear. And by the way, if you don't like your therapist, don't blame yourself—find another one. As in any relationship, the chemistry has to be good for healing to occur.

One technique that can be helpful when stress levels are high is to ask yourself, "What is one action step I can take to reduce my stress levels?" That might simply mean taking a walk in a beautiful place or getting two key things done on your to-do list. Sometimes it's just a matter of getting to bed earlier, spending relaxing time with loved ones, or reducing commitments. For some it may be a hot bath or a meal at a favorite restaurant.

Stress causes a variety of biochemical imbalances in the body. The following herbs and supplements may be helpful in managing stress.

Panax Ginseng and Ashwagandha

Ginseng is used to remedy all sorts of ailments in Chinese medicine. Try 150 mg of standardized extract three times a day to relieve anxiety. See an acupuncturist if you would like some help with herbal prescriptions for anxiety or other problems. Ashwagandha is an Ayurvedic herbal medicine; try 500 mg three times a day.

Calcium and Magnesium

Sometimes insomnia or anxiety can be caused by "universal" muscle tension, where it feels as if every muscle in your body is tense. People with this type of tension tend to get muscle cramps at night. When your grandmother gave you a glass of milk before bedtime, she was wisely giving you a dose of calcium to relax your muscles and ease you into sleep. Magnesium regulates calcium uptake by cells, so take a magnesium and calcium combination for the greatest effect. You can try a combination of 600 mg calcium and 300 mg magnesium before bed.

Treating Depression Naturally

Before getting into specific methods for treating depression naturally, let's first ask whether being down in the dumps or anxious for a few days now and then is cause for medication. We human beings are emotional creatures, and we naturally have our up times and our down times. Our down times can also be the universe's way of pointing out to us that something needs fixing. If we push ourselves back up with a pill without treating the cause, pretty soon we'll be depressed or anxious regardless of what we're taking.

If you're going through a down cycle, be sure to take time for yourself to be reflective about your life. Is there something in your relationship with yourself or someone else that needs healing? Do you have activities in your life that are important and meaningful to you? Have you been getting enough sleep? Are you taking a prescription drug that can cause anxiety or depression? How's your diet? Have you tried an elimination diet to find out if you're allergic to anything? All of these can be factors in anxiety and depression, as are major life changes such as children leaving home, divorce, major illness, and the death of a loved one.

Being anxious or depressed isn't fun—we've all been there—but coming back into emotional balance can be a valuable exercise in learning how to take care of yourself better and keeping your life on track. Most of the time these negative states of mind are caused by some combination of physical, emotional, mental, or spiritual troubles, so it pays to check in with yourself at every level.

In North America and Europe, we tend to believe all the TV ads that tell us we're not OK unless we're always vivaciously energetic, laughing, happy, and ready to party at all times. In truth, what most of us need in our lives is more balance. Not wildly happy, not terribly sad, but balance. Being in balance could be experienced as a state of calm well-being, or peacefulness. Depression and anxiety are two extremes of being out of balance, but oddly enough, they tend to have similar root causes, and many people bounce back and forth between the two.

It's also natural to be depressed if you are in the midst of grieving over the death or serious illness of a loved one, a divorce, a job loss, or another significant life event. In these cases, we sometimes can use some help, and when those times roll around, you're way ahead if you start with natural remedies.

Don't forego a discussion with your medical team and your pharmacist about herbs and supplements for anxiety and depression, especially if you are taking any prescription drugs. Some evidence suggests that St. John's wort may counteract the effects of oral contraceptives and could interact harmfully with blood-thinning medicines.

Omega-3 fatty acids from fish oil are very important for people with depression. A large body of research strongly links a lower omega-3 to omega-6 ratio in the diet to greater risk of depression and anxiety. Higher doses than generally required for overall good health are recommended for depression—somewhere around 2.8 to 3 grams per day of EPA and docosahexaenoic acid (DHA). Refer to Andrew Stoll's book, *The Omega-3 Connection*, for more on this.

An Important Note

Use St. John's wort, *or* S-adenosylmethionine (SAM-e), *or* 5-HTP. Don't use more than one of these neurotransmitter-altering natural remedies at the same time to treat your depression, and don't use any of them along with an SSRI, an SRNI, an MAOI, or a tricyclic antidepressant. We just don't know enough about how these substances interact with one another and how their additive effects might tweak neurotransmitter activity.

S-Adenosylmethionine (SAM-e)

SAM-e is a nutrient important for many processes in the body, including the production of neurotransmitters that strongly affect mood and well-being. It is made in the body, but the conversion of methionine to SAM-e is suspected to be impaired in depressed people. Studies show that this supplement is more effective than placebo, bringing significant reductions in depressive symptoms. Europeans have been using SAM-e as a prescription drug for depression for a couple of decades, and it's available over the counter in the United States. Try 200 mg twice a day for a few days; then increase to 400 mg twice a day. (Don't use this supplement if you suspect you might be bipolar or have a manic tendency, because SAM-e can worsen these problems.) The only (rare) side effects reported are nausea and vomiting.

Tryptophan

The amino acid tryptophan, a precursor to melatonin and the neurotransmitter serotonin, is a safe and effective sleep remedy. It can also be a wonderful remedy for anxiety and depression. Years ago, tryptophan was pulled off the market in the United States by the FDA when a contaminated batch from Japan caused death and illness in dozens of people. The illness it caused had nothing to do with the effects of uncontaminated tryptophan. In truth, tryptophan is very safe—far safer than sleeping pills and antidepressants, which it was competing with in a big way when it was pulled off the market. It's a good bet that tryptophan was pulled from the market to protect the profits of the big drug companies, not to protect your health. Ironically, tryptophan is still included in baby formulas and nutritional powders for senior citizens because it is an essential amino acid, but you can't get it by itself as a supplement in the United States. You can, however, purchase it in a form called 5-hydroxytryptophan (5-HTP) for use as a natural insomnia, anxiety, and depression remedy.

Tryptophan's effect on the brain is similar to that of drugs such as Prozac, except that it doesn't have the side effects, dangers, and withdrawal problems those drugs have; it's much less expensive; and it's probably more effective. One of tryptophan's primary effects on the brain is to reduce anxiety, which is often the culprit in insomnia. For the same reason, it is often quite effective for treating depression, especially if there is an anxiety component to it.

The usual recommended dose of 5-HTP is 150 to 300 mg per day.

If you are taking one of the SSRIs (Prozac, Paxil, Celexa, Luvox, or Zoloft), don't use tryptophan at the same time. Agitation, restlessness, aggressiveness, high body temperature, diarrhea, and cramping can result.

St. John's Wort

St. John's wort, which has been used medicinally for many centuries by the Chinese, the Greeks, the Europeans, and the American Indians, is well known for its positive effect on anxiety, insomnia, depression, and a physical illness that has long been associated with stress: heart disease. It also seems to be effective as a treatment for SAD. This herb has been extremely well studied in Europe and found over and over again to be as effective as the SSRIs in treating depression and as the benzodiazepines in treating anxiety. You may need to take it for a couple of weeks before it starts taking effect.

Several studies comparing prescription antidepressants with the herbal remedy St. John's wort have shown the latter to be as effective as the former against clinical depression. The encouraging results of these studies have inspired further research into the possible uses of St. John's wort. Some of the most interesting work has revealed its effectiveness against premenstrual syndrome (PMS) and as a gentle remedy for depression and other psychological problems in children.

Researchers at the University of Exeter's Department of Complementary Medicine in England gathered a group of 19 women who had PMS but who were otherwise in good mental and physical health and had not undergone any treatment for their PMS symptoms. These women were interviewed, completed daily symptom ratings for one menstrual cycle, and were medically screened before receiving an official PMS diagnosis. They then took 300 mg of St. John's wort daily (standardized to 900 mcg of hypericin) for two complete menstrual cycles. Daily symptom ratings were completed throughout the two months, and other tests of depression and anxiety levels were administered periodically. The womens' PMS symptom scores decreased 51 percent, with more than two-thirds showing at least a 50 percent improvement.

Children are being treated with SSRIs and Ritalin at an alarming rate these days. It's important that research be done on natural remedies for depression and anxiety in children so that fewer parents feel compelled to give their children these dangerous drugs. A group of German researchers investigated the use of St. John's wort in 101 children under the age of 12, giving them 300 to 1,800 mg daily for four to six weeks. Seventy-two percent of the physicians who followed the progress of these children rated the herb's effectiveness as good or excellent after two weeks; after four weeks, this rating was given by 97 percent of those physicians; and at the study's end, 100 percent approved of the job St. John's wort was doing for the study's young subjects. None of the subjects experienced adverse effects.

Before you turn to SSRIs or antianxiety drugs for treatment of your own PMS or of a child's psychological problems, consider trying a course of St. John's wort. Take it in the dose recommended on the container. If you are coming off an SSRI such as Prozac and want to try St. John's wort, allow a three-week period in between so you don't end up with serotonin syndrome (a dangerous condition where too much serotonin remains in the synapses).

B Vitamins

The B vitamins together and separately play important roles in nerve and brain function and in relaxing muscles. If you are older and not absorbing nutrients as well as you might be, your body may not be able to use the B vitamins in your food. It's important to include the B vitamins in a multivitamin. If you're having trouble with leg cramps at night, an extra 50 mg of vitamin B_6 an hour before bed may help. Some people are cured of restless leg syndrome by taking an extra 400 mcg of folic acid before bed.

The B vitamins play an essential role in our neurological health, and yet most adult Americans are deficient in these vitamins. Although each of the B vitamins plays some role in brain function, vitamin B_{12} is best known for its ability to combat depression. For years alternative health professionals have given vitamin B_{12} shots as part of an overall treatment program for people who are extremely stressed out or depressed. Until recently this practice has been pooh-poohed, but now more and more M.D.s are jumping on the B_{12} bandwagon.

If you want to try B_{12} as an antidote for stress or depression, it's important to know that it's not well absorbed when you take it orally (by mouth), which is why it is given in the form of injections. However, there are B_{12} supplements you can buy at your local health food store that are sublingual (dissolved under the tongue) and intranasal (in

the nose). You'll want to take about 1,000 mcg (1 mg) at least every other day to treat depression.

Amino Acids

Many alternative health care practitioners have had great success treating depression with amino acids. Amino acids are the building blocks of protein and play a vital role in the production and regulation of brain chemicals. Most of the new "personality" drugs have much the same effects on brain chemistry as the amino acids tryptophan, tyrosine, and phenylalanine. These substances affect the brain's production of serotonin, a neurotransmitter that affects our moods. However, please try the simpler solutions such as nutrition and exercise first for treating depression—it's always preferable to begin with the most simple, down-to-earth solutions.

Although amino acids are safe, especially when compared to the prescription drugs, don't take more than the recommended dose unless it's recommended by a health care professional, and monitor yourself carefully to track if and how they affect you (keeping a daily diary of how you're feeling works well). The stimulating amino acids such as tyrosine and phenylalanine can cause irritability in some people.

If you have chronic, recurring depression, work with a health care professional. If you are already taking a prescription drug for depression, please do not take amino acids for it without consulting your doctor.

If you, your physician, or health care professional wants to know about amino acids in detail, read the book *The Healing Nutrients Within: Your Guide to the Best-Stocked Drugstore of All—the Human Body* by Eric R. Braverman, M.D. (Basic Health Publications, 2003). Your doctor may want to check out the 120-page-plus reference section. Very few prescription drugs have been so thoroughly tested.

Tyrosine

The amino acid tyrosine is fairly well established through research and the experience of hundreds of alternative health care practitioners as a safe and effective remedy for depression. Tyrosine is the precursor to some of our most important neurotransmitters, so it is an important part of our brain's nutrition. It is also a precursor to adrenaline, thyroid hormones, and some types of estrogen. It has been shown to lower blood pressure, increase sex drive, and suppress appetite. L-dopa, which is used to treat Parkinson's disease, is made from tyrosine.

Start with 500 mg three times a day with meals. If that doesn't work, try 1,000 mg. The most you should take without consulting a health professional is 1,500 mg a day. Although tyrosine is considered to be one of the safest amino acids, it can trigger a migraine headache in some people and shouldn't be used in conjunction with MAOIs.

Phenylalanine

The amino acid phenylalanine is the precursor to tyrosine and has been used in numerous studies to successfully treat depression. Many supplement manufacturers will combine tyrosine and phenylalanine, but vitamin B_6 should be added to this combination for better use.

This amino acid should be avoided by people who have phenylketonuria (PKU), a genetic defect in the body's ability to process and use phenylalanine. This defect can cause severe retardation. If it is caught early enough, retardation can be avoided with a phenylalanine-free diet. Some researchers believe that many children who are hyperactive or have learning disabilities are suffering from a mild form of PKU. Because there are a small number of women whose phenylalanine levels fluctuate when they are pregnant, this amino acid should be avoided if you are pregnant, just to be on the safe side.

The most common source of phenylalanine these days is the artificial sweetener aspartame (NutraSweet). Every time you use aspartame, you get some phenylalanine and aspartic acid. However, it's better to take phenylalanine in a supplement because we don't know enough about aspartic acid and its side effects, or what it does in combination with phenylalanine. You can take up to 500 mg of phenylalanine three times a day.

Phenylalanine has been reported to raise blood pressure, so if you have high blood pressure, please monitor it carefully or consult your doctor. Phenylalanine gives some people headaches. A few studies suggest that phenylalanine may promote the growth of cancerous tumors. So if you have cancer, this should not be your antidepressant of choice, and please avoid the aspartame!

Chapter 16

Diabetes Drugs, Obesity Drugs, and Their Natural Alternatives

I f you have adult-onset (type 2) diabetes and your physician isn't working with you to aggressively treat the disease with diet and exercise, then you are simply being manipulated by the medical industry and used as a cash cow. The vast majority of type 2 diabetes, especially when it is caught early, can be very successfully treated with diet, exercise, and supplements, but most conventional physicians won't take that course. Instead they prescribe drugs that control the symptoms without treating the underlying disease, putting you on a road to certain illness and disability.

The Food and Drug Administration (FDA) is approving new types of diabetes drugs on a regular basis—it's a huge and rapidly growing market, and everyone wants a piece of the pie. A few years ago, a slick, full-color, four-page advertisement appeared in a pharmacy magazine and began with the headline, "The Diabetes Consumer: Shops More. Spends More. Shops the Whole Store." The headline on the following page read, "Maximize Your Profits with Diabetes Category Management." It went on to predict "dramatic growth" in the diabetes market.

The ad went on to explain that a diabetic customer spends about $2,500 more in a pharmacy each year than the average customer, and listed some 26 products needed by a diabetic, including insulin, syringes, cotton swabs, and blood glucose monitors.

Pharmacy costs for a diabetic don't take into account the cost of regular visits to the physician and the cost of the side effects of diabetes. Diabetics are two to four times more likely to have heart disease or a stroke. They also represent one-third of kidney dialysis patients, and they suffer from impotence, loss of vision, increased susceptibility to infections, and loss of sensation in the hands and feet. These costs line the pockets of physicians and hospitals. Any way you look at it, a person with diabetes is a financial boon for physicians, drug companies, and pharmacies. The rapidity with which unsuspecting patients are prescribed diabetes drugs can be dizzying, and the consequences can be dire.

Once you are diagnosed with type 2 diabetes, your physician is pressured, from many directions, to put you on diabetes drugs to control blood sugar. This ensures that you will need to visit your physician frequently to renew your prescription and guarantees the drug company and pharmacy a lifetime customer. All of the diabetes drugs have side effects, and all of them lose their effectiveness over time, guaranteeing the drug-dependent diabetic the life-

threatening side effects of both the drugs and the disease.

This wouldn't be such shameful behavior if it weren't for the fact that adult-onset diabetes is one of the most preventable of all chronic diseases and is highly treatable and reversible with diet and exercise. Taking the right nutritional supplements and herbs improves the picture even more.

Some 90 percent of adult-onset or type 2 diabetes, also known as non-insulin-dependent diabetes, is caused by poor eating habits, obesity, and lack of exercise. Three-quarters of those diagnosed with type 2 diabetes can avoid insulin injections and other drugs by losing weight, but most physicians believe that it's too difficult to help patients lose weight and eat properly, so they are most likely to recommend (pay lip service to) weight loss and exercise while simultaneously writing you a prescription for a diabetes drug.

Diabetes is such a profitable business that physicians will put "prediabetic" patients, with only marginally high blood sugar, on diabetes drugs before trying weight loss and exercise. The logic is that the drug will control blood sugar until the patient gets his or her act together and makes the necessary lifestyle changes because the earlier high blood sugar is controlled, and the more it is controlled, the less likely a person is to suffer from the side effects of diabetes. While this is very true, there's no comparison between the safety and effectiveness of lifestyle changes versus diabetes drugs when it comes to long-term health and quality of life—the drugs are the first step onto a deadly drug treadmill. The only comparison that makes diabetes drugs look good is the patient who is obese, eating poorly, and not getting any exercise and who does not make any lifestyle changes.

Diabetes drug side effects are also a classic case of what happens when doctors focus on changing the numbers (e.g., glucose, insulin) without paying attention to the big picture. Over and over again, diabetes drug studies show that while the drug controls the numbers, the patients taking it have an increased risk of heart disease and death, and those who survive tend to have a poor quality of life. Controlling diabetes numbers in a patient who continues to eat poorly and not exercise is an exercise in futility and failing health.

Giving a prediabetic patient drugs without directly helping him or her make lifestyle changes should be considered malpractice. Any physician or health organization that doesn't vigorously, consistently, and insistently work with a diabetic patient to lose weight (without weight loss drugs, preferably), eat healthy foods, and exercise is not in the business of healing—they are in the business of pushing drugs. Diabetes drugs should never, ever be a substitute for a healthy lifestyle.

But the truth is, in the end it's up to you. Your physician and health care organization have many patients and limited time, and they can't force you to do anything. Only you can make the changes necessary to avoid the lifetime of ill health created by diabetes. If you get on diabetes drugs and stay on them without addressing the underlying causes of the diabetes, the disease will inevitably progress, with its serious side effects. The only way to avoid the progression of diabetes is to bring the body back into balance.

In countries where people eat a diet low in fat and sugar and high in whole foods such as unrefined grains and fresh fruits and vegetables, diabetes is almost nonexistent. When people from these countries move to the United States, their diabetes risk skyrockets. Tragically, as "nutrition-free" Western processed and fast foods are introduced to third-world countries, their rates of diabetes are rapidly rising.

The government's Agency for Healthcare Research and Quality (AHRQ) estimates that if Americans don't change their ways, roughly 86 percent of those ages 18 and older may be overweight or obese by 2030. The cost of caring for this sickly

Are Prescription Drugs Causing Your Low Blood Sugar?

If you are diabetic or your blood sugar is unstable, and you are suffering from hypoglycemia or hyperglycemia, you should be aware of those substances that can lower your blood sugar:

Alcohol	Lithium
Allopurinol (Lopurin, Zyloprim)	Mebendazole
Ampicillin	Monoamine oxidase inhibitors (MAOIs)
Bromocriptine	Phenylbutazone (Butatab, Butazolidin)
Chloramphenicol (Chloromycetin)	Probenecid (Benemid, Probalan)
Clofibrate (Abitrate, Atromid-S)	Salicylates (aspirin)
Fenfluramine (Pondimin, pulled off the market)	Tetracycline
Indomethacin	Theophylline

population will approach a trillion dollars annually, or one out of every six health care dollars.

CAUTION!

If you have diabetes, notify your physician if any of the following occurs:

- Hyperglycemia: excessive thirst or urination
- Hypoglycemia: fatigue, excessive hunger, profuse sweating, or numbness in the extremities
- Miscellaneous: fever, sore throat, rash, or unusual bruising or bleeding
- Severe stomach pain

Diabetes Drugs

Examples of Alpha-Glucosidase Inhibitors

Acarbose (Precose)
Miglitol (Glyset)

This is a relatively new type of diabetes drug that works by blocking enzymes that normally break down carbohydrates. This drug can cause unpleasant stomach and digestive problems such as cramps, gas, and diarrhea, and can make existing intestinal problems worse.

What Does It Do in Your Body? Slows the digestion of carbohydrates in the small intestine, which reduces the amount of glucose (sugar) that is released into the blood after eating.

What Is It Prescribed For? Lowering blood sugar levels. This drug is intended to be supplemental therapy to diet and exercise.

What Are the Possible Side Effects? The most common side effects occur in the digestive system, including abdominal pain, diarrhea, and gas.

These drugs can impair kidney function and have caused cancerous kidney tumors in rats. They can cause hypoglycemia, or low blood sugar levels, so if you're taking it, be sure to have a readily available source of dextrose on hand to counteract hypoglycemia.

CAUTION!

Think Twice About Taking This Drug If . . .

- You have kidney problems of any kind.
- You have serious intestinal problems.
- You are exposed to stress such as fever, trauma, infection, or surgery.

What Are the Interactions with Food? Take this drug orally with the first bite of your main meal.

What Nutrients Does It Throw out of Balance or Interact With? Vitamin B_{12}.

What Else to Take If You Take This Drug. A supplement of vitamin B_{12}, sublingually.

Examples of Insulin

Insulin injection (Insulin, Humulin R)
Insulin injection, concentrated (Concentrated Regular)
Insulin zinc suspension, extended ultralente (Humulin U Ultralente)
Insulin zinc suspension, lente (Humulin L)
Isophane insulin suspension and insulin injection (Humulin 70/30, Humulin 50/50)
Isophane insulin suspension NPH (Novolin N)
Insulin glargine (Lantus)
Insulin aspartate (Novolog, Novolog Mix 70/30)

Adult-onset diabetes is usually a disease of excess sugar in the bloodstream and an impaired ability to use the hormone insulin to carry the sugar out of the blood and into the cells. In rare cases, it may be caused by the inability of the pancreas to make insulin. At one time, insulin was thought to be the savior of diabetics: simply inject it into the body to replace what isn't there. But diabetes is always more complicated than a pancreas that doesn't make insulin.

Most people with type 2 diabetes actually make plenty of insulin but have insulin resistance, a condition where their cells are resistant to using it. But the pancreas keeps getting the message that there isn't enough insulin and keeps producing it. Excess insulin causes its own problems, including high blood pressure and poor cholesterol levels (low HDL and high LDL), increasing the risk of complications as the disease progresses. This is why it is so important that even insulin-dependent diabetics reduce their need for insulin as much as possible through good management of blood sugar levels using diet, supplements, and exercise.

What Does It Do in the Body? Insulin is taken to replace the insulin that should be produced by the pancreas but is not produced at all or is not produced sufficiently. Insulin regulates blood sugar levels in the body.

What Is It Prescribed For? People who cannot survive without prescribed insulin for blood sugar regulation, which is mostly type 1 diabetics.

What Are the Possible Side Effects? Allergic reactions such as rashes, shortness of breath, fast pulse, sweating, a drop in blood pressure resulting in dizziness or light-headedness, as well as insulin shock.

If insulin is injected, redness, swelling, and itching at the site can occur. Open sores at the site of injection can occur. Also, if injec-tions happen at the same site several times, fat may accumulate at the site and inhibit insulin absorption.

CAUTION!

Think Twice About Taking This Drug If . . .

You have an insulin resistance or allergy. There is almost never a reason to prescribe insulin to a type 2 diabetic. Be sure your physician has a good reason if this is the case.

What Are the Interactions with Food? Coffee decreases the amount of insulin and length of time it is in your system.

What Nutrients Does It Throw out of Balance or Interact With? Blood sugar, vitamin B_{12}.

What Else to Take If You Take This Drug. Supplement of sublingual vitamin B_{12}.

Examples of Sulfonylurea Drugs

Acetohexamide (Dymelor)
Chlorpropamide (Diabinese)
Glimepiride (Amaryl)
Glipizide (Glucotrol)
Glyburide (Micronase, Glynase PresTab, DiaBeta)
Tolazamide (Tolinase)
Tolbutamide (Orinase)

These oral drugs (taken by mouth) lower the amount of sugar in the bloodstream by stimulating the pancreas to make more insulin. They decrease the liver's production of glucose, a simple sugar, and they make cells more sensitive to insulin, improving the uptake of insulin and sugar for energy. The downside of these drugs is that they increase the risk of dying of heart disease, one of the most common side effects of diabetes, and they tend to cause weight gain, one of the causes of diabetes! They can also cause hypoglycemia (low blood sugar) by removing too much sugar.

Less serious but frequent side effects are digestive upsets such as nausea, vomiting, heartburn, gas, diarrhea, and constipation.

What Do They Do in the Body? Lower blood glucose.

What Are They Prescribed For? Non-insulin-dependent diabetes mellitus (also called adult-onset or maturity-onset diabetes, ketosis-resistant diabetes, and type 2 diabetes). In addition, they are sometimes prescribed as temporary adjuncts to insulin therapy to improve diabetic control.

What Are the Possible Side Effects? Digestive-system reactions are common. They include nausea, heartburn, and diarrhea. These drugs can suppress the immune system and cause anemia, liver and kidney impairment, and jaundice.

The effectiveness of these drugs decreases over time, eventually resulting in a complete failure of the drug to control glucose—yet another reason to control your blood sugar with diet, exercise, and supplements!

Flushing of the face when taken with alcohol may occur, as can water retention—particularly if you have congestive heart failure or liver cirrhosis. These drugs can also cause weakness, ringing in the ears, fatigue, dizziness, and headache.

CAUTION!

Think Twice About Taking These Drugs If . . .

- You have diabetes complicated with a high count of ketones.

- You are diabetic and pregnant.
- You have heart problems. Diabetic patients using this drug were two-and-a-half times more likely to die from cardiovascular problems.
- You have liver or kidney problems.
- You are elderly, debilitated, or malnourished.
- Your adrenal or pituitary glands are not operating sufficiently.

What Are the Interactions with Food? Food delays absorption of these drugs by about 40 minutes. These drugs are more effective if you take them 30 minutes before eating food.

Do not drink alcohol with these drugs—particularly chlorpropamide and tolbutamide. Symptoms of this interaction can be dizziness, weakness, mental confusion, collapse, and coma.

What Nutrients Do They Throw out of Balance or Interact With? These drugs lower levels of vitamin B_{12}.

What Else to Take If You Take These Drugs. Sublingual vitamin B_{12}.

Miscellaneous Diabetes Drugs

Metformin (Glucophage)

Metformin is an oral diabetes drug that lowers blood sugar by suppressing glucose production in the liver and increasing the sensitivity of cells to insulin. Unlike the sulfonylurea drugs, it does not stimulate the production of insulin, so there is less chance of hypoglycemia, and it tends to cause weight loss, not weight gain. Like all of the oral diabetes drugs, digestive discomfort is a common side effect. It can also impair kidney and liver function and shouldn't be used by people who use alcohol excessively.

What Does It Do in the Body? It decreases liver glucose (sugar) production, decreases intestinal absorption of glucose, and increases uptake and use of glucose.

What Is It Prescribed For? To lower blood glucose levels in patients with non-insulin-dependent diabetes.

What Are the Possible Side Effects? Low blood sugar if you don't eat enough calories, if you exercise strenuously and don't supplement with additional caloric intake, if you drink alcohol, or if you take another glucose-lowering drug with metformin.

Digestive problems can occur with this drug, including diarrhea, nausea, vomiting, abdominal bloating, gas, and loss of appetite.

Lactic acidosis is a rare but serious metabolic complication where too much of the drug accumulates in the body. It is fatal in 50 percent of the cases. It usually happens in people with kidney impairment.

This drug can increase your chances of dying from cardiovascular problems by two and a half times.

CAUTION!

Think Twice About Taking This Drug If...

- You have kidney disease or dysfunction.
- You have cardiovascular problems.
- You have inadequate vitamin B_{12} or calcium intake.

What Nutrients Does It Throw out of Balance or Interact With? Vitamin B_{12}.

What Else to Take If You Take This Drug. Sublingual vitamin B_{12}.

Rosiglitazone maleate (Avandia)
Pioglitazone HCl (Actos)

These drugs were approved in 1999. Both belong to a class of antidiabetes drugs called thiazolidinediones and are usually taken with sulfonylureas, insulin, or metformin. They can also be used without other diabetes drugs.

What Do They Do in the Body? They lower blood glucose by increasing insulin sensitivity. They decrease the production of sugars by the liver and enhance the action of insulin, helping it move more glucose out of the bloodstream and into the cells. They do not increase insulin secretion from the pancreas.

What Are They Prescribed For? The treatment of type 2 diabetes.

What Are the Possible Side Effects? In May 2007, the *New England Journal of Medicine* reported that an analysis of dozens of studies on Avandia (Avandamet or Avandaryl when mixed with other diabetes drugs) showed that taking the drug significantly increased the risk of heart attack and death. Around the same time, the FDA issued a "safety alert" based on the same research. In December 2007, the *Journal of the American Medical Association* released the results of a large study showing that older patients treated with thiazolidinediones (Avandia and Actos) had a 60 percent increased risk of congestive heart failure, a 40 percent increased risk of heart attack, and a 29 percent increased risk of death. Those are *huge* increased risks! Finally, in February 2008, the FDA issued a black-box warning about the risks of using these drugs, but still didn't remove them from the market.

This is a classic case where a drug effectively changes the numbers, lowering insulin and glucose levels, but has a good chance of killing the patient in the process—"the treatment worked, but the patient died."

Here is an adapted excerpt from Avandia's "Medication Guide":

Avandia can cause serious side effects, including:

New or Worse Heart Failure

- Avandia can cause your body to keep extra fluid (fluid retention), which leads to swelling (edema) and weight gain. Extra body fluid can make some heart problems worse or lead to heart failure. Heart failure means your heart does not pump blood well enough.
- If you have severe heart failure, you cannot start on Avandia.
- If you have heart failure with symptoms (such as shortness of breath or swelling), even if these symptoms are not severe, Avandia may not be right for you.

Other side effects of Avandia may include edema (fluid retention), breathing problems, weight gain, fatigue, and other types of heart problems.

The FDA has issued a warning that older women who take Avandia or Actos are at a significantly higher risk of fracturing a bone.

Other side effects of these drugs can include accidental injury, anemia, back pain, diarrhea, edema, weight gain caused by edema, macular (eye) edema, fractures, fatigue, high blood sugar, low blood sugar (rosiglitazone), aggravated diabetes, muscle pain, throat irritation, tooth disorders (pioglitazone), headache, sinusitis, and upper respiratory tract infection (rosiglitazone and pioglitazone).

CAUTION!

Think Twice About Taking These Drugs If . . .

- You have liver disease. These drugs are similar to troglitazone (Rezulin), the diabetes drug that caused multiple cases of liver failure and was pulled from the market.
- You are premenopausal and have not been ovulating. These drugs, when given to women who are insulin resistant, can cause ovulation to resume, and pregnancy can result.

Ultimately, given all of these hazards, we're not sure why a physician would prescribe these drugs at all.

Exenatide (Byetta)

Byetta is a fairly new injectable diabetes drug that has the potential to take the place of insulin for type 2 diabetics because it doesn't tend to lower blood sugar excessively the way insulin can and because it promotes weight loss in most people who take it. Is it a magic bullet? No such luck. Side effects are listed later in this section, and remember, drugs tend to look a lot better in the first few years they are released, because long-term side effects haven't yet emerged. This may turn out to be a useful drug, but at this time you should consider yourself a guinea pig if you're taking it.

What Does It Do in the Body? It behaves much like human glucagon-like peptide-1 (GLP-1), which plays a role in regulating glucose metabolism and insulin secretion by stimulating insulin secretion in the pancreas and lowering blood glucose. It also suppresses the release of glucagon, which blocks the liver's ability to convert fat to sugar and can also reduce liver fat content.

What Is It Prescribed For? Byetta is prescribed for the treatment of type 2 diabetes, usually in combination with other drugs such as metformin.

What Are the Possible Side Effects? Here's the bad news: after Byetta had been on the market about three years, the FDA began to get reports of sudden and severe pancreatitis in patients taking it, resulting in serious illness and a handful of deaths. Severe abdominal pain and vomiting can be symptoms of acute pancreatitis.

In rodent testing, Byetta appeared to be associated with benign tumors of the thyroid.

This drug may make kidney disease worse.

This drug is not recommended for people with gastrointestinal disease. In the drug trials, 57 percent of those taking it experienced nausea, 17 percent experienced vomiting, and 8.5 percent experienced diarrhea. Those are extremely high percentages. Reportedly these side effects improve over time. Other side effects can include rash, flatulence, loss of appetite, sour stomach, belching, heartburn, indigestion, dizziness, headache, and feeling jittery. Patients taking Byetta had more episodes of hypoglycemia than those taking metformin or a sulfonylurea drug.

CAUTION!

This is a new drug. Please consider yourself a guinea pig if you take it. This drug can interact dangerously with many other drugs, and because it hasn't been on the market very long, new interactions will emerge over time. Be very cautious about taking any new prescription or over-the-counter drug or supplement if you're taking this drug.

What Are the Interactions with Food? Even though this is an injection, Byetta works much better when taken at least 30 minutes before eating.

Sitagliptin (Januvia)

This is another new diabetes drug that works by increasing levels of human glucagon-like peptide-1 (GLP-1), which plays a role in regulating glucose metabolism and insulin secretion. Although this drug is currently said to have fewer side effects than other diabetes drugs, it's new, which means we don't yet know the full extent of its side effects, especially long-term. You should consider yourself a guinea pig if you're taking it.

What Does It Do in the Body? It helps control blood sugar by stimulating insulin secretion in the pancreas and lowering blood glucose.

What Is It Prescribed For? This drug is prescribed for blood sugar control in type 2 diabetes.

What Are the Possible Side Effects? Side effects can include hypoglycemia, serious hypersensitivity reactions (anaphylaxis, angioedema, rash, urticaria, and exfoliative skin conditions, including Stevens-Johnson syndrome), common cold symptoms such as stuffy nose, upper respiratory infection, and headache.

Repaglinide (Prandin)

What Does It Do in the Body? This drug stimulates the pancreas to make more insulin. It is meant to be taken with meals to reduce blood sugar spikes after eating. It acts quickly and loses its effect quickly.

What Is It Prescribed For? This drug is prescribed for blood sugar control in type 2 diabetes.

What Are the Possible Side Effects? Hypoglycemia, sinusitis, rhinitis, bronchitis, nausea, diarrhea, constipation, vomiting, dyspepsia, musculoskeletal pain, arthralgia, back pain, headache, paresthesia, chest pain, and urinary tract infection.

Nateglinide (Starlix)

What Does It Do in the Body? Nateglinide is a D-phenylalanine derivative that lowers blood glucose levels by stimulating insulin secretion from the pancreas. It is fast-acting, and its effect doesn't last long; it is meant to help control blood sugar at mealtimes.

What Is It Prescribed For? This drug is prescribed for blood sugar control in type 2 diabetes.

What Are the Possible Side Effects? Side effects can include hypoglycemia, upper respiratory infection, back pain, flu symptoms, dizziness, arthropathy, diarrhea, accidental trauma, bronchitis, coughing, and hypersensitivity reactions (rash, itching, and urticaria). Jaundice, cholestatic hepatitis, and elevated liver enzymes have been reported—all symptoms of a damaged liver. Symptoms of hypoglycemia can include blurred vision, cold sweats, dizziness, fast heartbeat, fatigue, headache, hunger, lightheadedness, nausea, and nervousness. Like all diabetes drugs, this drug can be hard on the liver.

CAUTION!

This is a relatively new drug. Please consider yourself a guinea pig if you take it. New side effects and long-term side effects will undoubtedly emerge over time.

Obesity Epidemic

Adult-onset diabetes and obesity go hand-in-hand. Most people with type 2 diabetes or insulin resistance—a condition with the potential to progress to full-blown diabetes—are overweight. Weight loss dramatically improves insulin resistance, but many diabetics who struggle to lose weight are caught in a vicious cycle: chronically high insulin levels prime their bodies to store away any available calories as fat, and the fatter they get, the worse their insulin resistance becomes and the higher their insulin levels go to try to overcome that resistance. Eventually the pancreas becomes exhausted from the effort and can no longer maintain any semblance of blood sugar balance. That's when insulin becomes necessary.

Metabolic Syndrome: The Disease of the New Millenium

We now have a medical term in common usage for the cluster of problems caused by poor diet and obesity: *metabolic syndrome*. The term has actually been in use in medical research since the mid-1960s, but it wasn't widely recognized or accepted by the medical community until a few years ago.

Metabolic syndrome describes an obese person with central or abdominal obesity (a fat stomach) who also tends to have a poor cholesterol profile, high blood sugar and insulin and the attendant insulin resistance, high blood pressure, and clogged arteries—in other words, diabetes or heart disease is waiting to happen.

Hormonally, a woman with metabolic syndrome tends to have high androgen (male hormone) levels, high estrogen levels (the fat cells are making estrogen from androgens), high cortisol, and low thyroid—in other words, breast cancer waiting to happen.

Men with metabolic syndrome tend to have low testosterone and high estrogen—in other words, prostate problems waiting to happen.

Both men and women with metabolic syndrome are more prone to inflammation, which predisposes one to heart disease, arthritis, and headaches.

Diet Sodas Increase the Risk for Metabolic Syndrome

Published in the journal *Circulation*, a study of more than 9,500 middle-aged men and women whose health was tracked for nine years found what was expected: the typical Western diet high in red meat, white flour, and fried foods increased the risk of metabolic syndrome by nearly 20 percent. What surprised the researchers was the finding that those who consumed diet soda—even one can a day—increased their risk of developing metabolic syndrome by 34 percent compared to those who didn't drink diet soda.

Following these findings, nutrition researchers now theorize that the sweet taste of artificially flavored foods stimulates the pancreas to make insulin in preparation for the onslaught of sugar it thinks is coming. Insulin without a job (carrying sugar into cells) is dangerous, causing inflammation and causing the body to store fat more readily. The intensely sweet taste of diet sodas combined with caffeine seems to be habit forming, but this would be a great one to let go of. One way to wean yourself away from diet sodas is to mix a small amount of fruit juice (e.g., pomegranate juice) with some carbonated water.

Over the past three decades, the number of obese Americans has more than doubled. Sixty-one percent of American adults are overweight,

Health Problems Related to or Aggravated by Obesity

Birth defects	Kidney cancer
Breast cancer in women and men	Liver disease
Carpal tunnel syndrome	Low back pain
Chronic venous insufficiency	Obstetric and gynecological complications
Daytime sleepiness	Osteoarthritis of the knee and hip
Deep vein thrombosis	Pain
Endometrial cancer	Pancreatitis
End-stage kidney disease	Respiratory dysfunction
Gallbladder disease	Rheumatoid arthritis
Gastrointestinal cancers (esophagus, stomach, colorectal)	Sleep apnea
	Stroke
Gout	Surgical complications
Heart disease	Type 2 diabetes
High blood pressure	Urinary stress incontinence
Impaired immunity	Wound infection
Infertility	

meaning they weigh up to 30 pounds more than they should. Some 26 percent of the adult American population is more than 30 pounds over their ideal weight—in other words, they're obese. It's estimated that by the year 2030, roughly 86 percent of Americans ages 18 and older may be overweight or obese.

The health problems related to these extra pounds are costing the health care system at least $93 billion a year, and by the year 2030 they could cost nearly a *trillion* dollars a year.

Even more worrisome is the fattening of American children. According to the Centers for Disease Control and Prevention, 32 percent of American schoolchildren are overweight or obese. These children are developing type 2 diabetes and heart disease, life-threatening chronic diseases previously seen only in adults. According to pediatric endocrinologist Naomi Neufeld, M.D., overweight children are 20 to 30 percent heavier today than they were 10 years ago.

Extra weight and obesity are independent risk factors for many of the chronic diseases that affect Americans today. This means that even if you have no other risk factors for these diseases, simply being fat will still significantly increase your risk of developing them. Obesity also aggravates a number of other conditions.

While diabetes is one of the major risks inherent in being overweight, you can avoid many other conditions by staying within a healthy weight range. Men who are 20 percent over their desirable weight have a 20 percent increased likelihood of dying from all causes. They are 10 percent more likely to die from stroke, have 40 percent greater risk of gallbladder disease, and have double the risk of developing diabetes. For a man between ages 19 and 35, at 25 to 35 percent over ideal weight, the risk of dying from all causes is 170 percent—almost

double—that of a man of ideal weight. At 40 percent above desirable weight, the likelihood of dying from diabetes complications skyrockets 400 percent, and the risk of dying from stroke rises 75 percent.

Adults between the ages of 20 and 45 who are overweight are six times more likely to have high blood pressure. For every 10 percent increase in body weight over ideal, there is a 20 percent increase in the incidence of heart disease, a 6.5 mm Hg increase in blood pressure, a 12 mg/dL increase in blood cholesterol levels, and a 2 mg/dL increase in fasting blood sugar levels (the higher this number, the greater the risk of developing type 2 diabetes). Overweight men are much more likely to develop colorectal cancer, while heavy women are at increased risk of uterine and ovarian cancers. Women who are abdominally obese—who carry their excess weight in the upper body rather than in the hips and thighs—are at greater risk of breast cancer.

If you're uncertain about whether you fall into the category of "overweight" or "obese," calculate your body mass index (BMI): Multiply your weight in pounds by 703; then divide the result by your height in inches squared. If your BMI is 25 to 29.9, you're overweight; if it's over 30, you're obese.

Ninety-five percent of people who do manage to lose weight end up gaining it back again; those few who do manage to maintain weight loss have to work very, very hard at it. The human body is designed to gain weight; so to lose it, you're going to have to work against this natural design. Humans have evolved over millennia of food scarcity, and the body that readily stores food away as fat is actually better adapted for survival when food is not plentiful—which has been the case for most of human history.

In today's environment, where high-calorie, low-nutrition, toxin-filled junk food is so much more available, popular, and affordable than natural, organic whole foods, it's harder than ever to lose weight and keep it off. It's tough to resist the appeal of carbohydrate- and fat-filled comfort foods when life gets stressful. Once you have grown accustomed to the tastes, textures, and convenience of processed foods, it may seem impossible to make the shift to whole foods prepared in your own kitchen, but with some attention and awareness, you can reacclimate yourself to the tastes and textures of wholesome foods.

The news stories about new obesity theories often do little more than add to the difficulty. Is it a slow metabolism? Is it a genetic glitch that you can't control? Will any one diet or exercise program change the way your body works enough to help you lose weight? What is it that makes one person gain pound after pound on a typical American diet, while another who lives on super-sized portions of fast food and sweets stays thin as a rail? The short answer, in the words of the American Obesity Association, is this: "Once attributed mainly to lack of will power, obesity is now understood to result from a complex interaction of genetic, metabolic, behavioral, and environmental factors." In other words, no single factor causes obesity, and no single magic bullet is going to cure it.

Just about everyone can control their weight by eating smaller amounts of healthier foods and getting plenty of exercise. The bottom line is that it really is about the food—that's why the various stomach-shrinking surgeries are so successful. If you're not going to shrink your stomach (which we don't recommend unless the problem is severe), then exercise is essential. And you don't need to look like the models on the exercise machine infomercials to be healthy. You don't need to be thin, slim, or buff. Almost everyone gains weight as they age, and that's fine—you don't need to look like a 20-something to be healthy, either. In fact, recent research has shown that it's more important to be fit than to conform to an "ideal" body weight.

We list the following weight loss drugs primarily to illustrate how dangerous they are. We do not recommend them—period. It's not worth the risk, and not one of them has been shown to keep weight off. There is no safe magic pill for losing weight.

Weight Loss and Appetite Control Drugs

Examples of Anorexiants

Benzphetamine HCl (Didrex)

Diethylpropion HCl (Diethylpropion, Tenuate, Tenuate Dospan)

Phendimetrazine tartrate (Phendimetrazine, Bontril, Plegine, Bontril Slow-Release, Dital, Dyrexan-OD, Melfiat-105 Unicelles, Prelu-2, Rexigen Forte)

Mazindol (Mazanor, Sanorex)

Phentermine HCl (Phentermine, Ionamin, Fastin, Adipex-P, Obe-Nix 30)

What Do They Do in the Body? They suppress appetite and increase metabolic rate and blood pressure.

What Are They Prescribed For? As a short-term (8- to 12-week) adjunct to a regimen of weight loss based on caloric restriction. In some instances, a physician may prescribe intermittent courses of therapy, with three to six weeks on and half of the treatment period off before starting the drug again.

What Are the Possible Side Effects? Palpitations, tachycardia, arrhythmias, high blood pressure, low blood pressure, fainting, pain, pulmonary hypertension (the potentially fatal problem that got Fen-phen recalled after several people died), changes in electrocardiogram readings (diethylpropion only), overstimulation, nervousness, restlessness, dizziness, insomnia, weakness, fatigue, malaise, anxiety, tension, euphoria, elevated mood, drowsiness, depression, agitation, tremor, confusion, lack of coordination, headache, change in libido, dry mouth, unpleasant taste, nausea, vomiting, abdominal discomfort, diarrhea, constipation, stomach pain, urinary problems, impotence, menstrual problems, testicular pain (mazindol only), bone marrow and blood cell abnormalities, eye irritation, blurred vision, hair loss, muscle pain, chest pain, excessive sweating, clamminess, chills, flushing, fever, and growth of breasts in males.

Like the amphetamines sold on the street, these drugs are addictive, and everyone who uses them for long enough eventually develops tolerance. Increasing the dosage in response to tolerance is a very bad idea.

Going off these drugs can cause dizziness, fatigue, and depression. Use caution when driving or performing other tasks that require you to be alert.

CAUTION!

Don't Take These Drugs If . . .

- You have heart disease.
- You have high blood pressure.
- You have hyperthyroidism (overactive thyroid).
- You have glaucoma.

- You tend to be anxious or agitated.
- You have a history of drug abuse.
- You take MAOIs or stopped taking them less than 14 days ago.
- You are taking another drug that has stimulant effects on the central nervous system.
- You have any kind of psychological disturbance. These drugs can make it worse.
- You are epileptic. Some patients have had increased seizures while taking diethylpropion.
- You tend to have low blood sugar (hypoglycemia). Mazindol increases muscle glucose uptake, which can cause a hypoglycemic episode.
- You are sensitive to tartrazine. Asthma and other allergic reactions can result.

What Are the Interactions with Food? Take these drugs on an empty stomach. If mazindol causes gastrointestinal irritation, it can be taken with food.

Stay Away from Phenylpropanolamine (PPA)

The stimulant drug phenylpropanolamine (PPA) is the active ingredient in several diet aids (Phenoxine, Dexatrim Pre-Meal, Maximum Strength Dexatrim, Phenyldrine, Control, Unitrol, Acutrim 16 Hour, Acutrim Late Day, Acutrim II Maximum Strength, Spray-U-Thin). These drugs were available over-the-counter until research linked PPA to dramatic increases in the risk of stroke in people under the age of 50. They are now available only by prescription. Avoid these drugs and any others that contain PPA.

Sibutramine (Meridia)

What Does It Do in the Body? It reduces appetite by inhibiting the reuptake of the neurotransmitters dopamine, norepinephrine, and serotonin, in effect increasing their levels in the brain. This is a dangerous drug that has caused at least 50 deaths, and it doesn't even work very well. Why is it still on the market?

What Is It Prescribed For? Management of obesity, including weight loss and maintenance of weight loss.

What Are the Possible Side Effects? Heart attack and death may be side effects of this drug. Dry mouth (in 17.2 percent of patients), insomnia (in 10.7 percent of patients), rapid heartbeat, sudden drops in blood pressure, migraine, high blood pressure, palpitations, dizziness, nervousness, anxiety, depression, sleepiness, central nervous system stimulation, mood swings, anorexia, constipation (in 11.5 percent), increased appetite, nausea, upset stomach, stomach inflammation, vomiting, menstrual problems, urinary tract infection, thirst, edema, muscle pain, joint pain, runny nose, throat irritation, increased cough, laryngitis, changes in sense of taste, ear pain, headache (in 30.3 percent, compared with 18.6 percent of placebo patients), back pain, flu syndrome, injury accidents, abdominal pain, chest pain, neck pain, and allergic reaction.

CAUTION!

Think Twice About Taking This Drug If . . .

- You have a history of drug addiction. This drug can be addicting.
- You have a history of seizures. This drug could increase your chances of having them.

- You have high blood pressure. Sibutramine raises blood pressure by an average of 1 to 3 mm Hg (systolic and diastolic) and raises heart rate an average of four to five beats per minute. Higher doses cause more pronounced increases.
- You have glaucoma.
- You have kidney or liver disease.

CAUTION!

Don't Take This Drug If . . .

- You are taking other weight loss drugs or MAOIs.
- You have any type of cardiovascular disease.
- You could become pregnant. Be sure to use adequate contraception while taking Meridia; it has been shown to cause birth defects in lab animals.

Don't combine sibutramine with other drugs that raise blood pressure, such as decongestants or cold, cough, and allergy medicines that contain pseudoephedrine, ephedrine, or PPA.

What Are the Interactions with Food? The effects of sibutramine are increased by alcohol. Avoid alcohol while using this drug.

Orlistat (Xenical, Alli)

This drug prevents a significant portion of dietary fat from being absorbed into the body. Instead, the fat passes right through. The side-effect profile of this drug is daunting, with potentially embarrassing gastrointestinal problems occurring in up to 27 percent of patients (see the later section on side effects). Other side effects such as rash, headache, depression, and decreased immunity are likely the direct result of decreased absorption of essential fatty acids and fat-soluble vitamins such as A, D, and E. As the long-term consequences of using this drug come to light, gallstones are emerging as a serious side effect.

What Does It Do in the Body? Orlistat is a lipase inhibitor. It inhibits the activity of an enzyme that breaks down fats before they are absorbed through the walls of the intestines. This prevents the absorption of about 30 percent of the fat taken in through the diet.

What Is It Prescribed For? Management of obesity, including weight loss and weight maintenance. It is also prescribed to reduce the risk of regaining weight that has been lost.

What Are the Possible Side Effects? Gallstones are a serious possible side effect. Digestive side effects include oily spotting (in 26.6 percent of patients); flatulence with discharge (in 23.9 percent); urgent need to defecate (in 22.1 percent); fatty, oily stools; increased defecation; and fecal incontinence. Most side effects were dramatically reduced in the second year of treatment, but they still affected between 1.8 and 5.5 percent of patients using orlistat. Side effects include headache, anxiety, depression (starting in the second year of treatment), dizziness, dry skin, rash, abdominal pain or discomfort, gum disease, infectious diarrhea, nausea, rectal pain/discomfort, tooth disorders, vomiting, arthritis, back pain, joint disorders, muscle pain, menstrual irregularities, vaginitis, increased incidence of flu, respiratory tract infections, fatigue, eye irritation, sleep problems, and urinary tract infection.

CAUTION!

- While taking orlistat, it is important to adhere to a low-fat diet (less than 30 percent fat) to avoid fecal incontinence and diarrhea.

- This and other weight loss drugs should not be used by anyone with a history of eating disorders, such as anorexia nervosa or bulimia.

What Are the Interactions with Food? Orlistat should be taken with meals.

What Nutrients Does It Throw out of Balance or Interact With? In patients with normal baseline vitamin levels before using orlistat, after the use of orlistat vitamin A levels were low in 2.2 percent, vitamin D levels were low in 12 percent, vitamin E levels were low in 5.8 percent, and beta-carotene levels were low in 6.1 percent. When fats are flushed through the system without being broken down, fat-soluble vitamins go along with them.

What Else to Take If You Take This Drug. A high-potency multivitamin containing vitamins A, D, and E, and beta-carotene, along with an essential fatty acid supplement. Take them between doses of orlistat.

Natural Alternatives to Diabetes and Weight Control Drugs

There are many safe, natural, and effective ways to help control blood sugar and shed excess weight without drugs. For most diabetics, these two changes go hand-in-hand. If you are overweight but don't know whether you have diabetes or are at risk for it, make sure you are evaluated by a physician to rule it out; knowing you have diabetes or insulin resistance will help you make the right changes to move back toward health. The Six Core Principles for Optimal Health are your cornerstone for healthy weight and stable blood sugar, with an emphasis on exercise, the reduction of processed foods and sugar, and—yes!—vegetables, preferably fresh and organic and not overcooked.

The high-carbohydrate diet traditionally recommended by the American Diabetes Association is proving not to be the answer for many diabetics. If you are a type 2 diabetic who is overweight and insulin resistant, it may be important for you to cut way back on carbohydrates. When you do eat them, stick to complex carbohydrates with plenty of fiber such as whole grains, vegetables, and legumes (e.g., beans). Sugar and simple carbohydrates (e.g., white flour, pasta, potatoes, corn, and bananas) create spikes in blood sugar and insulin production, and your goal is to keep both insulin and blood sugar on an even keel. Beans are especially good foods for balancing blood sugar.

Many people who struggle with their weight have been trying to lose excess pounds with the government-approved high-carbohydrate, low-fat, low-cholesterol diet, and the result has been temporary losses followed by a gain larger than what was lost. We now know that this type of diet can cause or worsen blood sugar ups and downs that lead to carbohydrate cravings. We also know that the average low-fat diet—laden with processed foods that have the fat removed and flavor added back in with sugar and artificial flavorings—are notoriously unsatisfying. Such diets inevitably lead to overconsumption of high-carbohydrate foods, which can pack a lot of empty calories. Those calories are stored as fat, especially in a body that is insulin resistant and has high insulin levels. The book *The Zone* by Barry Sears (HarperCollins, 1995) provides good, in-depth coverage of a balanced diet for insulin and weight control.

We'd like to make a point too often missed by the trend-hungry diet industry: the healthfulness of your diet involves much more than its carbohydrate, fat, or protein content. A high-carb diet made up of bread, cake, cookies, sodas, and the occasional piece of fresh fruit is a very different thing from a high-carb diet made up of brown rice, beans, vegetables, and fruits. A high-protein diet made up of processed meats (ham, bologna, bacon), processed cheese, and sugar-laden yogurt is quite different from one made up of lean meats, eggs, tofu, and fish accompanied by plenty of fresh veggies.

As you read about the supplements that can help stabilize your blood sugar, keep in mind that they will affect your blood sugar, so they shouldn't be used without very close monitoring if you have diabetes. You should be able to find all of these supplements at your health food store. If you are not diabetic, many of the diabetes supplements could be helpful for you. If you are diabetic and obese, the supplements recommended for weight control could assist you in your efforts to keep weight—and, by proxy, insulin levels—within healthy limits. While under a doctor's care, make sure he or she knows about all of the supplements you're using.

An Ayurvedic, Chinese, or naturopathic doctor will work very closely with diabetics, prescribing a variety of herbs and supplements depending on the health of the patient. If you have unstable blood sugar or are diabetic, please work closely with one of these types of physicians, or an M.D. or D.O. (doctor of osteopathy) willing to use herbs and nutritional supplements. In the "Resources and Recommended Reading" section of this book, you'll find an organization that will refer you to an alternative health care professional in your area.

Chromium and Niacin: Partners in Blood Sugar Control

Chromium is one of your key supplements when you need better blood sugar control. The people who make those awful bottled "natural" fruit drinks and teas aren't going to like this, but it's possible that the steep rise in our consumption of high fructose corn syrup has contributed to the rise in diabetes by depleting chromium. (As our consumption of high fructose corn syrup has risen 250 percent in the past 15 years, our rate of diabetes has increased approximately 45 percent in about the same time period.) According to studies done at the Agriculture Department's Human Nutrition Research Center, fructose consumption causes a drop in chromium, raises LDL "bad" cholesterol and triglycerides, and impairs immune system function—yet another great reason to read labels and avoid processed foods.

According to researchers, giving people with elevated blood sugar a chromium supplement will result in a significant drop in blood sugar in 80 to 90 percent of those people. Please don't be scared away from chromium by media reports about its potential dangers. Taking chromium picolinate supplements of 200 to 600 mcg daily is not the same as giving rats 5,000 to 6,000 times that dose every day, nor is it the same as factory workers breathing chromium dust. It is estimated that 90 percent of Americans are actually deficient in chromium, and at the recommended doses it is very safe and very effective in helping stabilize blood sugar as well as helping burn fat during exercise and producing lean muscle tissue.

The other nutrient necessary to help insulin do its job of ushering sugar into cells is niacin (vitamin B₃). Niacin works with chromium and should be taken in the form of inositol hexanicotinate with enough to give you 100 mg of niacin daily to start with. For example, one brand of 500 mg tablets of inositol hexanicotinate yields 400 mg of inositol and 100 mg of niacin. You can gradually raise the dose if needed, up to 400 mg of niacin daily.

Other Important Supplements for Stable Blood Sugar

Vanadium, a trace mineral taken in the form of vanadyl sulfate, helps insulin work more efficiently. That may be why it also lowers cholesterol and triglyceride levels. Long-term high doses of vanadium are not recommended, but you can use it to help stabilize your blood sugar and then cut back. Start with 6 mg daily and work your way up to 100 mg daily until you get results. Once you begin having results, stay at that dose for up to three weeks and then taper back gradually to 6 to 10 mg daily.

Studies now link a **vitamin D** deficiency with diabetes, immune function, and bone loss. It may be that vitamin D deficiency is a factor in the onset of diabetes and that a supplement of vitamin D could help reverse the disease. Take 1,000 to 2,000 IU daily, and spend at least 15 minutes per day in the sun, with skin exposed and without sunblock.

Zinc (10 to 15 mg daily), selenium (100 to 200 mcg daily), and manganese (10 mg daily) all play a role in regulating blood sugar and should be included in your daily multivitamin. Many diabetics are deficient in magnesium, which is key to a healthy heart, so be sure you're getting 400 to 800 mg daily in a supplement.

Recent studies have shown that both **vitamin E** and **vitamin C** significantly improve glucose (sugar) tolerance in type 2 diabetics. In fact, two independent studies have shown that low blood levels of vitamin E are correlated with a four times higher risk of diabetes. In a study published in the *Journal of Clinical Investigation*, researchers at Harvard who gave diabetic patients intravenous vitamin C found that it significantly improved blood vessel dilation and function. Since impaired blood flow is one of the primary causes of diabetes complications, this is significant information. It's a good idea for almost everyone to take 1,000 to 2,000 mg of vitamin C daily, but if you are diabetic, you may want to double that amount. (Vitamin C can give false readings on some types of glucose tests, so consult with your physician or pharmacist about which form of glucose testing works best with vitamin C.) Make sure you're getting your bioflavonoids with the vitamin C. The bioflavonoids in grapeseed extract and ginkgo biloba help strengthen blood vessels and improve blood flow to the extremities.

Calcium, long known to be important for bone health, may also help with weight loss, according to recent research by scientists at the University of Vermont. Women who increased their calcium intake by as little as 130 mg a day showed an increased rate of weight loss compared to women whose calcium intake didn't increase. In-depth studies of fat-cell function have shown that when calcium intake is too low, a hormone that causes bones to demineralize is released. This same hormone affects fat cells, too, by prompting them to store more fat. Other research has shown that the amount of calcium stored in fat cells plays an important role in regulating how much fat they store or burn. Mice bred to be obese and plumped up on a high-fat, high-sugar diet were then put on a calorie-restricted diet. Some of the mice received calcium supplementation. Those with extra calcium in the diet lost 42 percent of their fat weight, while those receiving no extra calcium only lost 8 percent! One of the study's authors, Jean Harvey-Berino, Ph.D., advises that taking at least 1,000 mg of supplemental calcium per day is a good way to enhance weight loss.

Essential fatty acids (EFAs) are especially essential for people with unstable blood sugar, making it very important to cut out the EFA-blocking hydrogenated oils found in chips, baked goods, and nearly all processed foods. Research has shown that diabetics given evening primrose oil for a year had improved nerve function, while those on a placebo became worse. Other research has shown that diabetics

on a high monounsaturated oil diet (e.g., olive oil, canola oil, avocados) had lower triglycerides and better levels of blood glucose and insulin than those on a primarily high-carbohydrate diet. Eating plenty of fresh, organic vegetables, a variety of whole grains, and fish should give you a good base of EFAs over the long term. Limiting hydrogenated fats and refined carbohydrates will help the essential fats you take in to go down the proper pathway for better health.

Ginseng has been used by the Chinese for centuries to help control diabetes, and recent studies confirm that it can reduce fasting blood glucose as well as improve mood and help in weight reduction. Herbalist Donald Brown recommends a standardized extract with a 5 to 7 percent ginsenoside content. More or less can throw blood sugar off rather than bring it into balance. For this use, ginseng is probably best taken as a liquid extract.

One of the **Ayurvedic herbs** of choice in India for lowering blood sugar, now available in the United States, is called *Gymnema sylvestre*. There is also some evidence that *Gymnema sylvestre* actually reverses damage to certain cells in the pancreas that can be destroyed by diabetes. You can find it at your health food store. Be sure to tell your health care provider that you are taking this herb, because if you are taking diabetes drugs they may need to be adjusted.

An extract of a cucumber-like vegetable called **bitter melon** (*Momordica charantia*) has potent blood-glucose-lowering action. Bitter melon is eaten as a medicinal food in many parts of the world.

Banaba (*Lagerstroemia speciosa*) is a plant that grows wild all over the Philippines, and it is commonly used there as a folk remedy for diabetes. Scientists all over the world are studying its active component, corosolic acid, to better understand why it balances blood sugars so well. In one study, diabetic rats were fed the yolks of eggs from chickens that had been fed banaba, and their high blood sugar was normalized. Research has found that banaba also significantly decreases the amount of lipid (fat) accumulated in the liver. In one study, banaba was found to increase glucose transport into cells just like insulin, but at the same time, it had a suppressive effect on the creation of more fat cells. Banaba may be a very useful plant for the prevention and treatment of high blood sugar and obesity in type 2 diabetics.

Turmeric, a spice often used in the East, and the more familiar spice cinnamon have both shown tremendous potential in helping regulate blood sugar. Richard Anderson, Ph.D., tested these spices in a test tube and found that they tripled insulin's ability to metabolize sugar. Studies indicate that fenugreek is another spice that can aid you in controlling your sugar levels. In addition, maitake mushrooms have been found to help maintain correct sugar levels. Green tea, berries, and the herb rosemary can all improve insulin sensitivity.

Supplements for Weight Loss

The following supplements aren't specifically for diabetics, but they can be helpful for those who wish to lose weight. They are almost all derived from plants, and many have a long history of safe medicinal use.

Phaseolus vulgaris is derived from the common white kidney bean. It contains a substance that inhibits the activity of the alpha-amylase enzyme. Alpha-amylase is responsible for breaking down carbohydrates in the digestive tract, and inhibiting it helps slow or decrease the absorption of carbohydrates through the intestinal wall.

Foods That Raise Blood Sugar

Carrots
Oatmeal
Oranges
Potatoes
Processed cereals
Raisins
Refined grains (white bread, pasta)
Sugar, molasses
Sweet corn
Yams

It's believed that the neurotransmitter serotonin plays a powerful role in appetite control. SSRIs and other neurotransmitter-affecting drugs dampen appetite due to increases in serotonin availability in the brain.

Garcinia cambogia contains hydroxycitric acid, which has been found to increase the availability of serotonin in the brain almost as much as SSRI drugs do. It has also been found to decrease body fat synthesis. Unlike SSRIs, this plant extract is nontoxic, with side effects occurring only at doses far exceeding recommended dosages (5,000 mg [5 g] per kilogram—that would be equivalent to 350 grams for a 155-pound [70 kg] man). Interestingly, *Garcinia cambogia* also appears to protect against NSAID-induced ulcers, increasing the stomach lining's defenses against erosion and slightly decreasing the volume and acidity of digestive juices. Dosages will vary by brand; follow the instructions on the container.

Coenzyme Q10 (CoQ10) is made in the body and is needed within each cell to spark tiny cellular "engines" called mitochondria. Within the mitochondria, fuel—carbs, fats,

Good Foods for Stable Blood Sugar

Apples	Artichokes
Asparagus	Basmati rice
Beet greens	Broccoli
Brown rice	Brussels sprouts
Buckwheat	Cauliflower
Celery	Chicken
Chicory	Collard greens
Cranberries	Dandelion greens
Endive	Fava beans
Fish	Garlic
Grapefruit	Kale
Kidney beans	Leaf lettuce
Lean, white freshwater fish	Leeks
Lemons	Lima beans
Limes	Meat
Millet	Mung beans
Olive oil (small amounts)	Olives
Onions	Papaya
Parsley	Pears
Peppers	Persimmons
Pomegranates	Rye
Rye crisps	Sunflower seeds, raw
Swiss chard	Turkey

and sometimes proteins—are metabolized into energy. Research is showing that low CoQ10 levels are correlated with obesity and that boosting these low levels could also boost metabolism and weight loss. Try between 50 and 100 mg per day.

Making the Shift to Naturally Stable Blood Sugar

If you are struggling with unstable blood sugar and coping with a physician who just wants to put you on drugs, perhaps you can take some inspiration

from a woman named Susan. During an annual checkup with her physician, Susan was told she had high blood sugar and was given a prescription for an oral diabetes drug. She took the drug until she went on a lengthy vacation and ran out. Remembering the advice she had read in one of Dr. Mindell's books to cut out sugars, processed foods, and get plenty of exercise, she did just that while on vacation. She felt so great that she continued this regimen when she got back home and never renewed her prescription for the drug. A few months later, she went back to her physician, and her blood sugar was perfectly normal. A year later, her blood sugar was still normal, and she was in great health. Congratulations to Susan and to all of you who have taken charge of your health and are feeling better for it!

Ideally you should go off any drug under the supervision of a health care professional. As you change your diet, begin to exercise, and take the recommended supplements, your blood sugar will go down and stabilize. It is very important for you to track it daily and adjust any medications you're taking accordingly.

Supplements to Counteract the Harm Diabetes Can Do

Diabetes ages the body rapidly. The disease causes changes that, for all intents and purposes, presses the fast-forward button on your aging clock. Damage to the cardiovascular system, the kidneys, the eyes, and the nerves of the feet can lead to heart disease, stroke, impotence, kidney failure, blindness, and pain and numbness in the lower legs and feet.

Two reasons for this are (1) the dramatic increase in free radical production seen in diabetics, and (2) a process known as glycation, which is also amplified in people with the chronically high blood sugars seen in diabetes.

Free radicals are renegade electrons, formed during normal metabolism, that pull electrons from other molecules, causing damage to proteins and fats. These submicroscopic troublemakers can be stopped by antioxidants, but if there aren't enough antioxidants to go around, they can start chain reactions that powerfully contribute to accelerated aging and chronic disease. Also, most antioxidants actually become free radicals themselves once they've done the job of neutralizing a free radical, and they must be "replenished" by a different antioxidant to keep doing their good work. This is why it's important to get the full range of antioxidant nutrients rather than taking huge amounts of any single antioxidant.

Glycation describes the binding of glucose, the simplest form of sugar, to proteins. Think of how a turkey browns in the oven or look at some age spots on someone's skin to get a visual picture of this process. Glycated proteins can't do their jobs properly, and they contribute to the cellular breakdown that leads to dysfunctional organs and chronic disease.

A complete supplement program for people with diabetes should include supplements to counteract both free radicals and glycation. Antioxidants such as vitamins C and E and beta-carotene are a good start, as are more powerful free-radical snatchers such as green tea extract and grapeseed extract. Here are two more supplements that can keep you younger longer if you have diabetes.

Alpha-lipoic acid (ALA) is made in the body. Of all the known antioxidants, it's among the most versatile. It stops free radicals from damaging proteins and fats, and it "recycles" used-up vitamin C, vitamin E, and glutathione (another antioxidant that's made in the body). ALA is the only antioxidant proven to raise levels of glutathione within the cells. Take 50 to 125 mg twice daily.

L-carnosine is an amino acid found in high concentrations in the cells of the brain and muscles and in the lenses of the eyes. It has some effectiveness at blocking free radical damage, but its main strength is its ability to inhibit glycation. L-carnosine decreases glycation by binding with sugars before they have a chance to bind with proteins. It protects healthy proteins from being damaged by glycated proteins and helps prevent cross-linking, a process related to glycation that causes skin and other organs to lose flexibility and function. In studies on mice bred to age rapidly, L-carnosine extended life span by 20 percent. Test tube studies have shown that L-carnosine turns back the clock on aged cells, bringing back the appearance and function of youth. Take 50 mg daily.

Exercise: An Essential Part of Managing Diabetes and Controlling Weight

You cannot properly control adult-onset diabetes without a good exercise program. There's no getting around it. One of the most devastating side effects of diabetes over time is failing circulation to the extremities, causing numbness, tingling, loss of sensation, and sometimes even the loss of a limb. Exercise is essential for keeping circulation strong. Exercise is also an indispensable part of any weight loss program. A study of successful weight loss veterans—people who lost weight and kept it off—found that all of them exercised for an average of an hour each day.

The recent news that more than half of America is overweight inspired the Institute of Medicine (IOM), an independent advisory agency that reports to the government on health issues, to put together an 800-plus-page volume devoted to redefining the diet and exercise requirements for healthy weight and avoidance of lifestyle-related illnesses. Its basic conclusions and recommendations concerning exercise were that Americans need to engage in at least 60 minutes of exercise every day, not the 30 to 60 minutes, three to five times a week previously recommended, and that Americans need to pay more attention to the intensity of their workouts, making sure that they are expending enough energy to stave off weight gain or induce weight loss.

Once you're at an optimum weight, you will probably be able to eat slightly more than you did while losing weight, as long as you continue to exercise. In a study published in the August 2002 issue of the journal *Endocrinology*, obese rats were given a calorically restricted diet as their energy consumption was increased. They lost a significant amount of weight within five months. When food intake was increased after the weight was lost, they maintained their new weight as long as they continued to exercise.

The IOM's recommendation of one hour of moderate physical activity daily is double the 1996 recommendation given by the U.S. Surgeon General. With more than 60 percent of Americans not in a regular exercise program and 25 percent completely sedentary, the notion that people will adhere to this recommendation is quite far-fetched.

If you absolutely don't have 60 minutes a day to exercise, keep in mind that you can split up your activity into more manageable chunks. For example, you can take a 20-minute walk with your dog in the morning, a 20-minute walk on your lunch break, and another 20-minute walk in the evening to tally up your 60 minutes. If you would much prefer to watch TV than exercise, purchase equipment that will enable you to log your workout while watching your favor-

ite programs. Make it as easy and pleasurable as you can, but do it. You'll feel better, you'll live longer, and there will be more life in your years. Once you're used to doing it daily, it will just become part of your life and won't seem like such a chore.

Intensity is as important an element of your workouts as duration (the amount of time you spend doing a workout) and mode (the form of exercise you choose). Intensity is a tricky thing to measure; for someone who hasn't worked out before, a low-intensity workout can feel excruciatingly difficult, and for a highly trained athlete, a high-intensity workout can feel like a game of croquet. Your experience of intensity also varies according to the mode of exercise you choose. Non-weight-bearing exercise such as swimming and stationary cycling will often feel more intense at your target heart rate than weight-bearing exercise. You have to work harder to get your heart rate up because you don't have the added work of supporting your own body weight. If at all possible, include weight-bearing exercise in your regimen. It's better at strengthening bones and muscles. If you're heavy, keep in mind that the more you weigh, the more energy (calories) you'll expend during a weight-bearing workout.

Intensity is, most simply, the rate at which you expend energy. If you take an hour-long walk along a flat sidewalk at 2.5 miles per hour—only a little faster than window-shopping pace—you might expend 200 calories. If you speed up to a brisk four miles per hour and walk in a hilly area, you could conceivably expend more than twice that amount of caloric energy. Intensity affects your metabolic rate both during and after exercise. When you exercise at a moderate intensity rather than a low one, your body will continue to burn calories above and beyond those you burn doing everyday things. This elevated post-exercise energy consumption can last anywhere from a few hours to a whole day, depending on how hard you exercise.

Some overachievers go over the top with intensity. They exhaust themselves too quickly to keep up the pace, and they often end up overtraining—a situation that leads to pulled muscles, injuries, and a weak immune system. Additionally, they end up working out at a level that uses the mostly quickly available carbohydrate energy, so stored fat remains socked away while carbohydrate stores are burned as fuel. Blood sugars drop, causing light-headedness and weakness—symptoms referred to by athletes as "bonking"—and carbohydrate cravings result. High-intensity workouts can also cause a rush of the stress hormone cortisol. This rush of cortisol and other energizing body chemicals is the source of "runner's high." The catch is that day after day of high cortisol requirements can deplete the adrenal glands, which in turn leads to chronic fatigue, dampened immunity, worsening allergies, and other unpleasant symptoms. In the end, going overboard with intensity will work against a weight-loss program, because you'll have uncontrollable carbohydrate cravings and likely will incur an injury or illness that will make you unable to work out.

You can include time spent doing weight training in your daily exercise allotment. Keep in mind that if you can't meet the goal of logging an hour a day, you shouldn't just give up on exercise altogether. Something is always better than nothing. If you can't walk for an hour, walk for 20 minutes instead. If you have physical problems that preclude long bouts of aerobic exercise, try stretching exercises, yoga, or qi gong. If you are housebound by weather and want to get some aerobic exercise, find an exercise program on TV, clean your house from top to bottom, or put on your favorite dancing music. The best exercise is whatever is fun and easy for you to do every day.

Chapter 17

Drugs for Eye Diseases and Their Natural Alternatives

Your eyes are a window to more than just your soul. Unhealthy eyes can reveal ill health even before signs of illness emerge in other parts of the body. The condition of the tiny blood vessels that nourish the eye is a good indicator of the health of the blood vessels throughout the rest of your body. For example, if the tiny blood vessels in your eyes are broken or leaking, you can be sure that same process is under way in your larger arteries. If your eyes are dry enough to require rewetting drops, chances are the rest of your body is low on important nutrients needed to make lubricating tears, or you have an allergy caused by an overstressed immune system. Vision-stealing diseases such as glaucoma, cataracts, macular degeneration, and diabetic retinopathy are often caused or precipitated by a combination of exposure to toxins and poor nutrition.

What Causes Eye Disease?

Glaucoma can be caused by long-term use of steroid drugs or by overconsumption of optic nerve toxins such as aspartame and monosodium glutamate (MSG). Drugs used to treat glaucoma are designed to lower pressure in the eyeball. Much like the medical approach of bombarding the body with cholesterol-lowering or blood-pressure-lowering medication at the cost of general health and well-being, this tactic doesn't always help more than it hurts.

Macular degeneration is the most common cause of blindness in adults over 50. Unlike glaucoma, macular degeneration doesn't result in complete blindness but instead causes loss of central vision. In advanced stages of this debilitating eye disease, most of the visual field is blurred beyond recognition, rendering the person legally blind. The macula is a part of the retina that's particularly vulnerable to damage from the sun and poor nutrition. Because darker eyes have more dark pigment to filter out ultraviolet rays, brown-eyed people are at lower risk than those with blue, green, or hazel eyes. No medical treatment can stop this disease from progressing, and no drug can do any more than slow its progression. Laser surgery is a last resort, but it is done only on people in whom the disease is very advanced, because it carries the risk of making vision worse. Fortunately, a lot can be done nutritionally to prevent and control macular degeneration.

Cataracts are another very common vision problem. Clouding of the lens of the eye can be caused by too much sun exposure, an unhealthy diet over the years, heavy smoking, or diabetes. The lens loses its flexibility as we age, and focusing becomes more difficult. (Ever notice how many people who never needed glasses in their adult lives are suddenly wearing them when they hit 40?) The lens yellows and becomes very cloudy, blurring vision and causing uncomfortable glare from bright light.

Diabetic cataracts result from an accumulation of excess sugar in the lens. Cataracts make it impossible to see color accurately. Faces may become difficult to recognize, and family members may mistakenly think the person has become senile. Elderly people who fall and break a hip may have missed seeing the step they tripped on because of cataracts. There aren't any drugs for the treatment of cataracts; surgical removal of the clouded lens is the treatment of choice. It's a very simple surgery that almost always yields excellent results, especially when a new, synthetic lens implant replaces the old lens.

Diabetic eye disease is common in both type 1 (insulin-dependent) and type 2 (non-insulin-dependent) diabetes. Blood vessels throughout the body are more prone to clogging with fatty deposits in diabetics. Their risk for heart disease, peripheral vascular disease, and stroke is considerably higher than in the rest of the population. The blood vessels that feed the retina are especially at risk. When these vessels are unhealthy, the retina can't get the nourishment it needs. The body tries to get blood to the area by actually sprouting new blood vessels to bypass the clogged ones. The new blood vessels grow over the retina, causing blindness. Laser surgery and vitrectomy (where blood that has leaked into the eyeball is "vacuumed" out) are the only medical treatments available for diabetic retinopathy, and by the time these are needed, the disease is advanced. Good nutrition and the right supplements can do a great deal to keep things from going that far.

What Causes Irritated Eyes?

Itchy, runny, allergic, bloodshot, dry, gritty, or burning eyes are common complaints for which

Common Drugs That Can Cause Eye Problems

Antihistamines can cause sensitivity to the sun and cause dry eyes.

Blood thinners (e.g., heparin, Coumadin) can cause retinal hemorrhage.

NSAIDs (e.g., aspirin, ibuprofen, naproxen) used long term can cause cataracts, dry eyes, and retinal hemorrhages.

Preservatives in eyedrops can cause eye irritation (e.g., red eye).

Impotence (erectile dysfunction) drugs (e.g., Flomax) can cause floppy iris syndrome, which interferes with cataract surgery, color perception changes, blurry vision, and increased light sensitivity.

Adrenergic agents, beta-2-adrenergic agonists, and anticholinergic agents, which include some of the blood pressure drugs, asthma and allergy drugs, and impotence drugs, can cause dilation of the pupils and angle-closure glaucoma.

Glucocorticoids (e.g., prednisone, cortisol, asthma drugs) can increase pressure in the eye and lead to open-angle glaucoma, and can lead to cataracts and optic nerve damage.

Tamoxifen, the breast cancer drug, can cause damage to the retina.

Amiodarone, a drug used to treat irregular heartbeat, can cause multiple eye problems, including changes in color vision.

Rosiglitazone (Avandia), the diabetes drugs, can cause macular edema (swelling of the retina).

Prozac can cause dilated pupils, double vision, blurred vision, dry eyes, eye pain, eyelid infection, cataracts, glaucoma, ptosis (eyelid droop), and an inflammation of the iris (iritis).

Birth control pills can cause dry eyes and color vision disturbances.

we tend to buy over-the-counter eyedrops. It's estimated that over 30 million Americans complain of dry eyes. Smog, chemical irritants, contact lenses (which can pull moisture off the eyes), low humidity, cigarette smoke, dust, wind, sun, air-conditioning, heaters, chronic crying (which dilutes the viscous tear film that keeps moisture in), and droopy lower eyelids (which can allow tears to evaporate too quickly) are common causes of dry eye. People who suffer from arthritis tend to have dry eyes. In Sjögren's syndrome, which affects mostly women over the age of 40, the eyes and mouth become very dry. Tooth decay and severe eye discomfort can result.

A long list of medicines can cause dry eyes, and benzalkonium chloride, a preservative used in most eyedrops, may make dry eyes worse. If you are taking any type of medication and are suffering from dry eyes, be sure to check the package insert to find out if one of the drug's side effects is dry eyes or vision problems. Aspartame (NutraSweet) has also been shown to cause dry eyes.

Prescription and Over-the-Counter Drugs for the Eyes

Examples of Sympathomimetic Glaucoma Drugs

Apraclonidine (Iopidine)
Brimonidine (Alphagan)
Dipivefrin (Propine)
Epinephrine (Epifrin, Glaucon)

What Do They Do in the Body? These drugs increase the outflow of fluid (aqueous humor) from the eyeball. They also reduce the production of aqueous humor.

What Are They Prescribed For? Decreasing eye fluid pressure in people with ocular hypertension or glaucoma.

What Are the Possible Side Effects? The following are drug-specific side effects:

• **Alphagan.** Ten to 30 percent of those who use this drug have dry mouth, blood congestion in the eyes, burning and stinging, headache, blurred vision, feeling of having something stuck in the eye, fatigue or drowsiness, inflamed eyelash follicles or eyelids, eye allergy symptoms, and itching of the eye. Other side effects include staining or erosion of the cornea, increased sensitivity to light, redness or swelling of the eyelids or conjunctiva, aching or dry eyes, eye irritation, tearing, upper respiratory problems, dizziness, gastrointestinal problems, weakness, whitening or hemorrhage of the conjunctiva, abnormal vision, muscle pain, lid crusting, abnormal sense of taste, insomnia, depression, high blood pressure, anxiety, palpitations, nasal dryness, and fainting.

• **Epinephrine.** These drops tend to cause a lot of stinging and burning, which may lessen over time. Other side effects include eye pain or ache, headache, allergic reaction on eyelid, swelling or change in color of the conjunctiva, change in color of the cornea, eye irritation, deposits on the conjunctiva or cornea (with long-standing use), headache, palpitations, rapid heartbeat or other cardiac arrhythmias, high blood pressure, and faintness.

• **Dipivefrin.** This is turned into epinephrine in the body and has most of the same adverse effects, but is less irritating to the eyes.

• **Apraclonidine.** Blood congestion in the eyes, eye itching, discomfort and tearing, swelling of the eyelids, and feeling of having something stuck in the eye. Many other side effects have been reported, but they are rare.

Preservatives Commonly Used in Eyedrops

A preservative used in glaucoma and other eyedrops, benzalkonium chloride, has been shown to worsen dry eyes and to actually be toxic to the cells of the cornea. Look for preservative-free artificial tears. If you have to use glaucoma eyedrops, you'll be exposed to benzalkonium chloride; they aren't made without preservatives.

Thimerosal is another eyedrop preservative that can cause problems. It isn't hard to find thimerosal-free drops, but again, if you have to use a certain prescription eye drug, you may not have an alternative. If your eyes become dry while using these drugs, try our nutritional and lifestyle prescriptions to relieve dry eye symptoms.

CAUTION!

• Most of these drops contain a preservative called benzalkonium chloride, which can be absorbed by soft contacts. Take out lenses before using glaucoma drops, and wait at least 15 minutes before putting them back in.
• If you have clinical depression, Buerger's disease, Raynaud's phenomenon, orthostatic hypotension (drastic dips in blood pressure when you sit up from lying or stand up from sitting), diabetes, hyperthyroidism, bronchial asthma, or kidney or liver impairment, you should be cautious when using any sympathomimetic eyedrop.
• Those with high blood pressure, cerebrovascular disease (clogging of blood vessels in the brain that can lead to stroke), or heart disease should use caution, as these drugs can cause blood pressure to rise slightly.

- Elderly people are especially vulnerable to side effects from these drugs.
- Sympathomimetic drugs can cause fatigue or drowsiness, and most of these drugs alter vision temporarily; be careful while driving.
- Brimonidine (Alphagan) may lose its pressure-lowering effect over time, so your eye pressure should be checked regularly.
- Epinephrine can cause attacks of narrow-angle glaucoma. Your eye doctor should check to be sure you are not at risk for this before starting you on epinephrine.
- If you have had a lens removed from one of your eyes due to cataract, epinephrine can cause damage to the tiny spot on the retina called the macula. If you have a rapid loss of vision in that eye, stop using epinephrine right away.
- Don't wear soft contacts while using epinephrine. Your lenses could change color.
- If you are using dipivefrin (Propine) and miss a dose, don't try to "catch up" on a missed dose by taking two at once.
- You should not use apraclonidine (Iopidine) if you are taking monoamine oxidase inhibitors (MAOIs). Iopidine's effectiveness may decrease over a month's time. Some people who take Iopidine are hypersensitive and suffer from blood congestion in the eye, itching, general discomfort, tearing, feeling of having something stuck in the eye, and swelling of the eyelids and conjunctiva. If you have these problems, you need to try a different drug.

• **Brimonidine.** Central nervous system depressants such as alcohol, barbiturates, opiates, sedatives, or anesthetics can have additive effects with Alphagan. You may not be able to tolerate your usual number of drinks, or your sleep or pain pills may really knock you out. Beta-blockers (both ophthalmic and systemic) and other high-blood-pressure drugs, as well as cardiac glycosides such as digoxin, can add to the reductions in pulse and blood pressure that can occur with brimonidine.

• **Apraclonidine.** This drug may reduce pulse and blood pressure, and many cardiovascular drugs also have this effect. Pulse and blood pressure should be checked frequently if these drugs are combined.

Examples of Beta-Blocker Eyedrops

Betaxolol (Betoptic, Betoptic S)
Carteolol (Ocupress)
Levobunolol (AKBeta, Betagan Liquifilm)
Metipranolol (OptiPranolol)
Timolol (Timoptic, Timoptic-XE)
Levobetaxolol (Betaxon)

What Do They Do in the Body? When used as eyedrops, these drugs decrease the rate of production of aqueous humor (fluid) in the eyeball.

What Are They Prescribed For? Lowering of intraocular pressure in glaucoma.

What Are the Possible Side Effects? Headache, depression, heart rhythm irregularities, fainting, stroke or cerebral ischemia (insufficient oxygen going to parts of the brain), and cardiovascular effects such as heart rhythm changes, heart attack, stroke, heart failure, cardiac arrest (usually in elderly people who already are at risk for heart attack, stroke, heart failure, and other cardiovascular problems), palpitations, nausea, bronchospasm, respiratory failure, masking of low blood sugar in those with insulin-dependent diabetes, inflammation of the cornea, drooping of the upper eyelid, vision disturbances, and double vision have occurred with all of the ophthalmic beta-blockers.

• **Carteolol (Ocupress).** Eye irritation, burning, tearing, blood congestion in the conjunctiva, swelling, blurred or cloudy vision, sensitivity to light, decreased night vision, eyelid inflammation, abnormal staining or sensitivity of the cornea, decreased blood pressure, shortness of breath, weakness, dizziness, insomnia, sinus inflammation, and changes in sense of taste.

• **Metipranolol (OptiPranolol).** Eye irritation, eyelid dermatitis or inflammation, blurred vision, tearing, brow ache, abnormal vision, sensitivity to light, swelling, allergic reaction, weakness, high blood pressure, heart attack, heart rhythm irregularities, angina, nausea, runny nose, shortness of breath, nosebleed, bronchitis, coughing, dizziness, anxiety, depression, sleepiness, nervousness, arthritis, muscle pain, and rash.

• **Levobunolol (AKBeta, Betagan).** Burning and stinging, eyelid inflammation, and decreased corneal sensitivity.

• **Timolol (Timoptic, Timoptic-XE).** Eye irritation, conjunctivitis, eyelid inflammation, decreased corneal sensitivity, vision disturbances such as double vision, dizziness, fatigue, lethargy, hallucinations, confusion, shortness of breath, aggravation of myasthenia gravis, hair loss, change in color of fingernails, hypersensitivity resulting in rash, itching, weakness, impotence, decreased libido, electrolyte imbalances, diarrhea, and tingling of the extremities.

• **Levobetaxolol (Betaxon).** Slow heart rate, high blood pressure, low blood pressure, rapid heart rate, anxiety, dizziness, vertigo, hair loss, dermatitis, psoriasis, diabetes, hypothyroidism, constipation, upset stomach, breast abscess, cystitis, gout, increased cholesterol and triglyceride levels, arthritis, tendonitis, transient discomfort or blurred vision when instilling drops, cataracts, respiratory problems, ear pain, ringing in the ears (tinnitus), changes in sense of taste, headache, and increased risk of infection.

CAUTION!

Think Twice About Taking These Drugs If . . .

• You have bronchial asthma or chronic obstructive pulmonary disease (COPD).
• You have a heart rhythm disorder called sinus bradycardia (very slow heart rate), or if you have second-degree or third-degree atrioventricular block.
• You have congestive heart failure or have ever had cardiogenic shock.

These eyedrops can be absorbed in large enough amounts to cause the systemic reactions seen with beta-blocker pills. Fatal asthma attacks in asthmatics and cardiac failure in those with heart disease have been reported with use of beta-blocker eyedrops.

Beta-blockers can increase the risks of surgical anesthesia, potentially causing pronounced dips in blood pressure during surgery. If you are having heart surgery, beta-blockers can make it harder to restart your heart.

If you are diabetic, please remember that beta-blockers may mask the symptoms of dangerously low blood sugar. Symptoms of hyperthyroidism (including very rapid heartbeat) may also be masked.

If your physician has ever told you that you have cerebrovascular insufficiency (too little blood flowing to parts of the brain), be aware that beta-blockers can worsen the problem.

The accepted wisdom used to be that eye-drops and other topical medications wouldn't enter the bloodstream enough to affect the rest of the body, but we now know that's not true. If you're taking any type of drug that interacts with the beta-blockers (see Chapter 10), you should be watchful for adverse reactions.

Oral (usually given to lower blood pressure) and topical beta-blockers (for glaucoma) used together can become overwhelming to the body. Dangerous adverse side effects become much more likely.

What Else to Take While Taking These Drugs. Take 200 to 600 mg of chromium to help boost "good" HDL cholesterol while using beta-blocker eyedrops.

Examples of Direct-Acting Miotics

Carbachol (Miostat)
Pilocarpine (Isopto Carpine, Pilocar, Piloptic, Pilostat, Adsorbocarbine, Akarpine, Pilopine HS)

What Do They Do in the Body? When applied to the eye, they cause the pupils to constrict. This allows more aqueous humor (fluid) to flow out of the back of the eyeball.

What Are They Prescribed For? Lowering of intraocular pressure in glaucoma.

What Are the Possible Side Effects? The following are drug-specific side effects:

• **Carbachol.** Transient stinging and burning, clouding of the cornea, blisters on the cornea, inflammation of the iris after cataract extraction, retinal detachment, inflammation of the ciliary bodies and conjunctiva, spasm of the ciliary bodies (which makes vision less acute), headache, salivation, gastrointestinal cramps, vomiting,

diarrhea, asthma, fainting, heart rhythm irregularities, flushing, sweating, stomach distress, a feeling of tightness in the bladder, low blood pressure, and frequent need to urinate.

• **Pilocarpine.** Transient stinging and burning, tearing, spasm of the ciliary bodies (which makes vision less acute), blood congestion of the conjunctiva, headache, inflammation of the cornea, nearsightedness (especially in younger people when first starting with this drug), blurred vision, difficulty adapting to darkness, poor dim light vision (especially in those with cataracts), hypertension, very fast heartbeat, airway tightening, fluid in the lungs, excessive salivation, sweating, nausea, and vomiting.

CAUTION!

Think Twice About Taking These Drugs If . . .

• You have acute iritis, acute or anterior uveitis, secondary glaucoma (with some exceptions), pupillary block glaucoma, or acute inflammatory disease of the anterior chamber.
• You have an abrasion on your cornea. This makes excessive penetration of the medication carbachol more likely.
• You have recently had a heart attack, or if you have heart failure, asthma, stomach ulcer, hyperthyroidism, gastrointestinal spasm, urinary tract obstruction, Parkinson's disease, hypertension, or hypotension. Use caution when using direct-acting miotics.

Before starting to use these drugs, you should be sure your ophthalmologist gives you a thorough eye examination. Some people are more susceptible to retinal detachment than others, and miotics can cause this to happen in those people.

CAUTION!

- Use caution while driving at night. Miotics affect your ability to see in the dark.
- In susceptible people, miotics can bring on attacks of angle-closure glaucoma.

What Else to Take While Taking These Drugs. Take 1,000 to 3,000 mg a day of the bioflavonoids quercetin and rutin.

Examples of Cholinesterase-Inhibiting Miotics

Demecarium (Humorsol)
Echothiophate (Phospholine Iodide)
Physostigmine (Eserine Sulfate)

What Do They Do in the Body? Cause complete, rapid shrinking of the pupil of the eye.

What Are They Prescribed For? Lowering of intraocular pressure in ocular hypertension or glaucoma.

What Are the Possible Side Effects? Iris cysts, burning, watering of the eyes, twitching of the eyelid, redness of the conjunctiva and ciliary bodies, headache, nearsightedness and blurring, retinal detachment, cataract, nausea, vomiting, abdominal cramps, diarrhea, urinary incontinence, fainting, sweating, excessive salivation, difficulty breathing, heart problems, and thickening of the conjunctiva. Deterioration of the nasal canals and tear ducts can occur with long-term use.

Cysts may grow on the iris of the eye treated with these drugs. These can grow large enough to interfere with vision. They usually shrink or disappear when the drug is stopped. You should

have regular eye exams to be sure you aren't developing any iris cysts.

CAUTION!

Think Twice About Taking These Drugs If . . .

- You have active uveal inflammation or any inflammatory disease of the iris or ciliary body.
- You have glaucoma associated with iridocyclitis.
- You have any kind of angle-closure glaucoma. Don't use echothiophate. The other drugs in this class can also aggravate angle-closure glaucoma.
- You have myasthenia gravis. If you are taking cholinesterase inhibitors to control it, using topical cholinesterase inhibitors puts you at greater risk for adverse effects.

Overexcitability of the vagus nerve (vagotonia), asthma, gastrointestinal spasm, stomach ulcer, very slow heartbeat or low blood pressure, recent heart attack, epilepsy, and Parkinson's disease all put you at greater risk of problems with cholinesterase-inhibitor eyedrops.

The shrinking of the pupil (miosis) caused by this drug limits your ability to adapt to darkness. Use caution while driving at night.

You should discontinue these drugs three to four weeks before having eye surgery.

Avoid contact with carbamate or organophosphate insecticides and pesticides while using cholinesterase inhibitors. (Avoid such substances no matter what!)

Succinylcholine, a general anesthetic, can cause respiratory and cardiovascular collapse in people using these drugs. If you are going to have surgery, be sure to tell your doctor that you are taking these drugs.

What Else to Take While Taking These Drugs. Take 1,000 to 3,000 mg a day of the bioflavonoids quercetin and rutin.

Examples of Prostaglandin Analogues

Bimatoprost (Lumigan)
Latanoprost (Xalatan)
Travoprost (Travatan)
Unoprostone isopropyl (Rescula)

What Do They Do in the Body? These drugs resemble chemicals made in the body called prostaglandins. The body's natural prostaglandins increase the outflow of fluid from the eyeball, and these drugs enhance this effect.

What Are They Prescribed For? Lowering of elevated intraocular pressure in ocular hypertension or glaucoma. They're used in cases where other medications don't work or are not as effective as they need to be.

What Are the Possible Side Effects? Blurred or abnormal vision, blood congestion in the conjunctiva, increased pigmentation in the iris, dry eye, and sensitivity to sun.

The following are drug-specific side effects:

• **Latanoprost.** Burning, stinging, feeling of having something stuck in the eye, eye itching, corneal inflammation, excessive tearing, eye pain, eyelid swelling, eyelid redness, eyelid pain or discomfort, conjunctivitis, double vision, upper respiratory infection, muscle pain, joint pain, back pain, chest pain, angina, rash, and allergic reaction.

• **Travoprost.** Eyelid inflammation, cataract, corneal inflammation, blood congestion below the conjunctiva, tearing, accidental injury, back pain, anxiety, arthritis, slow heart

rate, bronchitis, colds, depression, stomach upset, gastrointestinal disorders, hypercholesterolemia, high or low blood pressure, increased likelihood of infection, pain, prostate disorders, sinusitis, urinary incontinence, and urinary tract infection.

• **Bimatoprost.** Eyelash growth or darkening, eye itching, eye burning, feeling of having something stuck in the eye, excessive tearing, eye pain, eyelid redness, eye discharge, allergic conjunctivitis, increased colds and upper respiratory infections, headache, abnormal liver function tests, weakness, and abnormal hair growth.

• **Unoprostone isopropyl.** Itching, increase or decrease in length of eyelashes, eyelid disorders, feeling of having something stuck in the eye, tearing disorders, eyelid inflammation, cataract, corneal lesions, eye discharge, eye pain, irritation, vitreous disorders, flu syndrome, accidental injury, allergic reaction, back pain, bronchitis, increased cough, diabetes mellitus, dizziness, headache, high blood pressure, insomnia, throat inflammation, pain, runny nose, and sinusitis.

CAUTION!

• Latanoprost and travoprost may cause a permanent change of eye color from blue, green, or hazel to brown. The change happens gradually, with pigment darkening from the pupil outward.
• Don't use these drugs while wearing contact lenses. Benzalkonium chloride, a preservative used in many eyedrops, can accumulate on lenses.
• Don't use these drugs within five minutes of using any eyedrop containing thimerosal.

Miscellaneous Glaucoma Drugs

Dorzolamide (Trusopt)

What Does It Do in the Body? Dorzolamide is a carbonic anhydrase inhibitor. Inhibition of this enzyme system causes the eye to make less aqueous humor (fluid).

What Is It Prescribed For? Lowering of intraocular pressure in ocular hypertension or glaucoma.

What Are the Possible Side Effects? Bitter taste in the mouth; burning, stinging, and discomfort in the eye right after medication is used; inflammation of the cornea; symptoms of eye allergy; blurred vision; tearing; dryness; increased sensitivity to light; headache; nausea; skin rashes; and calcium deposits in the urinary tract (urolithiasis).

CAUTION!

Facts to Consider Before Taking These Drugs:

- Dorzolamide is a sulfa drug, similar to sulfa antibiotics. When it's used topically, enough is absorbed into the bloodstream to bring on the same adverse reactions that can occur with sulfa antibiotics. Some people have severe reactions to these drugs, which have in a few cases been fatal. Be alert for any signs of hypersensitivity, including itching, rash, swelling of the eye sockets, difficulty breathing, and blood congestion in the conjunctiva or sclera (part of the tough covering over the eyeball).
- If you have any kind of kidney impairment, you should not use dorzolamide. Those with less than full liver function should use this drug with caution.

- Don't use these drops while wearing soft contact lenses. They contain benzalkonium chloride, which can be absorbed into lenses.

Eyedrops for Allergies and Other Types of Eye Irritation

Examples of Ophthalmic Vasoconstrictors

Naphazoline (Allerest Eye Drops, Clear Eyes, Degest 2, Naphcon, Allergy Drops, VasoClear, Comfort Eye Drops, Maximum Strength Allergy Drops, AK-Con, Albalon, Nafazair, Naphcon Forte, Vasocon Regular)
Oxymetazoline (OcuClear, Visine L.R.)
Phenylephrine (Paredrine)
Tetrahydrozoline (Collyrium Fresh, Eye-Sine, Geneye, Mallazine Eye Drops, Murine Plus, Optigene 3, Tetrasine, Visine)

What Do They Do in the Body? In low concentrations sold over-the-counter, these drugs cause the blood vessels in the eyes to constrict. They stimulate the sympathetic nervous system and so are sometimes called sympathomimetics.

What Are They Used For? Relief of eye redness and irritation.

What Are the Possible Side Effects? Stinging when first instilled, blurred vision, pupil dilation, increased redness, irritation, discomfort, inflammation of the cornea, tearing, increased intraocular pressure, palpitations, heart arrhythmias, high blood pressure, heart attack, burst blood vessels in the lungs or brain, stroke, headache, blanching, trembling, sweating, dizziness, nausea, nervousness, drowsiness, weakness, and high blood sugar. (The more serious of these tend to happen with prescription-strength doses, not the over-the-counter varieties.)

CAUTION!

Facts to Consider Before Taking These Drugs:

- Don't use these drugs if you have narrow-angle glaucoma or a predisposition to this problem.
- Overuse of these drugs can cause eye redness or rebound congestion.
- If you have high blood pressure, diabetes, hyperthyroidism, cardiovascular problems, or hardening of the arteries, you are at greater risk for side effects.
- Phenylephrine can cause floaters in the aqueous humor of elderly people. It can also temporarily blur or destabilize vision, so be cautious when driving or performing hazardous tasks.

Examples of Ophthalmic Corticosteroids

Dexamethasone (AK-Dex, Decadron Phosphate, Maxidex)

Fluorometholone (Fluor-Op, Flarex, FML, FML Forte, FML S.O.P.)

Medrysone (HMS)

Prednisolone (Pred Mild, Econopred, AK-Pred, Inflamase Mild, Econopred Plus, Pred Forte)

Rimexolone (Vexol)

Tobradex, a combination steroid and antibiotic

What Do They Do in the Body? Decrease inflammation.

What Are They Prescribed For? Allergic conjunctivitis, corneal inflammation (keratitis, including herpes zoster keratitis), iris inflammation (iritis), inflammation of the ciliary bodies that control pupil size (cyclitis), treatment of injuries to the cornea, and some forms of eye infection.

What Are the Possible Side Effects? Raising of intraocular pressure with optic nerve damage (glaucoma), loss of some visual ability, formation of cataracts, eye infections including ocular herpes simplex, perforation of the eyeball, worsening of fungal infections of the eye, stinging or burning when drops are instilled, blurred vision, discharge, discomfort, eye pain, feeling of having something stuck in the eye, blood congestion, and itching.

With longtime use or high doses of steroid eyedrops, enough can be absorbed into the bloodstream to cause systemic side effects. Corticosteroid drugs can also cause an outbreak of intestinal or vaginal candida (see Chapter 14).

CAUTION!

Think Twice About Taking These Drugs If . . .

- You are having an outbreak of herpes virus of the cornea (herpes simplex keratitis).
- You have any fungal eye disease.
- You have ocular tuberculosis.
- You have just had a foreign object removed from your cornea.

While using steroid eyedrops, you should have frequent exams to be sure you aren't developing elevated eye pressure or cataracts. Any steroid drug can mask signs of infection. See your eye physician regularly to nip dangerous infections in the bud.

Examples of Over-the-Counter Antihistamine Eyedrops

Antazoline (Vasocon-A)

Pheniramine Maleate (Naphcon-A, AK-Con-A, Opcon-A)

What Do They Do in the Body? Block the actions of histamine in the eye. All products containing these drugs also contain the decongestant naphazoline.

What Are They Used For? Temporary relief of itchy, watering eyes caused by allergies.

What Are the Possible Side Effects? Burning, stinging, and discomfort when instilled. Ophthalmic antihistamines may also cause pupils to dilate.

CAUTION!

Think Twice About Taking These Drugs If . . .

You are at risk for angle-closure glaucoma.

Natural Alternatives to Eye Drugs

First let's talk about your eyes and the sun. Despite all the bad press it's getting lately, sunshine is a nutrient essential for the health of your eyes and the rest of your body. Sunlight striking the retina keeps it active, much like exercise keeps your body fit. It stimulates the glands to produce hormones that regulate our waking and sleeping cycles, fluid balance, and mood. Vitamin D is made by your body and stored in your liver when you go out in the sun. If there's a shortage of vitamin D, calcium metabolism in your body is thrown off, and bones begin to deteriorate.

On the other hand, too much sunlight can do you harm. Ultraviolet rays are invisible to our eyes but can cause cataracts; skin cancer; temporary blindness from glare off sand, snow, or water; growths on the eyes called pterygia; macular degeneration, and melanoma on the back of the eyeball. Sunlight causes an increase in the rate at which harmful free radicals are produced in the eye, which can contribute to getting eye diseases that can make you go blind.

Put on Your Shades

The first step to take in prevention of cataracts and macular degeneration is to invest in a pair of sunglasses that block 100 percent of ultraviolet rays. The best sunglasses also filter out some blue light. You can buy sun goggles that fit over your prescription glasses. A hat with a brim should accompany you out into the sunshine. You don't have to be fanatical about it unless you already have severe eye disease, because your eyes need some ultraviolet light. The majority of the time you spend outdoors, however, you should be wearing these sun-protection accessories.

Nutrition for Healthy Eyes

People with eye diseases such as glaucoma, cataracts, and macular degeneration can often prevent or slow the disease with some dietary changes and the right supplements. The mainstay of an eye-healthy diet is a wide variety of fresh vegetables (especially the deep green, leafy variety), fruits, and whole grains, complemented by good protein sources such as deep-water fish, eggs, chicken, and turkey. Red meat is OK, but not every day. Eggs are loaded with sulfur, a mineral your body needs to make glutathione, an antioxidant substance essential for eye health. Asparagus, onions, and garlic are also good sources of sulfur. Deep-water fish is rich in vitamins D and A, and in docosahexaenoic acid (DHA), an essential fatty acid. Especially good foods for healthy eyes include berries, watermelon, and carrots for their bioflavonoids and carotenoids, any foods rich in vitamin C such as citrus fruits and kiwi, as well as foods rich in essential fatty acids such as almonds, olive oil, and avocados.

Of course, the more you avoid refined, processed foods loaded with sugar, white flour, hydrogenated oils, artificial flavorings, and colorings, the healthier your whole body will be. While you replace "bad" fats like artery-clogging hydrogenated vegetable oils with the "good" fats listed, try to keep daily fat intake below 30 percent of total calories.

Fish oils improve circulation in the tiny blood vessels of the eye. Whatever you can do to keep your blood vessels healthy ensures that the retina and optic nerve cells get plenty of oxygen and nourishment.

Avoid optic nerve toxins such as aspartame, MSG, steroid drugs, tranquilizers, the antidepressants lithium and MAOIs, antibiotics, and cigarettes.

Vitamins for Healthy Eyes

Certain nutrients are more important to good eye health than others. If you have an eye disease or are at risk for one, please supplement your daily vitamins with the following:

- Vitamin C, at least 1,000 mg a day, with bioflavonoids
- A mixed carotenoid supplement
- Vitamin E, 400 IU
- Vitamin A, 10,000 IU a day
- Quercetin and rutin are bioflavonoids that help keep your retinas healthy; try 1,000 to 1,500 mg a day.
- Magnesium at bedtime, between 300 to 400 mg
- Coenzyme Q10 is a great circulation booster, 90 to 200 mg a day
- Carnitine can help boost the heart's pumping power and get more nourishment to your optic nerves and retinas; up to 500 mg three times daily.
- Selenium, a mineral with powerful antioxidant and antiviral potential, protects cell membranes from being destroyed by free radicals; 200 mcg daily.
- N-acetyl cysteine (NAC), an amino acid, helps keep your body's antioxidant defenses strong and increases the production of glutathione; 500 mg two to three times a day. There is good research to back up the use of NAC for eye disease.
- Those with macular degeneration or cataract should get 10 to 15 mg of zinc a day, either in a multivitamin or a separate supplement.

Natural Remedies for Eye Diseases
Glaucoma

- **Forskohlii.** If you have glaucoma, you can try an herbal remedy that's been used in India for centuries and is now backed up by scientific research. Derived from the coleus plant, forskohlii relaxes blood vessel walls to relieve high blood pressure and high intraocular pressure. Look for capsules or eyedrops of forskohlii.

- **Omega-3.** You can supplement omega-3 fish oils in capsules or liquid form; DHA, an essential fatty acid found in fish oil, is an important component of the optic nerve lining. Take care to ensure that fish oil supplements haven't gone rancid. Keep them in the fridge, and use a brand that contains a natural preservative such as vitamin E.

- **Vitamin B$_{12}$**, 1,000 to 2,000 mcg taken intranasally or sublingually, can help slow vision loss from glaucoma.

Macular Degeneration

- **Lutein and zeaxanthin.** If you have been diagnosed with macular degeneration, start taking a lutein and zeaxanthin supplement right away. Lutein and zeaxanthin are protective yellow pigments that cover the macula and protect it from light damage. These carotenoids are found naturally in foods such as spinach, collard greens, and kale. Supplements are usually derived from marigold petals. Make an effort to take them at different times from your multivitamin if it contains beta-carotene, because they can block each other's path into the body. Also eat beta-carotene-rich foods and foods rich in lutein and zeaxanthin at different meals.

Diabetic Eye Disease

Diabetics should use 1,000 to 1,500 mg of quercetin and 200 mcg of chromium a day. **Quercetin** inhibits an enzyme that may be directly responsible for the formation of sugar cataracts, while **chromium** helps balance blood sugar.

To slow the progression of cataracts, include plenty of tofu, eggs, asparagus, onions, garlic, carrots, cantaloupe, yams, corn, and leafy greens in your diet. Make sure you're getting 50 mg of **riboflavin** in your multivitamin, or add an extra riboflavin supplement. Please don't hesitate to have cataracts extracted if you feel your quality of life is being compromised. These days it's a relatively risk-free surgery.

For control of diabetic retinopathy, control of diabetes is essential. Check blood sugars at least four times a day, and keep levels in the range your physician has recommended. A diet rich in colorful vegetables, fruits, and whole grains, moderation in the drinking of alcohol and intake of sugar and refined flour, daily exercise, and maintenance of a healthy weight are all important for the diabetic.

See Chapter 16 for details on natural alternatives to diabetes drugs.

Diabetics shouldn't use a multivitamin with iron, because iron can increase the formation of free radicals. (Daily iron for any adult over the age of 30 or for men at any age is not recommended.)

Eye Allergies

Those who see a doctor with the complaint of itchy, watery, allergic eyes are generally pre-

Drugs That Can Cause Dry Eyes

Antihistamines

Atropine

Benzodiazepine tranquilizers (Valium, Xanax)

Beta-blockers (taken by mouth or as eyedrops)

Codeine

Decongestants (taken by mouth or as eyedrops)

Diuretics

Glaucoma eyedrops (some)

Isotretinoin

Methotrexate and other cancer drugs

Morphine

Scopolamine

Tricyclic antidepressant (Elavil)

scribed antihistamine, decongestant, or steroid eyedrops. An eye doctor can distinguish eye allergy from dry eye by checking for small bumps along the lower eyelid. These drugs can be useful for temporary symptom relief, but it's important to support your body nutritionally with the goal of reducing or eliminating the need for eyedrops. These drugs have too many side effects to justify their use for more than a couple of days at a time. See Chapter 12 on allergy drugs for details on natural remedies.

Aside from supporting your body nutritionally, your best strategy for avoiding allergies is to determine what irritates your eyes and try your best to avoid exposure. Women may need to change to a different kind of eye makeup or stop using it altogether. Hair sprays or gels, perfumes, certain eyedrops, or contact lens solutions can cause allergic reactions in some people. Fumes from copy machines, laser printers, and so-called air fresheners (fakegrances) can have a strongly irritating effect, too.

The following supplements may help:

- **Quercetin** can be very helpful in decreasing allergic inflammation. Take 1,000 to 2,000 mg a day, and eat plenty of red onions, brussels sprouts, red apples, bell peppers, asparagus, and kale.
- **Vitamin B$_6$** taken with **omega-6 essential fatty acids** (found in evening primrose oil) can also take the edge off of eye allergies.
- **Vitamin C** (1,000 to 2,000 mg a day) can also help relieve allergic inflammation.

Dry Eyes

Before you turn to constant use of artificial tears to relieve dry eyes, try to improve your eyes' ability to keep themselves moist. Here are some tips for treating dry eyes:

- Buy a humidifier and use it whenever you turn on the heater or air-conditioner in your home.
- Avoid smog, ozone, fumes, and perfumes.
- Don't use products that contain aspartame (NutraSweet).
- Wear wraparound sunglasses outside to keep tears from evaporating.
- Soft contacts can cause dry eyes, so keep glasses around to wear when your eyes feel uncomfortable.
- Try to blink more.
- If you work at a computer, arrange your workspace so that you are looking slightly downward at the screen, lids lowered.
- Don't use a lot of eye makeup.
- Check to be sure your glasses aren't pulling your lower lids away from your eyes.
- Use only preservative-free eyedrops (preservatives can actually worsen dry eyes).
- Eat more fruit, vegetables, walnuts, and cold-water fish.
- Evening primrose oil capsules (500 to 1,500 mg per day), 1,000 to 2,000 mg of vitamin C, and 50 mg of B$_6$ can also help relieve eye dryness.

Chapter 18

Drugs for the Prostate and Their Natural Alternatives

More than 20 percent of all American men over the age of 50 will develop prostate problems of some kind, and 1 in 11 will develop prostate cancer. By the time they are 70, over 50 percent of American men will have an enlarged prostate gland, and by the time they are 80, the number will go up to 85 percent. This amounts to an epidemic of prostate problems, and once again it looks like poor eating habits and excessive estrogen in the environment are the biggest culprits. What "modern" medicine has to offer you if you have prostate troubles are drugs and surgery that are only sometimes effective and that often have side effects such as impotence and urinary dysfunction (with surgery, these side effects are permanent).

What Is the Prostate Gland?

The prostate is a gland in men located at the neck of the bladder and urethra (the tube through which urine and semen pass on the way out of the body). It's about the size of a grain of rice when you are born; by the time you're in your twenties, it's about the size and shape of a chestnut. Starting at puberty, the gland produces a milky fluid that mixes with semen during ejaculation.

The prostate stays about the same size until you reach the age when some male hormones begin to decline (in most men, in their fifties), and the prostate begins to grow again. This is called benign prostatic hypertrophy (BPH). If the gland grows too much, it begins to pinch the urethra, interfering with urination. Symptoms of an enlarged prostate can include dribbling during urination, a decrease in the size of the stream, frequent or difficult urination, and chronic discomfort in the abdominal area.

No Visible Progress in Prostate Treatment

There's not much good news to report on detecting prostate cancer or conventional medical treatment of prostate enlargement or prostate cancer, but there is useful new research about prostate risk factors.

According to a recently released report from the federal government's Agency for Healthcare Research and Quality (AHRQ), which reviewed 592 published articles and compared eight prostate cancer treatment strategies, "Not enough scientific evidence exists to identify any prostate cancer treatment as most effective for all men, especially those whose cancers were found by PSA testing." In essence, the AHRQ report says that we have no prostate cancer treatment that's consistently safe and effective, and that it's questionable whether many of the prostate cancers detected by the PSA test should even be treated.

Surgical and radiation treatments carry a high risk of permanent side effects such as urinary and rectal problems and impotence. One study showed that men who get external beam radiation treatment for prostate cancer have a 70 percent higher risk of rectal cancer than those who had surgery. The only treatment that causes these problems temporarily (vs. permanently) is androgen (male hormone) suppression with drugs, but the lack of hormones quickly increases the risk for diabetes and heart disease, similar to what happens when a woman gets a hysterectomy and loses her hormones. At best, androgen suppression is a temporary fix. When it's stopped, the cancer often comes back, and with a vengeance.

That leaves "wait and watch," which isn't a bad option if the cancer is small and localized, and if you can stand it. It's estimated that 80 to 96 percent of men have a bit of prostate cancer when they die, meaning it's a very slow-growing cancer that often does no harm. Thanks to research on prostate cancer risks, we have a pretty good idea of what blocks or feeds prostate cancer growth—more about that shortly.

The PSA Test

The PSA test isn't faring any better than prostate cancer hormone research and treatment. According to the AHRQ:

The lifetime risk of being diagnosed with prostate cancer has nearly doubled to 20 percent since the late 1980s, due mostly to expanded use of the prostate specific antigen (PSA) blood test. But the risk of dying of prostate cancer remains about 3 percent. Therefore, considerable overdetection and overtreatment may exist. The U.S. Preventive Services Task Force, a panel of outside experts convened by AHRQ that makes independent evidence-based recommendations, maintains there is insufficient evidence to recommend for or against PSA testing for routine prostate cancer screening. PSA tests can detect early-stage cancer when it is potentially most treatable but also lead to frequent false-positive results and identification of prostate cancers unlikely to cause harm.

Doctors like to say they have to treat all discovered prostate cancer because they don't know which ones will cause harm, but thanks to recent research on prostate cancer risk factors, we know a lot more about what drives prostate cancers to grow.

The Good News About Prostate Research

The good news about prostate research is that a lot has been done to examine non-hormone-related risk factors for both benign prostatic hypertrophy (BPH) and prostate cancer, including lifestyle, nutrition, and diet. This research gives us an abundance of information that can be used to prevent and treat prostate problems ranging from a little bit of trouble urinating to prostate cancer.

What Causes Prostate Enlargement?

Some scientists believe that when testosterone production declines, other male hormones synthesized from testosterone not only decline but are thrown out of balance, causing prostate enlargement. Unfortunately much of the research on this question has been done either with excessively high doses of testosterone or synthetic testosterones that can create numerous side effects, so it has given us few useful answers. We need studies done with real human testosterone in physiologic (the same as the body would make) doses.

Dihydrotestosterone (DHT) is a hormone synthesized from testosterone that is thought to contribute to prostate enlargement. The drug Proscar (finasteride) is supposed to keep testosterone from producing DHT. However, this drug has only been partially successful in treating prostate enlargement and has side effects, including a very high price tag. Adverse reactions may include impotence, decreased libido, and decreased volume of ejaculate (which most men don't think are minor problems!). The most frequent adverse effect of Proscar is breast enlargement, which is also not a minor problem.

Among Japanese men who traditionally eat a diet low in fat and high in soy products, prostate problems are rare, as is the case in other cultures that favor low-fat diets. However, a study of Japanese men who moved to Hawaii and presumably began eating a typically high-fat American diet showed that they had prostate problems at the same rate as Americans. A study of 51,000 American men between the ages of 40 and 75 who were followed for two to four years showed that prostate cancer was directly related to total fat consumption, with red meat showing the strongest association with advanced cancer. Another study in Italy comparing 271 men with prostate cancer to 685 men who did not have the disease concluded that a high dietary consumption of milk was a significant indicator of prostate cancer risk, even in men who also ate a lot of whole grains and fresh vegetables.

Other studies have linked prostate cancer to exposure to herbicides that are typically used in agriculture, forestry, and in cities and suburbs to control weeds. Many pesticides are potent estrogen mimics.

Western Lifestyles Create a Convergence of Risk Factors for Prostate Problems

If we wanted to make a sweeping generalization about prostate cancer, we could say that the biggest risk factor for both having it and dying from it is living in the United States, Canada, and most of Europe. Asian men have, by far, the lowest incidence of prostate cancer and the lowest risk of dying from it (unless they move to the United States—then it goes up). Our Western lifestyles increase prostate cancer risk pretty much the same way they increase breast cancer risk: we eat too many bad fats and sugars and not enough fiber and veggies, we don't exercise enough, we're too fat, and we're bombarded with xenoestrogens everywhere from pesticides and tap water to meat and perfumed garbage bags. This lifestyle leads to chronic inflammation.

Preventing Chronic Inflammation

Inflammation plays an important role in prostate cancer. One of the primary causes of inflammation in the prostate is too much of certain fats and oils. The saturated fat found in meat is one culprit. We want to emphasize that the key concept is excess; there's no evidence that having a steak, lamb chop, or bacon now and then does any harm. Ironically, the other fatty acid culprit is at the other end of the saturation spectrum— the omega-6 unsaturated oils such as corn, cot-

tonseed, safflower, and soybean. These are the oils found in chips, cookies, mayonnaise, salad dressings, and countless processed food products. The third culprit in prostate inflammation is (you guessed it) refined carbohydrates, especially the fatty carbs like French fries and the sweet carbs like cookies and doughnuts.

Both types of fatty acids (in excess) and refined carbohydrates cause the body to set up a multilayered defense system to break down and dispose of them. In the normal workaday world of the body, this is no big deal. But when you overload the system, it overcreates enzymes known as 5-LOX, COX-1, and COX-2. These enzymes, in turn, wreak all sorts of havoc further along the biochemical pathways. Part of the collateral damage of this havoc is inflammation—in the heart, the blood vessels, the joints, and the prostate in particular. In fact, not only does this havoc do damage, it actually feeds and protects cancer cells in the process. To add insult to injury, literally, it also pushes estrogens down more destructive pathways. Again, these are normal biochemical processes that run amok when they become overloaded. As we age we become increasingly susceptible to these types of inflammation and the DNA damage they cause, which can be the first step in the creation of a cancer.

Weapons Against LOX and COX

You can help your body reduce LOX and COX damage with some targeted supplement choices. The idea here, however, is not so much to try to help your body get over the shock of a burger and fries every other day, as to add a weapon to a prostate health arsenal that is already well stocked with overall good lifestyle choices. In other words, make the lifestyle changes and take these next suggestions as an extra layer of protection.

One of the easiest ways to block LOX and COX damage is to eat fish a few times a week or take fish oil supplements. Many people like flax oil as a source of beneficial oils, but we don't recommend it. It's so extremely unsaturated that unless you grind the seeds and eat them right away, it's pretty much guaranteed to be rancid, which is like throwing the doors wide open for LOX and COX damage. Even when you grind the seeds, flax still has to go through conversion processes in the body to have benefit. In the hardware or paint store, flax oil is known as linseed oil and is used as a wood varnish, a carrier for oil paints, and glazing putty. If you put a coat of linseed oil on wood and leave it in the sun, it'll harden in a few hours. That type of oxidation reaction is good for protecting wood but may not be so good for protecting the body. And yes, the lignans in flax are phytoestrogens that can be beneficial, but there are other ways to get lignans (whole grains, broccoli, pumpkin seeds, sesame seeds, soybeans, chia seeds).

Another way to combat LOX and COX damage is to take an anti-inflammatory drug such as aspirin or ibuprofen. Remember, though, that when taken regularly, these drugs carry the risk of gastrointestinal bleeding, which kills more than 10,000 people a year. Use them with discretion. If you have a sensitive stomach, this is probably not a good choice for you.

Some supplement formulas are specifically designed to douse LOX and COX inflammation. Most notable are New Chapter's Zyflamend and Life Extension's 5-Loxin. Zyflamend is a blend of herb and spice extracts that has been well researched and shown to have benefit. For details, please visit the New Chapter website.

And remember, our old friend estrogen is potently inflammatory in excess. It doesn't take much estrogen to make a man estrogen dominant, in this case meaning too much estrogen relative to testosterone and progesterone. In women and men, fat cells are estrogen factories, which is part of why obesity is a risk factor for prostate problems.

For more details on xenoestrogens and how to avoid them, please visit the "Resources and Recommended Reading" section at the back of this book.

Lifestyle Reminder

Just a reminder that you can take handfuls of supplements every day to keep your prostate healthy, but if you're overloading it with an excess of "bad" fats, sugar, and refined carbohydrates and not getting any exercise or sleep, they won't have much effect. Good prostate health requires a multifaceted approach with a healthy lifestyle, hormone balance, avoidance of xenoestrogens, and—last but not least—supplements as needed.

Drugs for Treating an Enlarged Prostate

Examples of 5-Alpha Reductase Inhibitors

Finasteride (Proscar)
Dutasteride (Avodart)

What Do They Do in the Body? They block or inhibit an enzyme called 5-alpha reductase, which converts testosterone to dihydrotestosterone (DHT), lowering levels of DHT in the blood serum.

What Is It Prescribed For? Symptoms of benign prostatic hypertrophy (BPH) or enlarged prostate.

What Are the Possible Side Effects? Liver damage, impotence, decreased libido, decreased volume of ejaculate, breast tenderness and enlargement, and rash.

CAUTION!

Think Twice About Taking These Drugs If . . .

You are having sex with a woman who might become pregnant. Any exposure to these drugs, even in minute amounts, can cause abnormalities in the male fetus; do not use. Give the natural remedies a good try before resorting to these drugs.

Examples of Alpha-1 Blockers

Alfuzosin (UroXatral)
Doxazosin (Cardura)
Prazosin (Minipress)
Tamsulosin (Flomax)
Terazosin (Hytrin)

What Do They Do in the Body? Alpha-1 blockers, also called alpha-adrenergic antagonists or alpha-adrenergic antagonists, help block the effect of the adrenal hormone norepinephrine (noradrenaline), which contracts smooth muscles and constricts small veins and blood vessels. This improves blood flow and helps the smooth muscles of the bladder neck and prostate to relax. These drugs (e.g., Cardura, Minipress, Hytrin) are also used to lower blood pressure, although these days they are usually not a first choice for treating hypertension.

What Are They Prescribed For? Symptoms of benign prostate hypertrophy (BPH), or enlargement of the prostate, such as reduced urine flow, urinary frequency, weak stream, hesitancy, and incomplete emptying.

What Are the Possible Side Effects? Dizziness is a common side effect of this drug, especially when it's first taken and when standing up from a sitting or lying down position. This can be dangerous in many situations, including driving. It may also predispose to falls when getting up at night to urinate, a common occurrence in men with prostate enlargement. Other side effects include fainting, excessively low blood pressure (this can cause dizziness), weakness, upper respiratory tract infection, headache, fatigue, edema (water retention), weight gain, rapid heartbeat, liver damage, increase in LDL (bad) cholesterol, runny nose, priapism (erection lasting more than four hours), rash, hives, itching, and flushing. Less frequent side effects include generalized pain, abdominal pain, indigestion, constipation, nausea, impotence, bronchitis, and sore throat.

CAUTION!

Think twice about using this drug if you have liver or kidney disease, as it could make it worse.

Natural Remedies for Prostate Enlargement

There are nutrients and herbs that can dramatically improve the symptoms of prostate enlargement in men over time. Your best bet is to find a formula that combines the following ingredients:

Zinc

Zinc is necessary for the proper function of the prostate gland. In men, higher concentrations of this mineral are found in the prostate than anywhere else in the body. A recent study looked at zinc supplementation in young men and found that when plasma zinc levels were low, there was a corresponding drop in testosterone. Many clinical studies have shown that zinc supplementation can reduce the size of the prostate gland, along with troublesome symptoms.

It's a good idea for all men to take 10 to 15 mg of zinc daily and include zinc-rich foods in the diet such as oysters (well cooked, please!), lamb chops, and wheat germ. Pumpkin seeds are a good source of zinc and are also rich in the amino acids alanine, glycine, and glutamic acid, which seem to have a positive effect in reducing the size of the prostate. A handful of dried pumpkin seeds a day is plenty. Please don't get pumpkin seeds that have been roasted in oil and salted—the oil is probably rancid and you don't need the extra salt. Plain roasted pumpkin seeds have a pleasant, nutty flavor. Pumpkin seed oil capsules are also available.

Selenium

Selenium is another important mineral in male hormone regulation that is found in large amounts in the prostate. Blood levels of both zinc and selenium are low in men who have prostate cancer. Men who live in areas where the soil is rich in selenium tend to have lower rates of prostate cancer. Rich sources of selenium are garlic, shellfish, grains, and chicken. If you're over the age of 50, you can supplement your diet with up to 400 mcg of selenium daily.

Pygeum Africanum

Pygeum africanum, an evergreen tree from Africa, is an important part of your healthy prostate program. The bark of this tree helps balance hormone levels and reduce prostate inflamma-

tion. It also improves the quality and quantity of prostate secretions.

Saw Palmetto

Saw palmetto is the most important prostate herb. An extract made from the berry of saw palmetto (*Serenoa repens*), also called sabal, a palm tree native to Florida, Texas, and Georgia, has been shown in numerous studies to reduce the urinary symptoms caused by prostate enlargement. Like the previously mentioned drugs, it is a 5-alpha reductase inhibitor that blocks the conversion of testosterone to dihydrotestosterone (DHT), which is associated with prostate enlargement. Unlike the previously mentioned drugs, this herb, taken as directed, has no reported side effects, seems to be more effective, and is significantly less expensive! It's also possible that it opposes or blocks estrogen. Look for a standardized extract from a reputable company.

The Healthy Prostate Program

The Six Core Principles for Optimal Health have all the elements of a healthy prostate diet. Here is where the special emphasis should be if you're a man over the age of 50:

Eat More . . .

Fiber
Fish oils or other sources of omega-3 fatty acids
Garlic
Hormone-free chicken (a good source of selenium)
Oysters or lamb chops every other week (a good source of zinc)
Pumpkin seeds

Soy products such as miso, tofu, and tempeh (or take in capsule form)

Drink More . . .

Clean water

Avoid . . .

Red meat (unless it is organic)

Vegetable oils and hydrogenated oils (trans fats)

Whole milk (yogurt is OK)

Supplements That Support a Healthy Prostate

Saw palmetto extract

Selenium

Zinc

Lycopene (carrots, tomatoes, tomato sauce)

Milk thistle (helps the liver clear excess hormones)

Vitamin D (men with prostate cancer tend to be low in vitamin D)

Melatonin (helps balance estrogen)

Chapter 19

Synthetic Hormones and Their Natural Alternatives

Hormones play innumerable roles in the everyday workings of your body. Lack of a single hormone can make the difference between well-being and life-threatening illness. Hormonal pathways and interactions are so complex that we have only a weak grasp of exactly how they work. The body uses hormones as one way to maintain homeostasis (balance) in all of its systems despite drastic changes in the environment. For example, your body goes from sleep in a toasty warm bed to rising, bathing, cooking, and eating an assortment of foods. On that same day, you might engage in vigorous exercise, have an emotional conflict with a loved one, relax in the sunshine, and see a sad movie. If you are working in a stressful profession, you might have to work capably while under considerable pressure. All of these activities in some way put a demand on the body to maintain balance.

You're probably most familiar with the steroid hormones progesterone, dehydroepiandrosterone (DHEA), the cortisones, the estrogens, and testosterone. All of these hormones are made from a hormone called pregnenolone, which is made from cholesterol. This is why the myth that all cholesterol is bad is a dangerous one. While your body can manufacture 75 percent of its own cholesterol, the remaining 25 percent comes directly from cholesterol that you eat. Cut out all cholesterol, and you're asking for a hormone imbalance.

When you drink a glass of juice, your blood sugar rises, and the hormone insulin, secreted by the pancreas, is required to bring it back down by ushering it into your cells. Thyroid hormones, which regulate how the body uses energy, are secreted by the thyroid gland in the neck. Adrenaline, the cortisones, and DHEA are a few of the hormones secreted by the adrenal glands. Your brain secretes the hormone melatonin in response to darkness, but it's also found in larger quantities in your intestines. Vitamin D, believe it or not, is really a hormone that regulates (among other things) how your bones take up minerals.

Your hormone or endocrine system is actually a group of systems that work via circulation. Hormones are secreted by glands into the bloodstream as the body demands them. For example, when you exercise, you use glucose, which your body can replace by activating cortisol, a hormone that allows you to manufacture more glucose in your liver. As these specialized molecules pass through the body, they are recognized by receptors on cells that fit them like a lock and key. Once the hormone locks on to the receptor, it causes the cell to behave in a generally

predictable way. For example, some estrogens can stimulate cell growth and testosterone can stimulate the growth of facial hair.

There are many ways your hormone systems can be thrown out of balance, which will in turn throw your health out of balance. Symptoms may be subtle or blatant. Chronic stress can cause the constant release of cortisol and adrenaline, hormones that were originally designed for occasional use only, under highly stressful circumstances such as hunting a woolly mammoth or fighting a bear for a cave. Routine exposure to bright lights late into the night has most likely thrown our melatonin levels out of balance. Environmental pollution is contributing to hormone imbalance, thanks to plastics and pesticides with molecules that resemble estrogen and fit into estrogen receptors, stimulating an estrogen-like response in the body. The millions of women who have undergone hysterectomies are plunged into instant hormone imbalance, even if their ovaries are intact. Nutritional deficiencies, which are widespread in the United States, especially among the elderly, can cause glands to atrophy and malfunction.

In an ideal world, we wouldn't need supplemental hormones. But because our environment is less than ideal, small amounts of natural hormone supplements can be safely used to help our bodies function optimally. Physiologic dosages of hormones are very small, just enough to restore balance. They are approximations of what the body itself would secrete under ideal conditions, and they are much safer and work better than pharmacologic doses, which are usually many times more than what the body would make itself.

The typical medical model advocates the "more is better" philosophy. In the case of hormones, this approach not only is ineffective but also can be counterproductive and harmful. Hormones are powerful agents designed for very specific use. The use of pharmacologic dosing (often with synthetic versions of the natural hormones our bodies make) has a lot to do with the negative outcomes in many medical studies of hormone replacement. The following recommendations for hormone supplementation involve only physiologic doses of the natural hormone.

What's Wrong with Synthetic Hormones?

Synthetic, not-found-in-nature hormones do not behave the same way in the body as natural or bioidentical hormones. A synthetic drug isn't one that was made in a lab, because they all are (most vitamins are, too); it is one that is not found in nature. Drug companies prefer that you take synthetic hormones not because they are better for you, but because they can be patented, so the companies can charge you more for them.

A natural substance cannot be patented, so drug company scientists take a perfectly good natural substance into the lab and add a methyl group here, an acetate group there, and voilà! They have created a drug that has many of the same effects as the natural substance but can be patented. Nowhere is there a better example of how tragically awry this practice has gone than in the realm of hormones.

John R. Lee, M.D., a pioneer in the use of natural progesterone cream, used to tell a story about a package he received in the mail from a woman who sent him copies of her medical charts and a letter pleading for help. Her physician had put her on a progestin (a synthetic progesterone) and then a few months later had taken her blood and measured her progesterone levels. According to her blood test, her progesterone levels hadn't risen at all, so he increased the dose of progestins. A few months later, the lab test still didn't measure any progesterone. Meanwhile, the woman was suffering terribly from the side effects of the progestin.

Dr. Lee pointed out to her that her physician was giving her a progestin but measuring for progesterone; since they aren't the same, of course it didn't show up on her blood tests! This confusion is rampant throughout the medical literature, where even in the most prestigious medical journals the terms *progesterone* and *progestin* are used interchangeably, and whole theories are advanced on the basis that testing one is the same as testing the other. The real victims of this mistaken identity are the women who are prescribed progestins. Thankfully, the research and medical communities are starting to become more aware and educated about natural hormones, and these errors are increasingly rare.

In case your physician wants to argue with you that progestins and progesterone are the same, you might remind him or her that progesterone is the first and foremost hormone necessary for a healthy pregnancy, while progestins taken during pregnancy can cause birth defects. Progestins almost universally make women feel awful, while progesterone almost universally makes women (who need it) feel better.

Synthetic estrogens aren't any better. For a while, the makers of Premarin were trying to convince women that the synthetic Premarin is a natural estrogen because part of it is made from the urine of pregnant mares. Horse estrogen is natural if you're a horse, but it's not natural if you're a human. There are actually several different types of estrogens, and horses have estrogens in their bodies that are unique to horses but foreign to the human body. Other estrogens appear in both horse and human urine, but the levels are very different. The relationship between the levels of the three human estrogens—estriol, estrone, and estradiol—in a woman's body makes a big difference in how she feels and in her state of health. A healthy young woman's ovaries make about 10 times more estriol, a weaker form of estrogen that doesn't promote cancer, than it does the stronger versions, estradiol and estrone. In estrogen derived from horse urine, estriol comprises a bit less than 50 percent of the total estrogen content, with an estrogen unique to horses comprising 22 percent and several other fairly strong estrogens making up the rest.

Marla Ahlgrimm, R.Ph., a pharmacist who specializes in providing individualized natural hormone combination creams, has noticed that women taking Premarin suffer more from breast tenderness, water retention, and high blood pressure than those taking natural estrogen.

From the mid-1980s, the use of combined estrogens and progestins for hormone replacement therapy (HRT) increased steadily. Women and their doctors believed—and many still believe today, despite powerful evidence to the contrary—that it is the only answer for uncomfortable menopausal symptoms. Physicians also believed for much of that time that HRT would protect women against heart attacks and osteoporosis without increasing their risks of breast cancer. Some studies showed that colon cancer and ovarian cancer risks were reduced by HRT. In the year 2000, approximately 38 percent of postmenopausal women in the United States were using HRT, usually made up of Premarin and some form of synthetic progestin.

It took a groundbreaking study published in the *Journal of the American Medical Association* to get the attention of conventional medicine. In 2001, the results of the large Women's Health Initiative (WHI), conducted by the government's National Institutes of Health (NIH), were made public. This study involved 16,601 healthy postmenopausal women and was stopped prematurely after five years (three years early) because it had become obvious that the risks of the study drug (Prempro and combination of Premarin and a progestin) far exceeded its benefits. After five years, those using the HRT had a 29 percent higher risk of breast cancer, a 26 percent higher risk of heart disease, and a 41 percent higher risk of stroke. Risk of colon cancer dropped by 36 percent and risk of hip fracture dropped by 24 percent, but these positive results were outweighed by the negatives. Most of these adverse events began to appear within two years of the study's beginning, with the breast cancer diagnoses appearing at about three years into the study. Since the WHI was published, millions of women have stopped their conventional HRT, and many have turned to natural or bioidentical hormones.

If at all possible, please avoid long-term use of birth control pills, which are also made from synthetic hormones. They suppress ovulation and increase the risk of stroke and breast cancer. It's just not worth it when so many other forms of birth control are available. Newer forms of hormonal birth control such as vaginal rings (NuvaRing), IUDs (Mirena), patches, and injections contain the same harmful synthetic progestins and/or estrogens found in conventional HRT and found by the WHI to be so harmful to so many women.

Methyltestosterone, a synthetic version of testosterone, has a long list of side effects that natural testosterone doesn't have.

When it comes to HRT, there doesn't seem to be any reason why anybody, anytime, would use synthetic hormones instead of natural hormones. It just doesn't make sense if your goal is optimal health.

Although most of the natural hormones are available by prescription, some are available over the counter. Only the most commonly used synthetic hormones are listed in the following section on replacement hormones. More important is the section "Using Natural Hormones," where you can learn about taking natural hormones.

Replacement Hormones

Examples of Estrogens

Synthetic estrogens: conjugated estrogen (Premarin), conjugated estrogen with a progestin (Prempro), estropipate (Ortho-Est, Ogen), ethinyl estradiol with a progestin (FemHRT), estradiol with a progestin (Activella)

Natural estrogens: estradiol patches (Alora, Climara, Vivelle, Estraderm), estradiol creams (Estrace), estradiol and estriol cream (Bi-Est), estradiol pills (Estrace), estradiol vaginal (Estring, Femring, Vagifem)

What Do They Do in the Body? Natural estrogens have dozens of effects on the body, including the development and maintenance of female sex characteristics such as the ovaries, uterus, and breasts. Estrogens given as HRT during menopause may relieve hot flashes, night sweats, and vaginal dryness.

What Are They Prescribed For? For HRT, usually for menopausal women and women who have had a hysterectomy. Many forms of birth control contain synthetic estrogens. See the following section on birth control. Estrogens are prescribed for the symptoms of menopause, including hot flashes, night sweats, and vaginal dryness.

What Are the Possible Side Effects? Natural estrogens given in small amounts and in balance with progesterone to menopausal women have few, if any, side effects. However, the synthetic estrogens, estrogens in high doses, and estrogens without progesterone can cause water retention, headaches (including migraines), irritability, mood swings, depression, fatigue, lack of libido, breast tenderness, breast and uterine cancer, gallbladder disease, strokes (they reduce vascular tone and strength), increased blood pressure, low thyroid function, cervical dysplasia, breakthrough bleeding, vision problems, asthma, premenstrual syndrome (PMS), and low cellular oxygen levels.

CAUTION!

Please avoid the synthetic estrogens altogether, and use natural estrogens: estradiol, estriol, and estrone.

What Nutrients Do They Throw out of Balance or Interact With? Excess estrogens and synthetic estrogens can block the action of thyroid hormone, leading to low thyroid symptoms with normal thyroid test results. Excess estrogens and synthetic estrogens also increase sodium retention, which causes water retention or bloating.

Excess estrogens and synthetic estrogens cause depletion of the B vitamins in general, but especially of folic acid and vitamin B_6, which can lead to elevated homocysteine levels, a major risk factor for heart disease; cervical dysplasia; and carpal tunnel syndrome. They also cause vitamin C to be cleared from the body more rapidly.

There is also some evidence that some types of birth control pills deplete the mineral zinc.

What Else to Take If You Take These Drugs. If you're taking small amounts of natural estrogens, along with natural progesterone to treat menopausal symptoms, you should be fine. If for some reason you're using synthetic drugs, it's important to take supplements of vitamin B$_6$ (50 mg daily), folic acid (400 mcg daily), and vitamin C (500 mg three times daily). You should also be taking vitamin E to offset the risk of blood clots and strokes that comes with taking estrogens. Make sure you're getting at least 5 mg of zinc in your daily multivitamin.

Examples of Progestins

Medroxyprogesterone acetate (Cycrin, Provera, Amen, Curretab)
Megestrol acetate (Megace)
Norethindrone acetate (Aygestin)
Norethindrone acetate with estradiol (FemHRT)

What Do They Do in the Body? The progestins are mainly used as pseudo-progesterones in HRT to offset the cancer-causing effects of estrogens, but these strange hybrid hormones also behave a little like androgens (male hormones) and steroids, and natural progesterone does not. For a more detailed explanation of what natural progesterone does in the body, turn to the section "Using Natural Hormones" at the end of this chapter.

What Are They Prescribed For? In addition to being used in HRT for menopausal women, progestins are used to stop abnormal uterine bleeding, to regulate irregular menstrual periods, in birth control pills, and to control endometriosis.

What Are the Possible Side Effects? The side effects of the progestins are so severe that many women refuse to take them, preferring the risks of unopposed estrogen to the unpleasantness of progestin side effects. Most doctors don't seem to realize that women can use natural progesterone, which has none of the side effects of the progestins. First and foremost, progestins can cause birth defects. They increase the risk of some types of strokes; they can cause loss of vision, migraine headaches, fluid retention, depression, weight gain, fatigue, back pain, and tender breasts; and they are hard on the liver. They can also cause insomnia, nausea, breakthrough bleeding, and amenorrhea (no menstruation). Like testosterone and other androgens, they can cause excessive hair growth where women don't want it, hair loss where they do want it, and a variety of skin problems and rashes, including acne. Progestins can also cause high blood sugar, reduced HDL ("good") cholesterol, raised LDL ("bad") cholesterol, and photosensitivity.

Like the cortisones, megestrol acetate actually increases appetite, can increase risk of respiratory infections, and may suppress adrenal function.

CAUTION!

Please don't use the progestins at all, either as HRT or in birth control pills. In rare cases, they may be useful to stop excessive breakthrough bleeding, but otherwise it's difficult to imagine why any physician who wanted to do the right thing would prescribe these drugs when he or she could prescribe natural progesterone.

Examples of Chemical Contraceptives

Drospirenone and estradiol (Yasmin)
Ethinyl estradiol and desogestrel (Desogen, Ortho-Cept)
Ethinyl estradiol and ethynodiol (Demulen)
Ethinyl estradiol and etonogestrel (NuvaRing)
Ethinyl estradiol and levonorgestrel

Ethinyl estradiol and norelgestromin (Ortho-Evra Patch)

Ethinyl estradiol and norethindrone (Genora, Loestrin, Nelova, Norethin, Norinyl, Ortho-Novum, Ovcon)

Levonorgestrel IUD (Mirena, Progestasert)

Medroxyprogesterone acetate (Provera, Depo-Provera injection)

Norethindrone (Ortho Micronor, Nor-QD)

What Do They Do in the Body? Oral contraceptives are either a combination of a synthetic estrogen, usually ethinyl estradiol, with a progestin, or a progestin alone.

What Are They Prescribed For? Birth control and to regulate menses. Some versions may be prescribed to control acne.

What Are the Possible Side Effects? Oral contraceptives can cause all of the side effects of the synthetic estrogens and the progestins, and they have their own unique profile of negative effects on the body. One of their most frequent side effects is breakthrough bleeding and spotting.

Oral contraceptives increase the risk of blood clots, stroke, heart attacks, liver cancer, gallbladder disease, and osteoporosis, especially in women already susceptible to those diseases. The risks are higher for women with high blood pressure or high cholesterol, obese women, diabetic women, and women who smoke.

The Ortho-Evra contraceptive patch earned itself an FDA black-box warning that estrogen levels are higher in women using the patch than in women using similar oral contraceptives, thus increasing the risk of potentially fatal blood clots. It's been known for at least a decade that when hormones are delivered through the skin such as in creams and patches, more hormone gets into the blood compared with hormones taken

orally (pill). When you take a hormone orally, a large percentage of it is dumped by the liver and excreted. Nevertheless, those who developed Ortho-Evra missed this basic tenet of hormone delivery and failed to reduce the estrogen dose in their patch, putting millions of women at risk of fatal blood clots. The patch is arguably a better delivery system than the pill, but it needs to be properly dosed.

The injectable Depo-Provera earned itself an FDA black-box warning because it significantly increases the risk of osteoporosis, probably by blocking the action of real progesterone, which plays a role in building bone.

Women who smoke absolutely should not use oral contraceptives—it is a deadly combination, especially in women over the age of 35. Oral contraceptives also increase the risk of arterial disease and vision loss, and controversial studies suggest they increase the risk of breast cancer, cervical cancer, and osteoporosis, especially when taken long term. Oral contraceptives can cause candida overgrowth (yeast infections), breast tenderness and lumpiness, and nausea.

Women going off them may be infertile, usually for a few months, but it can be permanent in older women.

CAUTION!

Please avoid these drugs altogether, and use an alternative form of birth control. If the only other choice is an unwanted pregnancy, then perhaps birth control pills should be an option, but they cannot be considered a safe drug.

What Nutrients Do They Throw out of Balance or Interact With? Primarily vitamins B_6 and folic acid. See the section on synthetic estrogens for details.

What Else to Take If You Take These Drugs.
Vitamin B$_6$ (50 mg daily), folic acid (400 mcg daily), and vitamin C (2,000 mg daily).

Examples of Synthetic Testosterone

Fluoxymesterone (Halotestin)
Methyltestosterone (Android, Testred, Virilon)
Testosterone cypionate, injection

Examples of Natural Testosterone

Androderm, patch
Androgel
Striant, buccal or in the cheek
Testoderm, patch

What Do They Do in the Body? Testosterone is the male hormone that develops the male genitals, increases metabolism and muscle, encourages the growth of hair, and deepens the voice.

What Are They Prescribed For? In men, a deficiency of testosterone, which may be caused by genetics, environment, or disease. They are used in women to treat metastatic breast cancer and postpartum breast pain and as hormone replacement when testosterone levels are low, as in hysterectomy.

What Are the Possible Side Effects? Although the effects of the synthetic testosterones are hard to separate out from the effects of real testosterone, you can probably safely assume that most of the side effects are caused by the synthetic testosterones or by excessive doses of real testosterone. Side effects can include hypercalcemia (too much calcium in the blood), liver damage, reduced ejaculatory volume, fluid retention, abnormal swelling of the breast in men, masculinization and menstrual irregularities in women, worsening of prostate enlargement and prostate cancer, acne, baldness, nausea, headache, aggressiveness, anxiety, and increased or decreased libido. They may also raise the risk of some types of cancer in women.

CAUTION!

Please don't use synthetic testosterone. If you need testosterone, use the real thing. See the discussion on testosterone in "Using Natural Hormones" later in this chapter.

Examples of Synthetic Glucocorticoids (Adrenal Hormones)

Beclomethasone, asthma inhaler, cream (Becotide, Qvar, Beconase, Vancenase)
Betamethasone, various creams, gels, and so on
Cortisone acetate
Deoxycorticosterone acetate
Dexamethasone (Decadron, Dexameth, Dexon)
Methylprednisolone (Medrol)
Prednisolone (Delta-Cortef, Orapred, Prelone)
Prednisone (Deltasone, Orasone, Panasol, Meticorten)
Triamcinolone (Aristocort, Atolone, Kenacort, Kenalog)

Examples of Natural Glucocorticoids

Hydrocortisone (Cortisol, Cortef)

What Do They Do in the Body? They are potent anti-inflammatory drugs that also play a role in regulating the immune system, appetite, and sodium balance in the cells. They play dozens of roles in the body having to do with metabolism and inflammation. See the section "Using Natural Hormones" for more information.

What Are They Prescribed For? Adrenal insufficiency, arthritis, lupus, psoriasis, allergies, eye inflammations, respiratory diseases such as bronchial asthma, Crohn's disease, multiple sclerosis, and other diseases that involve severe, chronic inflammation or overactive immune response.

What Are the Possible Side Effects? The gluco-corticoids have many very dangerous and destructive side effects, but many are due to the use of the synthetic versions of the drug and excessively high doses. Side effects and adverse reactions can include weight gain, osteoporosis, increased blood pressure, peptic ulcers, adrenal suppression, immunosuppression, increased susceptibility to bacterial and fungal infections, masking of bacterial and fungal infections, water retention, increased appetite, cataracts, glaucoma, steroid psychosis, muscle weakness, blood clots, pancreatitis, heartburn, thin and fragile skin, scaly lesions, headaches, dizziness, menstrual irregularities, increased sweating, and blood sugar imbalances.

People who take these drugs over a long period of time should never stop taking them abruptly. See your health care provider.

CAUTION!

Think Twice About Taking These Drugs If . . .

- You have high blood pressure.
- You have osteoporosis.
- You have ulcers, eye disease, or kidney or liver disease.
- You have a fungal infection.
- You are obese, elderly, or pregnant.

Examples of Thyroid Hormone Drugs

Levothyroxine, T4 (Synthroid, Levothroid, Levo-T, Levoxyl, Unithroid)
Liothyronine, T3 (Cytomel, Triostat)
Liotrix, T3 and T4, synthetic (Euthroid, Thyrolar)

Examples of Natural Thyroid Drugs

USP thyroid, dessicated beef or pork, T3 and T4 (Armour, Nature-Throid, Thyrar, Westhroid)

What Do They Do in the Body? Thyroid hormones regulate many types of metabolism in the body, including heart rate and strength of heartbeat, respiratory rate, oxygen consumption, body temperature, metabolism of food, growth, maturation, and enzyme activity.

What Are They Prescribed For? Thyroid hormone deficiency. (See the section "Using Natural Hormones" for more details on thyroid.)

What Are the Possible Side Effects? Side effects of a physiologic dose of USP thyroid in someone who is thyroid deficient are rare. Excessive thyroid can cause heart palpitations, rapid heartbeat, irregular heartbeat, angina, heart attack, tremors, headache, nervousness, insomnia, diarrhea, weight loss, menstrual irregularities, sweating, and intolerance to heat.

CAUTION!

Think Twice About Taking These Drugs If . . .

- You have diabetes. Work very carefully with your doctor.
- You have Addison's disease. Work very carefully with your doctor.

What Else to Take If You Take These Drugs. If you have hypothyroidism, it's a good idea to eat iodine-rich foods regularly, such as dried seaweeds (dulse, kelp).

Using Natural Hormones

Pregnenolone

Pregnenolone is a steroid hormone made from cholesterol. All the other steroid hormones, including progesterone, DHEA, the cortisols, the estrogens, and testosterone, are made from pregnenolone. Like progesterone, pregnenolone is not a sex steroid, meaning it doesn't have masculinizing or feminizing effects on the body, and it seems to be safe even in higher doses.

A flurry of research was done on pregnenolone in the 1940s, but the only clear effect it had was in relieving symptoms of rheumatoid arthritis. You can try 10 to 200 mg divided into three doses daily for arthritis and see if it helps. Give it at least three weeks to work. It is available as a supplement, over-the-counter.

More recent studies show that pregnenolone improves memory after learning, which makes sense because it has an excitatory effect on the brain and blocks GABA receptors, which play a role in blocking memory. Studies in rats and humans suggest that giving pregnenolone enhances the ability to learn and enhances memory. Other studies suggest that it improves sleep and reduces anxiety.

Even though pregnenolone is a precursor to all of the other steroid hormones, taking a pregnenolone supplement will not necessarily raise the levels of other hormones in the body. It might, but so far the evidence isn't in to indicate that this happens reliably.

Pregnenolone needs to be studied much more closely, but it is clearly of benefit for people who complain that they aren't retaining information when they learn something new. You can take up to 100 mg daily between meals for improving memory.

Progesterone

Progesterone is a steroid hormone with important effects nearly everywhere in the body. It is a precursor to all of the other steroid hormones except pregnenolone and DHEA, and it is made by the adrenal glands in both sexes and in a woman's ovaries. Progesterone is also made in the peripheral nervous system. It is an essential part of the Schwann cells that form the myelin sheath that protects nerves. Studies done with progesterone and brain injuries show that progesterone is effective in reducing the effects of a brain injury when given after an accident.

One of progesterone's biggest roles in a woman's biochemistry is opposing or balancing estrogen in the uterus and probably elsewhere. While estrogen stimulates cell growth, progesterone signals cells to mature and differentiate.

Women produce progesterone in their ovaries only when they ovulate. During months when they don't ovulate but still have a menstrual period, they may be estrogen dominant, a condition where estrogen levels aren't necessarily high, but there is no progesterone to balance its effects. This can cause PMS, and over time, according to Dr. John Lee, it can also cause fibroids, fibrocystic breasts, cervical dysplasia, and reproductive cancers. In his book *What Your Doctor May Not Tell You About Breast Cancer* (Warner Books, 2002), written with David Zava, Ph.D., and Virginia Hopkins, Dr. Lee makes a convincing argument in favor of estrogen dominance as an important risk factor for breast cancer. In women going through menopause, it can cause symptoms such as weight gain, irritability, mood swings, and headaches.

A woman's ovaries normally produce 20 to 30 mg of progesterone daily during the middle part of the menstrual cycle. Progesterone is made by the placenta in pregnant women in relatively huge quantities (as much as 300 mg daily in the last trimester). Much of postpartum depression may be caused by the plunge in progesterone levels.

At menopause, progesterone production in a woman drops even more than estrogen does, and women can often relieve menopausal symptoms using only a natural progesterone cream.

In a bizarre twist of conventional medicine working hand in hand with drug company marketing and advertising, progesterone has been all but forgotten in the rush to prescribe estrogen, and yet it is equally if not more important than estrogen in HRT.

Many premenopausal and menopausal women who use progesterone cream report that their hair becomes thicker, their libido comes back, and their vaginal dryness disappears.

Progesterone should never be confused with its synthetic cousins the progestins, such as Provera, which have many negative side effects. Natural progesterone is made in a laboratory, but it is the exact same molecule found in your body. The progestins have been altered to produce not-found-in-nature molecules that can be patented and sold at high prices. Women who take them generally report feeling awful, and their risk of dangerous side effects is very real. In contrast, women who use natural progesterone tend to be very healthy, and there are no known negative side effects at recommended doses.

If you are using HRT or contemplating it, please use natural progesterone and natural estrogens. The books *What Your Doctor May Not Tell You About Menopause* (Hatchette, 2004) and *What Your Doctor May Not Tell You About Premenopause* (Hatchette, 2005), by John R. Lee, M.D., and Virginia Hopkins, and *Dr. John Lee's Hormone Balance Made Simple*, by John R. Lee, M.D., and Virginia Hopkins (Hatchette, 2006) are classics that are recommended for all premenopausal and menopausal women. They will give you a very good sense of how your hormones work and how to balance them in a safe, natural way.

Progesterone cream works wonders for the majority of postmenopausal women; most feel dramatically better physically, mentally, and emotionally. It also works well for women of any age suffering from premenopause symptoms such as PMS, weight gain, mood swings, fibroids, and fibrocystic breasts.

In general, the best way to use progesterone is as a cream in a dose of 15 to 20 mg daily. We know that physicians prefer to give pills, but in this case the cream probably gives a more accurate dose. When taken orally, as much as 80 percent of the progesterone is processed by the liver and excreted, so you have to take 100 mg or more to get the dose you need. Depending on how your liver is working, you may get far more or far less than you need.

In a 2-ounce jar containing 800 mg of progesterone, a physiologic dose would work out to ¼ to ½ teaspoon per day. Only progesterone USP is natural progesterone.

Please be aware that some "wild yam" products may not contain any progesterone. They may contain diosgenin or dioscorea, but these will not convert to progesterone in the body.

It does not matter whether the progesterone cream is made from wild yam or soy—when they come out of the lab, they're both progesterone.

Don't think that more is better when it comes to dosing with hormones. If the recommended dose doesn't help your symptoms, then you need to do more detective work to find out what's causing the problem. *Dr. John Lee's Hormone Balance Made Simple* is a great book for tracking down the causes of hormonal imbalances.

You can buy a variety of progesterone creams over-the-counter, but if you don't understand how to use them, work with a health care professional. Please check the "Resources and Recommended Reading" section at the back of the book for sources of more detailed information on natural hormones and hormone balancing.

Dehydroepiandrosterone (DHEA)

Dehydroepiandrosterone (DHEA) is a steroid hormone manufactured in the adrenal glands. These prune-sized glands sit on top of the kidneys and are responsible for the secretion of over 150 hormones. The adrenal hormones are our major stress buffers, allowing us to adapt to whatever stresses our environment brings.

DHEA is the most abundant steroid hormone in the body. It acts as a precursor from which several other steroid hormones are made, including estrogens and testosterone, but not progesterone or the cortisols. It is an androgenic or male hormone. Only 5 percent of the body's circulating DHEA is in the active form; the remainder is joined to sulfur molecules (DHEAS) and serves as a reserve of the hormone that can be easily converted back to the active form.

DHEA production peaks between the ages of 20 and 25, with men having a higher peak than women. There is about a 2 percent decrease in blood levels for each year of life that follows. A large body of research, particularly on men, shows a clear relationship between this progressive drop in DHEA levels and diseases of aging, such as cardiovascular disease, diabetes, and some cancers. In other words, sick people have less DHEA in their bodies than well people do. Elderly people have less than young people, and elderly people with higher DHEA levels are healthier than those with low levels.

Several studies have shown that when DHEA is given to elderly subjects who started out with low levels, there is a sizable improvement in their sense of well-being. Both men and women with depression, some types of cancer, allergies, type 2 diabetes, or autoimmune diseases (such as rheumatoid arthritis) have low blood levels of DHEA. Researchers guess that raising DHEA levels can help prevent or treat these diseases. Some clinicians have reported success in treating patients who have lupus with DHEA.

DHEA may help prevent heart disease in men, but its effect on heart disease risk in women is much less promising. Most studies on this topic indicate that risk may even increase somewhat in women if it is supplemented in too high a dose. Here again, it's important to use a physiologic dose, or one close to what the body would produce naturally. In a woman, that would be less than in a man.

DHEA aids in the body's immune defenses against unwelcome invaders. One mechanism for this may involve DHEA's opposing actions to cortisol, a fight-or-flight hormone secreted by the adrenal glands when we are under stress. Cortisol suppresses some parts of the immune system. This makes sense if you're a caveman. If your body thinks you are in some kind of immediate danger, it wouldn't waste energy on building up the immune system during the crisis. This would be like deciding to cook dinner for the family in the kitchen of a house that's burning down. Modern life resembles the house that could catch fire at any moment; too dangerous to relax and cook a nourishing meal in, but not such an emergency that you have to escape immediately. Chronic stress (an almost inescapable part of life these days) leads to chronically elevated cortisol levels, which lessen our immunity against illness. The result of many years of constantly high cortisol levels can exhaust your adrenal glands, causing output of cortisol and DHEA to drop to unhealthy lows. This seems to be particularly true of women.

DHEA supplementation appears to enhance the youth-preserving effects of growth hormone, which will be addressed in detail later in this chapter. This may be one reason for DHEA's remarkable effect on well-being. In one study, a large dose of DHEA given before sleep to 10 healthy young men increased the amount of REM (rapid eye movement) sleep. REM sleep is the most restorative kind of sleep, and it is reduced in the elderly.

In a study of pregnant women, intravenous DHEAS (the sulfate form, the same form as the body's reservoir of DHEA) dilated a major eye artery, increasing blood flow. This points to a possible use of DHEAS as a blood vessel dilator that can improve circulation to the eyes.

It follows that raising DHEA levels could have powerful health-enhancing and youth-preserving effects. However, straightforward assumptions rarely work with hormones, and we can't assume that DHEA levels appropriate for a 25-year-old will be safe for a 75-year-old. That might be like putting a jet engine on an old biplane; it might fly really fast for a little while, but a crash is inevitable. We do recommend DHEA, especially for older men, but again, in moderate doses and with regular measurement of hormone levels. It's best to work with an alternative physician if you would like to use DHEA on a regular basis.

If you are a man over 40 years old and want to try DHEA, start out with 25 mg daily. If you are a woman, take 5 to 10 mg daily. Men can take up to 50 mg daily, but if you're taking that much, please get your blood or saliva levels tested at least every six months to make sure you're not overdoing it.

Because the end products of DHEA in women are primarily androgens (male hormones), women should monitor themselves carefully for any masculinizing effects of supplementation. If you notice loss of hair on the head or growth of hair on the face, acne, or weight gain around the midsection, cut back signifi-

cantly on the dosage. Chances are good that if you are experiencing these side effects, you will also begin to develop insulin resistance, a first step toward adult-onset diabetes. In men, DHEA has the opposite effect, actually improving insulin uptake. Women can experience benefit from DHEA supplementation with doses as low as 5 mg a day.

One of the reasons the medical establishment may be so cautious about DHEA is because in many of the studies, the doses given were quite high. The likelihood of negative side effects is much greater with higher dosing.

You should avoid DHEA altogether if you have or have had a hormone-sensitive cancer such as breast, ovarian, testicular, or prostate cancer. DHEA is a precursor to estrogen and testosterone, meaning that the body can manufacture those hormones from DHEA. Reproductive cancers in women seem to be largely driven by estrogen, so it makes sense not to boost levels of this hormone when you have this type of cancer.

Keep in mind that these recommendations are based on research, theory, and guesswork and are derived from what seems to be common sense and logic. In truth, we have a long way to go before we really understand how the steroid hormones interact with each other and their effects on cancer.

DHEA is not recommended for people under the age of 40, unless your levels are measurably low, as it can suppress your own natural hormone production. (Remember, more isn't necessarily better when it comes to hormones.)

For anyone using DHEA, a check of salivary levels of this hormone plus estradiol and testosterone every six months is a good idea.

Please don't take supplements derived from Mexican yam (*Dioscorea mexicana*) or wild yam

(*Dioscorea villosa*) thinking that you're getting DHEA, progesterone, or any other hormones. These products are often billed as DHEA or progesterone "precursors," which is patently false information. The reason that some manufacturers use diosgenin instead of the actual hormone is that it's much cheaper than the hormone.

While it is true that pharmaceutical-grade steroid hormone drugs are made from the diosgenin extracted from wild yam or soybeans, this all goes on in the laboratory, not in your body. Our bodies simply do not have the enzymes necessary to break down diosgenin into the steroid hormones. Many studies have been done trying to prove that diosgenin raises steroid hormone levels, using both blood and salivary hormone level testing, and not one has shown an effect. Don't waste your money on these products. If you want DHEA, take DHEA. If you want progesterone, take progesterone. It's also wise to purchase DHEA that says "pharmaceutical-grade" DHEA on the label.

Estrogens

Estrogens are the female hormones produced in the ovaries, adrenal glands, and fat cells of women and in much smaller amounts in the adrenal glands and fat cells of men. There are three predominant types of estrogens: estriol, estradiol, and estrone. These are the only natural estrogens on the market. Accept no substitutes! They come in oral, cream, and patch forms. Currently no commercial brand of estriol is available, but you can get it by prescription from a compounding pharmacist. Please read *Dr. John Lee's Hormone Balance Made Simple* for details on using estriol.

Estradiol and estrone stimulate the growth of breasts and the maturing of a girl's other reproductive organs. They are central to the menstrual cycle and stimulate the growth of tissue in the uterus each month. In excess, or without progesterone, they can cause weight gain, fluid retention, mood swings, depression, and can block thyroid function. They increase the risk of strokes and the risk of reproductive cancers. In postmenopausal women, androgens (male hormones) made by the ovaries and adrenal glands are converted to estrogen in the fat cells.

Women who are having menopausal symptoms such as night sweats, hot flashes, and vaginal dryness may benefit from some estrogen, but again it's only needed in small amounts. Taking small amounts of estrogen right around the time of menopause can also help prevent the large drop in bone density seen around that time, so if you are at risk for osteoporosis, it might be worth supplementing it for a few years. Please don't think of estrogen as a long-term replacement hormone unless you're very thin. Your fat cells and adrenal glands will make what you need, and you're getting dosed with it every time you're exposed to pesticides and plastics, which for most of us is many times daily.

There is a myth among physicians that women who have had their ovaries removed don't need progesterone along with their estrogen. What they don't realize is that estrogen alone frequently makes women feel as if they have permanent PMS. You'll feel dramatically better if you use both or even just progesterone cream. We now know that estrogen alone can increase your risk of breast cancer.

Estrogen is available by prescription only. If you decide you need some estrogen, use the smallest dose possible that will alleviate your symptoms.

Testosterone

This steroid hormone is produced in relatively large amounts in the testes of men and in much smaller amounts in the ovaries of women and the adrenal glands of both sexes. The typical secondary sex characteristics of men (deeper vocal tone, more abundant body hair, thicker skin, greater muscle mass, higher metabolism, and pattern baldness) are attributable to testosterone. There is a significant drop in both male and female testosterone levels in late life.

Studies of testosterone replacement in elderly men have shown increased libido and musculoskeletal mass and strength. In men, testosterone builds bone. Men who have had their testicles removed or who are using anti-androgenic drugs to treat prostate cancer have a much higher rate of osteoporosis and heart disease.

Testosterone replacement is worth trying in men if levels are measurably low or if there are symptoms of deficiency such as muscle wasting. In cases of unexplained weight gain, thinning skin, fatigue, or loss of muscle tone with aging, testosterone replacement could help. All forms of supplemental testosterone are only available by prescription. Ask your physician to give you a natural form, which can be taken as a pill, patch, cream, or sublingual drops. Please avoid the synthetic forms of testosterone such as methyltestosterone, as they have unpleasant and potentially dangerous side effects. Stick to the natural form, which means that the testosterone molecule looks identical to those produced in your own body. Take it in small, physiologic doses that mimic what your body would be producing on its own, which in men is about 5 mg daily, and in women 1 to 2 mg daily.

It is becoming increasingly evident that women, too, can benefit from natural testosterone replacement. Women who experience a dramatic downshift in their libido, including loss of sexual sensation in previously sensitive areas, difficulty in reaching orgasm, and drying and thinning of the vaginal walls that doesn't improve in response to natural estrogens, may want to try testosterone. Other possible symptoms of female testosterone lack are low energy, decrease in sense of well-being, thinning of pubic hair, skin dryness, and osteoporosis. Testosterone may often be the missing link in building bone in a postmenopausal woman.

Since testosterone is available only by prescription, you'll need to talk with your doctor about whether it is right for you. Testosterone is a very potent hormone that can cause undesirable side effects in doses that are even slightly elevated. Do not use testosterone if you could become pregnant.

It would be a mistake to try to achieve the testosterone levels you had as a young man or woman. The body of a 50-year-old is simply no longer equipped to handle such a hormone load. The goal is to have the symptoms of testosterone deficiency go away, not to feel like a 20-year-old again.

Thyroid Hormone

In every cell in your body, thyroid hormone plays a major role in regulating metabolic rate, your body's rate of energy production. The thyroid gland is located in the neck, with half of its 20-gram mass lying on each side of the trachea (windpipe). Lack of thyroid hormone causes a precipitous drop in your ability to expend energy, while too much of the hormone expends more energy than is necessary.

More thyroid tells the body to speed things up, causing you to breathe faster, use more oxygen, raise body temperature, have a faster heartbeat, have more blood pumping through the circulatory system, have quicker burning of calories, and have a higher production of enzymes. Symptoms of too much thyroid (hyperthyroidism) include rapid heartbeat, intolerance to heat, headache, irritability, nervousness, and sweating.

Symptoms of low thyroid hormone (hypothyroidism) are low energy, cold intolerance, especially cold feet and hands, unexplained weight gain, depression, dry skin, recurrent infections, headaches, and constipation. Although excess thyroid is relatively rare, thyroid deficiency affects up to 25 percent of American adults. Aging is one explanation, as the thyroid gland shrinks and becomes less active with age. Ten to 24 percent of cases of thyroid deficiency are missed by the blood test commonly used to screen for it. This is because blood tests measure thyroxine, or T4, which makes up 90 percent of thyroid gland secretion. Another form, triiodothyronine (T3), is a derivative of T4 and is the most active form. There are many people whose thyroid function would appear normal according to blood tests but who have trouble making the T4 to T3 conversion. Functionally, these people are thyroid deficient and their symptoms clear up when they are given thyroid supplementation. Sometimes a deficiency that doesn't show up when T4 and T3 are measured will show up when thyroid stimulating hormone (TSH) is measured. Elevated levels of TSH may indicate hypothyroidism.

Thyroid hormones, like many of the hormones made in your body, are important players in both physical and psychological health. Even slight imbalances in the production or activity of these hormones can have powerful adverse effects on emotional well-being. The physical symptoms of thyroid imbalance, in and of themselves, are often enough to cause depression and anxiety, which are then compounded by the fact that the hormonal imbalance itself can cause these psychological problems. Many thyroid patients report disturbing changes in their bodies, emotions, relationships, and ability to cope, even in instances of mild thyroid imbalance. Once they are properly diagnosed and treated,

a whole constellation of emotional and physical issues may be resolved at once.

Thyroid problems quite often masquerade as other health problems, including depression, anxiety, PMS, menopausal symptoms, obesity, and high cholesterol. This is especially true when the problems are low-grade, because most physicians aren't trained to spot subtle signs of thyroid disease. Some patients with thyroid imbalances end up getting Prozac, antianxiety drugs, or HRT. Estrogens are believed to have an aggravating effect on autoimmune thyroid disease, and drugs for anxiety or depression can cause symptoms of thyroid imbalance to worsen rather than improve.

Natural Methods for Increasing Thyroid Production. Deficiencies of zinc, copper, iron, selenium, and the amino acid tyrosine can prevent the thyroid from functioning properly. The absence of these nutrients also causes problems with the T4 to T3 conversion. Tyrosine is found plentifully in soy and in chicken, fish, and beef, or you can take it in supplement form, following directions on the container.

Chronic high cortisol levels due to excessive stress block the conversion of T4 to T3.

Iodine is an essential component of the thyroid hormones. Goiter, a disease that was once common in people living too far from the ocean to get fresh fish, manifests itself in the form of a swollen thyroid gland. This swelling occurs due to lack of iodine. Today most salt is iodized, and saltwater fish are readily available. You can also get iodine by eating sea vegetables (seaweed) such as dulse, wakame, kombu, and nori. You can take supplemental iodine (no more than 1,000 mcg a day should be used without a physician's prescription) if you think your thyroid gland needs extra help.

If stress relief and nutritional interventions don't work to relieve your symptoms or raise your basal temperature, see your physician. Thyroid hormone replacement may be necessary and can only be done by prescription. The closest thing you'll find to a natural thyroid is USP thyroid (e.g., Armour), which is a combination of T3 and T4 from cows or pigs in the ratios naturally found in the body.

Hydrocortisone (Natural)

This hormone is another classic example of drug company profits taking precedence over your health. When prednisone and the other synthetic, patentable, and much more profitable cortisone-type drugs were invented some 50 years ago, hydrocortisone was all but forgotten, and research on it came to a standstill.

Prednisone and the other synthetic cortisones are renowned for their nasty, life-destroying side effects. Yet, for many people who need them, low doses of cortisone or hydrocortisone, the natural forms of glucocorticoids, cause few or minimal side effects. If you are taking a synthetic cortisone and want a wonderful source of good information on cortisones, read the book *The Safe Uses of Cortisol* by William McK. Jefferies, M.D., FACP (Charles C. Thomas Publisher, 1996).

Cortisone and cortisol are important glucocorticoid adrenal hormones that regulate dozens of functions in the body, but especially inflammation and immune response. They are widely used to treat autoimmune diseases such as lupus and arthritis, because of their immune-suppressing properties, and severely inflammatory diseases such as Crohn's disease and psoriasis. They are also used to treat adrenal insufficiency, a condition of "tired" adrenal glands that aren't producing enough hormones. People with transplanted organs usually take cortisone-type drugs for life to suppress their body's rejection reaction.

A lot of low-level adrenal insufficiency, especially in women, is diagnosed as chronic fatigue. It's not severe enough to show up as Addison's disease, a severe deficiency of cortisone, but it is enough to cause chronic fatigue, low blood pressure, and chronic allergies. Again, if you think you might fall into that category, read Jefferies's book.

Taking hydrocortisone drugs can suppress your own adrenal function if you take too much over a long period of time. They should be used with great care, in the smallest possible dose to alleviate symptoms, over the shortest possible period of time.

Chronic stress over a long period of time is what usually causes tired adrenal glands, and rest is the best medicine. Licorice root in a tea or tincture form can also be helpful, as it supports glucocorticoid function. Some of the nutrients important to adrenal function include vitamin C, vitamin B$_6$, and vitamin E.

For more information on glucocorticoids, see the section "Replacement Hormones" earlier in this chapter.

Human Growth Hormone

The use of human growth hormone (HGH) as an antiaging hormone is very controversial and very expensive.

The pituitary gland lies at the base of the brain. One of the many hormones it secretes is somatotropin, more commonly known as growth hormone. Some of its effects are:

- Increase in lean muscle mass
- Decrease in fat mass
- Increase in size and functional capacity of organs

- Growth of endplates of bones, increasing their length (this is how children grow to adult stature), and with it the growth of collagen, a component in skin and other tissues
- Synergistic stimulation of thyroid hormone and DHEA

The physical transformation of tiny infant to small child to adult happens in large part due to plentiful growth hormone stimulation of the body's tissues. In the years since growth hormone was isolated, it has been used to help children with malfunctioning pituitary glands grow to normal size. Adults who are growth-hormone deficient because of pituitary tumors or other diseases have been helped a great deal with growth hormone replacement.

For each decade of adult life, growth hormone secretion drops 14 percent. People over the age of 60 are, for all intents and purposes, deficient in this hormone relative to youthful levels. As a result, as we age, organs shrink and work less effectively and lean mass is replaced by fat. Thyroid and DHEA production dwindle. It's no wonder scientists have begun to think that supplemental growth hormone might be one key to eternal youth.

Excess cortisol (due to stress) and excess insulin (seen in most cases of adult-onset diabetes) hamper growth hormone production. Lack of quality sleep also robs us of growth hormone's benefits: the most pronounced surge in growth hormone production occurs during deep sleep.

Giving growth hormone, growth hormone-releasing hormone (GHRH), and IGF-1 (insulin-like growth factor 1) to older adults has been shown to restore growth hormone blood levels to those of younger people. The expected positive changes in body composition are seen. In people with growth hormone deficiency caused by pituitary disease, administration of growth hormone had beneficial effects on bone, heart, thyroid, and psychological health. However, there is some indication in the research that the positive effects of growth hormone supplementation wear off after about two years.

At high doses, growth hormone can cause side effects, including fluid retention, carpal tunnel syndrome, worsening of adult-onset diabetes, and increased risk of heart failure. Since tumors use growth hormone to fuel their growth just as other cells within the body do, there is some concern that supplementation might increase the rate of growth of cancers. On the other hand, the evidence that growth hormone stimulates and strengthens the immune system may mean it can help fight cancer.

Growth hormone may be a good choice for those who are deficient, in small, physiologic doses that mimic what the body would produce naturally. Because it needs to be taken by injection and is financially out of reach for many, it is fortunate that there are several things you can do to enhance your body's own production of this youth-preserving hormone. Growth hormone secretion is stimulated after a meal rich in dietary protein. Growth hormone secretion can also be stimulated during a fast, as well as during and after exercise. Within a few months, a moderate program of weightlifting can produce increases in lean muscle mass equal to those produced by growth hormone injections.

Chapter 20

Drugs for Osteoporosis and Their Natural Alternatives

Although cardiovascular disease is the leading cause of death among American women, osteoporosis is the disease they are most likely to develop as they age. Four out of 10 white women in the United States will fracture a hip, their spine, or a forearm due to osteoporosis. As many as 5 out of 10 will develop small fractures in their spine, causing great pain and a shrinking in height. This amounts to 15 to 20 million people affected by a crippling and painful disease that is almost entirely preventable and reversible.

Osteoporosis is a gradual decrease in bone mass and density that can begin as early as the teen years. Bone mass should be at its peak in the late twenties or early thirties, but thanks in large part to a poor diet and lack of exercise, many women are already losing bone in their twenties. Bone loss occurs more rapidly in women than in men, especially right around the time of menopause, when an abrupt drop in estrogen and progesterone accelerates bone loss.

When you think of your bones, you may imagine a dead skeleton, but your bones are living tissue just like the rest of your body, and they need a good supply of nutrients and regular exercise. New bone is constantly being made, while old bone is being reabsorbed and excreted by the body. In fact, it's important for the old bone to go away so that the new, better quality bone can take its place. Our larger long bones, such as our arm and leg bones, are very dense, and they are completely replaced about every 10 to 12 years. Our less dense bones, such as our spine and the ends of our long bones, turn over every two to three years. Thus, as you can see, we always have the opportunity to be creating better bone for ourselves.

We all hear about how having enough calcium in the diet and taking estrogen can help prevent osteoporosis, but there is a much bigger nutritional and lifestyle picture to look at when we are talking about preventing this bone-robbing disease. The most important element of bones is minerals. Without minerals we don't have bones. The most important bone minerals are calcium, magnesium, potassium, phosphorus, and fluoride. Equally important is the balance between the minerals. Too much phosphorus or fluoride will create poor bone structure.

Without enough magnesium, the calcium can't be absorbed into the bone. Vitamins are also involved. For example, vitamin B_6 works with magnesium to get calcium into your bones. Vitamin D and vitamin K also help orchestrate the movement of calcium into bones.

The hormones testosterone, estrogen, and progesterone are also actively involved in the making and unmaking of bone. Testosterone and progesterone build bone, while estrogen slows bone loss.

In osteoporosis, the old bone is being taken away faster than new bone is being made, causing the bones to lose density and become thinner and more porous. The integrity and strength of our bones are related to bone mass and density. The bones of a woman with osteoporosis gradually become thinner and more fragile. A progressive loss of bone mass may continue until the skeleton is no longer strong enough to support itself. When that happens, bones can spontaneously fracture. As bones become more fragile, falls or bumps that would not have hurt us before can cause a fracture. Bone loss seems to be most severe in the spine, wrists, and hips. Unfortunately, there are usually no signs or symptoms of osteoporosis until a fracture occurs.

Early Signs of Osteoporosis

Gradual loss of height
Gum disease, loose teeth
Sudden insomnia and restlessness
Nightly leg and foot cramps
Persistent low back pain

Bone Mineral Density Testing

Menopausal women are a huge market for conventional medicine, and one relatively recent technology that has been used to scare millions of women into thinking they have osteoporosis when they really don't is bone mineral density (BMD) tests. These tests do not take into account the differing size of bones in large women and small women, so small women almost always come out showing low on BMD tests, while large women almost always come out looking OK, even when they aren't. The true usefulness of a BMD test is only in serial tests where you are comparing your own test results. This means that you should get a bone density test when you are in your thirties or forties and use that as a baseline to compare future tests against. That is the only real way you will know if you are losing bone. If you are petite, please do not be scared into taking Fosamax, Evista, or synthetic estrogens by a poor BMD level. The amazing truth about BMD is that no study has ever shown it to consistently and significantly correlate with fracture rate. Taking tranquilizer drugs that cause falls has a much higher correlation than does low bone density! This is likely because factors besides density affect the risk of fracture, including elasticity and toughness. BMD is used as a gauge of bone health not because it's the best test, but because doctors have a machine that measures it.

Should You Take Hormone Replacement Therapy to Prevent Osteoporosis?

There is a misconception that osteoporosis begins at menopause. In reality, bone mass begins declining in most women in their mid-thirties, accelerates for three to five years around the time of menopause, and then continues to decline at the rate of about 1 to 1.5 percent per year. Because bone loss accelerates at menopause, and because estrogen levels decline at menopause, conventional medicine has adopted the belief that osteoporosis is an estrogen deficiency disease that can be cured with estrogen replacement therapy. This is only partly true.

Your Risk of Osteoporosis Is Higher If You:

Are a woman
Have a family history of osteoporosis
Are white
Are thin
Are very short
Are very tall
Went into menopause early
Have a low calcium intake
Don't exercise
Smoke cigarettes
Drink more than two alcoholic drinks daily
Are on chronic steroid therapy (e.g., prednisone)
Are on chronic anticonvulsant therapy
Are taking drugs that can cause dizziness
Have hyperthyroidism
Eat too much animal protein (e.g., large servings or at more than two meals a day)
Use antacids regularly
Drink more than two cups of coffee daily

The missing pieces of this puzzle are diet and lifestyle, plus the bone-building hormone progesterone, which drops much more precipitously at menopause than estrogen does. (Progesterone refers to the natural hormone, not the synthetic progestins. See Chapter 19 for more detailed information on natural hormones.)

There is no question that estrogen can slow bone loss around the time of menopause, but the scientific evidence is very clear that after five to six years, bone loss continues at the same rate, with or without estrogen. A very large study, published in the *New England Journal of Medicine* (*NEJM*) in 1995, studied risk factors for hip fractures in white women. After following

How Aware of Osteoporosis Are You?

A Gallup poll sponsored by the National Osteoporosis Foundation found that:

- 75 percent of women believed they were familiar with osteoporosis.
- 80 percent were not aware that it was responsible for disabling fractures.
- 90 percent were surprised to learn that osteoporosis frequently causes death.
- 60 percent could not identify the risk factors of osteoporosis.

over 9,500 women for eight years, researchers found no benefit in estrogen supplementation in women over the age of 65.

In the *NEJM* study, risk factors for hip fractures included:

- Being tall (they fall farther)
- Poor overall health
- Previous hyperthyroidism (high thyroid)
- Treatment with long-acting benzodiazepines or anticonvulsant drugs (which made them dizzy, drowsy, and more likely to fall)
- Heavy coffee drinking (which depletes calcium)
- Lack of exercise
- Poor depth perception (which would naturally increase the tendency to fall)

Prescription Drugs for Osteoporosis

A number of pharmaceutical drugs are being used to treat osteoporosis, none of which work very well and all of which have unpleasant side effects. The most heavily prescribed prescription drugs for osteoporosis are the bisphosphonates—Fosamax, Didronel, Boniva, and Actonel. They all stop bone loss by powerfully inhibiting the resorption of old bone, which is the medical way of saying that they slow bone loss. The good news is that the bisphosphonates stop a cycle where bone is being lost faster than it is being replaced. The bad news is that when old, poor-quality bone is not taken away, new healthy bone cannot replace it. In other words, the inhibition of bone loss also inhibits bone building. Both are essential for healthy bones. BMD testing shows increased density, but this is only one measure of bone quality and occurs because the old bone is denser than new bone. That doesn't mean it's of good quality; in fact all indicators are that it's not. The increased BMD is due to increased mineralization of the bone, but increased bone mineralization eventually leads to increased brittleness.

Research into elasticity, a key component of healthy bone, showed that those taking a bisphosphonate had significantly reduced elasticity compared to a placebo. Other research showed that bisphosphonate treatment significantly reduced bone "toughness," a measure of the ability to resist breaking.

Another issue with the bisphosphonates is that suppression of bone resorption reduces the ability of the bone to repair itself. Normal wear and tear on the bones causes "microdamage," which in healthy bone is repaired when the damaged bone is resorbed and new bone is put in its place. The bisphosphonates inhibit this repair process, and the damage accumulates over time.

A group of bone researchers from the University of Texas Southwestern Medical Center reported on a group of nine patients, all taking a bisphosphonate long term, who had spontaneous fractures in unusual places. Up to two years later, some of the fractures had not healed. An examination of bone quality showed "severe depression of bone turnover" and thus a deterioration of the bone's ability to repair itself. The authors point out that in some of the patients, the bone turnover suppression may have been increased by taking estrogen (which also slows bone resorption) or glucocorticoids (e.g., prednisone).

Ironically, bisphosphonates also significantly deplete calcium, so much so that they are approved by the Food and Drug Administration (FDA) for treating hypercalcemia, or excess calcium.

The prestigious *British Medical Journal* published an article titled "Drugs for Pre-Osteoporosis: Prevention or Disease Mongering?" The article points out that

> Osteoporosis is a controversial condition. An informal global alliance of drug companies, doctors, and sponsored advocacy groups portray and promote osteoporosis as a silent but deadly epidemic bringing misery to tens of millions of postmenopausal women. For others, less entwined with the drug industry, that promotion represents a classic case of disease mongering—a risk factor has been transformed into a medical disease in order to sell tests and drugs to relatively healthy women. Now the size of the osteoporosis market seems set to greatly expand, as the push begins to treat women with pre-osteoporosis. These are women who are apparently at risk of being at risk, a condition known as osteopenia that is claimed to affect more than half of all white postmenopausal women in the United States.

The article concludes that ". . . we need to ask whether the coming wave of marketing targeting those women with pre-osteoporosis will result in the sound effective prevention of fractures or the unnecessary and wasteful treatment of millions more healthy women."

The drug companies that sell bisphosphonates keep coming out with studies showing that these drugs reduce the risk of fracture. However, their research leaves out many important bone health markers, dodges important questions, and uses questionable statistical juggling to prove their points. When drug researchers cherry-pick their questions, limit their answers, and fiddle with the numbers, patients become guinea pigs regarding long-term health risks. While long-term consequences are unfolding, the drug companies make millions, if not billions, of dollars. Thanks to incomplete research it will be years before we really understand the full long-term consequences of using bisphosphonates.

We do know, thanks to a large study published in the *Journal of the American Medical Association*, that there isn't any benefit to using bisphosphonates for more than five years. It's important to understand that once the bisphosphonates are deposited in the bones, they never go away. They're with you for life. We don't even know to what extent bone building can begin again after bisphosphonate treatment is stopped. As you'll read later, bisphosphonates come with other possible serious risks and side effects.

Boniva (ibandronate sodium) is an extremely high dose of bisphosphonate taken once a month. It's a new drug, so you are a guinea pig if you use it. We simply don't know what the long-term effects may be of taking that high a dose of a bone-turnover-suppressing drug. Furthermore, while Boniva has been shown to reduce the risk of vertebral (spinal) fractures, there is no evidence that it reduces the risk of nonvertebral fractures such as those of the hip, feet, and arms. Although vertebral fractures can be debilitatingly painful, hip fractures carry a high risk of death within a year after they occur.

Reclast (zoledronic acid) is a bisphosphonate given once a year by IV (in the vein). It is FDA approved for treating Paget's disease but is being aggressively marketed to postmenopausal women. We don't know the long-term consequences of long-term use of Reclast.

Bisphosphonates may be a reasonable short-term treatment to slow bone loss in extreme cases, but it's difficult to understand how their use can be otherwise justified. As you'll read later in this chapter, there are numerous safe and effective ways to slow bone loss and build bone. They involve more attention than taking one pill a month, but they address the underlying causes of bone loss.

Examples of Bisphosphonates

Alendronate (Fosamax)
Etidronate (Didronel)
Ibandronate sodium (Boniva)
Risendronate (Actonel)

What Do They Do in the Body? They slow bone loss by inhibiting the mechanism by which old bone is reabsorbed.

What Are They Prescribed For? They are prescribed for osteoporosis and osteopenia.

What Are the Possible Side Effects? Severe heartburn that can cause permanent damage to the esophagus, stress on the kidneys, impaired fertility, diarrhea, constipation, fever, low calcium, vitamin D deficiency, magnesium deficiency, flatulence, rash, headache, and severe

and sometimes incapacitating bone, joint, and muscle (musculoskeletal) pain.

A rare but terrible side effect of bisphosphonates has emerged recently, which is osteonecrosis of the jaw, or death of jawbone tissue. Most of the women who got this disease were on IV (in the vein) bisphosphonate to treat bone cancer.

Rats given high doses of these drugs developed thyroid and adrenal tumors.

CAUTION!

The long-term consequences of using these drugs are poorly studied.

What Are the Interactions with Other Drugs? Bisphosphonates may raise levels or prolong the effects of aspirin. This drug may increase the effects or prolong the action of ranitidine. These drugs may reduce the effects of antacids and calcium supplements.

What Nutrients Do They Throw out of Balance or Interact With? These drugs can cause a deficiency in just about every nutrient important to healthy bones, including calcium, magnesium, and vitamin D.

What Else to Take If You Take These Drugs. A good mineral supplement.

Miscellaneous Osteoporosis Drugs

Raloxifene (Evista)

What Does It Do in the Body? Raloxifene is a synthetic estrogen known as a selective estrogen receptor modulator (SERM), which means that it has some of the effects of an estrogen but not all. The goal of creating raloxifene was to have the estrogen property of slowing bone loss without the cancer-causing properties and other negative side effects of estradiol and estrone.

What Is It Prescribed For? Osteoporosis.

What Are the Possible Side Effects? Hot flashes, leg cramps, increased risk of blood clots in the veins, pain, rash, sweating, gastrointestinal problems, endometrial disorder, fluid retention, weight gain, muscle pain, sinusitis, pneumonia, laryngitis, flu syndrome, headache, and conjunctivitis. It can deplete the B vitamins, especially vitamin B_6, which is essential for a healthy nervous system.

CAUTION!

Raloxifene caused cancer in animals in dosages from 0.3 to 34 times the dosage level normally prescribed to postmenopausal women. In other words, a dosage equivalent to three-tenths of the dose used to prevent osteoporosis caused both benign and malignant cells to form in these animals. It's unnecessary to resort to a drug like this when natural hormones and other alternatives can do the job more safely.

Calcitonin-salmon (Calcimar, Salmonine, Osteocalcin, Miacalcin)

What Does It Do in the Body? This hormone is made by the thyroid gland that can temporarily slow bone loss. The long-term side effects are not well known, and its effectiveness diminishes rapidly after a few years.

What Is It Prescribed For? Osteoporosis.

What Are the Possible Side Effects? Flulike symptoms, back pain, respiratory problems such as cough and bronchitis, high blood pressure, angina, rapid heartbeat, irregular heartbeat, hyperthyroidism, numbness, insomnia, anxiety, dizziness, headaches, vision disturbances, swollen lymph glands, nausea, loss of appetite or increased appetite, dry mouth, diarrhea, rash, increased sweating, and tinnitus (ringing in the ears).

CAUTION!

This is an outdated drug that doesn't work very well. Please don't use it unless there's a very good reason.

Natural Remedies for Osteoporosis

Now that we know the process of preventing osteoporosis begins early in life, we are hearing about sugary drinks fortified with calcium for teenagers, antacids with calcium, and calcium supplements. Osteoporosis is not a calcium deficiency disease; it is a disease of excessive calcium loss. In other words, you can take all the calcium supplements you want, but if your diet and lifestyle choices are unhealthy, or you're taking prescription drugs that cause you to lose calcium, you will still lose more calcium from your bones than you can take in through diet.

In fact, getting adequate calcium is only a small part of the prevention picture. Please pass up the sugary drinks and antacids. The damage that refined sugar does to a growing teenage body or even an adult body far outweighs any benefit that might come from a little calcium supplementation. There is even some evidence that sugar depletes calcium, so the added calcium in these drinks may only be balancing out the damage done by the sugar. The same goes for antacids containing calcium. Since antacids tend to cause you to lose calcium, the added calcium may only offset that damage.

Although osteoporosis is not a calcium deficiency disease, you can rest assured that getting adequate calcium is an important factor in preventing osteoporosis. Some good food sources of calcium are snow peas; broccoli; leafy green vegetables such as spinach, kale, and beet and turnip greens; almonds; figs; beans (soybeans are the best); nonfat milk; yogurt; and cottage cheese. Please don't depend on milk to get your calcium. This is because milk has a poor calcium-to-magnesium ratio. Your body needs a certain amount of magnesium to get the calcium into your bones—without magnesium, calcium can't build strong bones.

In fact, magnesium deficiency may be more common in women with osteoporosis than calcium deficiency. Although many fruits and vegetables have some magnesium in them, especially good sources of magnesium are whole grains, wheat bran, leafy green vegetables, nuts (almonds are a very rich source of magnesium and calcium), beans, bananas, and apricots.

Trace minerals are also important in helping your body absorb calcium. Eating plenty of leafy green vegetables gives you calcium along with these helpful trace minerals. Boron and manganese are especially important. Foods that contain boron include apples, legumes, almonds, pears, and leafy green vegetables. Foods that include manganese include ginger, buckwheat, and oats. Be sure you're getting 1 to 5 mg of boron in your daily multivitamin or osteoporosis formula.

The organic matter in our bones consists mainly of collagen, the "glue" that holds together skin, ligaments, tendons, and bones. Zinc, copper, beta-carotene, and vitamin C are all important to the formation and maintenance of collagen in the body. If you're following the Six Core Principles for Optimal Health, you'll be getting plenty of these vitamins.

Japanese women have a significantly lower rate of osteoporosis than American women do, even though they tend to be smaller, and it's likely that their high consumption of soy products is a factor. Studies are showing that some aspect of soy—most likely, the phytoestrogens they contain—have bone-strengthening effects. Recent research published in the *Journal of Women's Health and Gender-Based Medicine* found that postmenopausal women who ate a lot of soy foods had greater spinal bone density than those who didn't. Adding soy products such as miso, tempeh, and tofu to your diet in moderate amounts may contribute to better overall health and stronger bones.

Progesterone, Testosterone, and Osteoporosis

John Lee, M.D., an internationally known expert on women's hormones, has suggested that one of the important factors in osteoporosis is a lack of progesterone, which causes a decrease in new bone formation. He and others have extensive clinical experience showing that using a natural progesterone cream will actively increase bone mass and density in women with significant bone loss and can reverse osteoporosis. These patients consistently show as much as a 29 percent increase in bone mineral density in three years or less of progesterone therapy. After treating hundreds of patients with osteoporosis over a period of 15 years, Dr. Lee found that those women with the lowest bone densities experienced the greatest relative improvement, and those who already had good bone density maintained their strong bones. Some of his patients were taking both progesterone and estrogen, which simultaneously encourages bone building and slows bone loss.

Postmenopausal women using a transdermal (on the skin) progesterone cream or oil should use the equivalent of 15 to 20 mg daily for three weeks out of the month, with a week off each month to maintain the sensitivity of the progesterone receptors.

Testosterone is also an important bone-building hormone in women. Please review the information in Chapter 19 about testosterone to find out if you might be a candidate for supplementation.

Nutritional Supplements for Osteoporosis

Calcium

Everyone should get at least 1,200 mg of calcium daily through diet, supplements, or a combination. Although you can easily get that much with a healthy diet, taking a calcium-magnesium supplement can be a wise form of health insurance for some women. In fact, calcium supplements can help slow bone loss in some women. To be incorporated into bone, calcium requires the help of enzymes, which require magnesium and vitamin B_6 to work properly. We tend to be more deficient in magnesium and B_6 than we are in calcium.

If you're female and over the age of 12, you should be taking at least 400 mg of calcium, combined with 200 to 400 mg of magnesium every day. If you can find a formula that also includes vitamin B_6, so much the better.

Sunshine Is the Best Medicine: Vitamin D

Vitamin D is another important ingredient in the recipe for strong bones because it stimulates the absorption of calcium. A deficiency of vitamin D can cause calcium loss. The best way to get vitamin D is from direct sunlight on the skin. Sunlight stimulates a chain of events in the skin leading to the production of vitamin D in the liver and kidneys. (This is why liver and kidney disease can produce a vitamin D deficiency.) Going outside for just a few minutes a day can give us all the vitamin D we need; yet many people don't even do that. They go from their home, to their car, to their office, and back home, without spending more than a few seconds outdoors. Many elderly people are unable to get outside without assistance, but their getting outside safely every day should be a priority for their caretakers.

Recent studies have shown that the RDA for vitamin D of 400 IU daily is far too low. Most Americans are deficient in vitamin D, which raises the risk of a number of cancers, including breast and colon cancer, as well as heart disease and osteoporosis. Most experts now agree that the average person should get 1,000 to 2,000 IU daily of vitamin D, as vitamin D_3 (not D_2), and should also spend 15 to 20 minutes a day in the sun, without sunblock. This being said, you should not get a sunburn. If you're not used to being in the sun, increase your exposure gradually.

Stomach Acid: Betaine Hydrochloride

As we age, we tend to produce less stomach acid. To be absorbed, calcium requires vitamin D and stomach acid. For this reason, it's important to avoid antacids and the H2 blockers such as Tagamet and Zantac, which block or suppress the secretion of stomach acid. Contrary to what the makers of heartburn and indigestion remedies would have you believe, the last thing in the world most people need is less stomach acid. Heartburn and indigestion are caused by poor eating habits and a lack of stomach acid. Ulcers are caused by a bacteria, not by too much stomach acid. (See Chapter 11 for more information

---

To Absorb Calcium and Build Bones We Need . . .

Exercise

Hydrochloric acid in the stomach

Magnesium

Progesterone (women) or testosterone (men)

Vitamin D

Vitamin K (found abundantly in deep-green leafy vegetables)

on preventing heartburn and indigestion.) A simple way to improve your calcium absorption may be to take a betaine hydrochloride supplement just before or with meals, to increase your stomach acid. You can find betaine hydrochloride at your health food store.

These Deplete Calcium and Magnesium

Alcohol
Lack of exercise
Lack of the hormone progesterone
    or testosterone
Phosphorus (found in soda)
Sugar
Too much protein

The Collagen Vitamins and Minerals: Zinc, and Vitamins A and C

Collagen is the tissue that makes up your bones. To build collagen, you need vitamin A (or beta-carotene), zinc, and vitamin C. Vitamin C is especially important, as it is the primary ingredient in the collagen matrix.

What to Avoid to Prevent Osteoporosis

We've known for decades that certain medications can contribute to bone loss. They include steroids such as prednisone, and calcium-channel-blocking drugs for hypertension such as Procardia and Norvasc. Now we can add three other classes of drugs to the list:

- Acid-suppressing drugs used for heartburn, such as Prilosec, Prevacid, and Nexium

- Selective serotonin reuptake inhibitor (SSRI) antidepressants such as Celexa, Zoloft, Prozac, and Paxil
- Diabetes drugs such as Avandia and Actos

Heartburn or Hip Fracture?

A major heartburn drug study examined the medical records of 13,000 people who had suffered a hip fracture and compared them with 135,000 similar people who had never had a hip fracture.

Those who had used the family of heartburn drugs known as proton pump inhibitors (PPIs) for more than a year had a whopping 44 percent higher risk of hip fracture. Those taking the drugs at the highest doses for the longest period of time had the highest risk of hip fracture. Critics of the study point out that so-called retrospective research looking back at medical records tends to be less accurate, but even if the PPI users had a 22 percent risk instead of 44 percent risk, it would still be a very high number.

It's theorized that the PPIs probably cause bone loss that leads to hip fracture by interfering with the absorption of nutrients that build bone, such as calcium and other minerals.

The PPIs can be a very useful short-term solution for stopping heartburn, but it's important to make the lifestyle changes that can prevent heartburn and get off the drugs.

Antidepressants

The research on SSRIs and bone loss is smaller but still important. A Canadian study was done at McGill University that began with a pool of 5,008 randomly selected people over 50 and followed them for five years. Of that group, 137 were taking SSRIs, and they were found to have 2.1 times the risk of bone fractures—in other words, double the risk of a fracture. Although this was a relatively small group taking the SSRIs, the researchers took into account many other risk factors for bone fractures and still got the same result. Some critics argue that people who are depressed fall more often, but the study showed that the SSRI users had "fragility" fractures, meaning broken bones caused by relatively minor incidents like falling out of bed—it didn't take much for their bones to break.

Diabetes Drugs

The FDA has issued warnings that women who take the type-2 diabetes drugs Avandia (rosiglitazone) or Actos (pioglitazone) have an increased risk of upper arm, hand, and foot fractures. Women taking these drugs had double the fracture risk of women taking other types of type-2 diabetes drugs.

Triple Prescription-Drug Bone-Loss Whammy

It's common to find senior citizens on multiple prescription drugs. Some of the most common include prednisone, calcium channel blockers, and PPIs—all now linked to bone fractures. There are many reasons to avoid prescription drugs in general, and now we can add bone loss to the list.

Break the Soda Habit

There's a good chance that one of the leading contributors to osteoporosis in the United States is carbonated soft drinks containing phosphorus. Research has shown a direct link between too much phosphorus and calcium loss. If you're guzzling down a couple of fizzy soft drinks a day, you're most likely creating bone loss.

Our other source of excessive phosphorus in the United States is eating too much meat. The average American gets more than enough protein, so for most of us it can only help to cut down on our meat consumption. A recent trend among those who love meat but don't love the consequences of too much fat and protein is to use meat as a garnish or flavoring in a meal, rather than as a major portion. Fill up on vegetables first and complex carbohydrates (whole grains, potatoes, rice, corn, beans) second, and use meat to enrich your meals. Beans are an excellent and nutritious source of protein and contain many important vitamins and minerals.

Coffee, Alcohol, and Cigarette Smoking

Here's yet another good reason to either give up coffee and alcohol or use them in moderation. And do you need to be told how important it is to stop smoking now? (It's never too late to reap the benefits of quitting smoking.) Each of these substances creates a negative calcium balance in the body. Substances called phytates and oxylates bind with calcium in the large intestine and form insoluble salts, rendering the calcium useless. The bone mineral content of smokers is 15 to 30 percent lower in women and 10 to 20 percent lower in men. Cigarette smoking is a significant risk factor for osteoporosis. Twice as many women with osteoporosis smoke as compared with women who do not have osteoporosis.

Aluminum

Don't take antacids with aluminum, and don't use aluminum cooking pots. It has been shown that small amounts of aluminum-containing antacids increase the urinary and fecal excretion of calcium, inhibit absorption of fluoride, and inhibit absorption of phosphorus, creating a negative calcium balance. The calcium is excreted instead of being used. Aluminum is also found in tap water, processed cheese, toothpastes, and white flour.

Diuretics

Diuretics are medicines that cause water loss in the body. Along with the water, you lose minerals, most notably calcium, magnesium, and potassium. They are commonly used in conventional medicine to treat high blood pressure, swelling of the lower legs, and congestive heart disease. People who use diuretics have a higher risk of fracture. If you need to use a diuretic, first try a gentle herbal one such as dandelion root in a tincture, capsule, or tea.

High-Dose Cortisone

A well-known risk for osteoporosis is long-term treatment with the synthetic cortisones such as prednisone. Since the cortisones are closely related to progesterone in their molecular structure, the theory is that they compete for the same receptor sites on bone-building cells. However, while progesterone gives bones the message to grow, the cortisones give bones the message to stop growing. If you must be on a cortisone, talk to your physician about using a low-dose natural cortisone called hydrocortisone rather than the synthetic cortisones. You can refer him or her to the classic book *The Safe Uses of Cortisol* by William McK. Jefferies, M.D., FACP (Charles C. Thomas Publisher, 1996).

Fluoride Is Bad for Your Bones

The common and seemingly irrefutable wisdom is that cavities in the United States have been greatly decreased by the addition of fluoride to our drinking water and our toothpaste. But it's not true, and fluoride is most likely doing a great deal of harm.

The original studies that were supposed to show how well fluoridated communities did are highly suspect. The original U.S. Public Health study on fluoridation was supposed to compare hundreds of communities, but the final study included only a few dozen, presumably those that fit the desired profluoridation profile. And even those were flawed. For example, two towns in Michigan were compared for dental cavities, but those children studied in the fluoridated community were from families with higher incomes, received regular dental checkups, and agreed to brush their teeth twice a day. It wouldn't seem strange that they would have a lower rate of cavities, with or without fluoride. "But," you may be protesting, "I had lots of cavities when I was a kid, and my kids hardly have any. It must be due to fluoride." Not so. In both fluoridated and unfluoridated areas in North America and Europe, the decline in tooth decay has been the same for 30 years. This even holds true for entire countries in Europe that have never had fluoridated water or toothpaste.

What has changed is that dental hygiene has improved, nutrition has improved, and access to dental care has improved. Studies do show a strong correlation between higher rates of tooth decay and lower economic status.

Japan and all of continental Europe either rejected the fluoride concept from the beginning or have stopped the practice. Most of Great Britain has also discontinued the practice, and Australia and New Zealand are in the process of reversing the trend. A 1994 study of virtually all New Zealand schoolchildren showed no benefit in dental health in fluoridated communities.

What's so bad about fluoride? There is good, solid evidence in reputable studies that fluoridated drinking water increases your risk of hip fractures by 20 to 40 percent. For a while, it was thought that fluoride might actually help prevent osteoporosis. But long-term studies with hundreds of thousands of people proved the wisdom of checking things out thoroughly. There is a clear correlation between bone fractures and fluoridation. It turns out that while fluoride does create denser bone, it is poor-quality, structurally unsound bone that is actually more prone to fracture over the long term.

So much fluoride has been put into our water and toothpaste over the past 30 years that levels in our food chain are very high. While eating a normal diet the average person exceeds the recommended dose. Fluoride is a potent enzyme inhibitor that interferes with enzymes in the body, particularly in the lining of your intestines, causing stomach pain, gas, and bloating. This enzyme-inhibiting effect also interferes with thyroid gland function. Some studies indicate that fluoride damages the immune system, leading to autoimmune disorders and arthritis. There is also evidence that communities with fluoridated water have a higher incidence of heart disease and higher rates of bone cancer in young men. Some 30 percent of children in fluoridated communities have fluorosis, a malformation of tooth enamel that causes discoloration (usually chalky white patches) and brittleness. This is a permanent change in the teeth that has also been associated with abnormal bone structure.

Advocates of putting fluoride in toothpaste and mouthwash argue that it is not swallowed and therefore not ingested. However, fluoride is absorbed through the mucous membranes of the mouth, and young children do not have control over their swallowing reflex. There have been numerous reports of children poisoned by ingesting high levels of fluoride through school fluoride mouthwash programs or fluoridated toothpastes full of sweeteners that kids want to swallow. Who knows how many stomachaches, in kids and adults alike, have been caused by unknowingly ingesting too much fluoride?

Please avoid fluoride in all forms, including toothpastes. This substance has crept into every link in our food chain, and the evidence is that even without fluoridated water and toothpaste, we're getting a higher dose than is safe or recommended in our daily diets.

Avoiding Fluoride in Your Water

You can be thankful if you live in an unfluoridated community, because it's not easy to get rid of fluoride in your tap water. Distillation and reverse osmosis are the only two reliable methods for removing fluoride. Other water filters may work at eliminating fluoride for a short period of time, but fluoride binds so strongly and quickly to filter materials such as charcoal that the binding sites become fully occupied after a short time. The best ways to avoid fluoride are to stay away from toothpastes and mouthwashes that contain it. (You can also become politically active and begin to educate your community about the harmful effects of fluoride.)

If you are at a high risk for osteoporosis, it may be worth spending the money on a reverse osmosis water purification system.

Exercise for Strong Bones: Use 'Em or Lose 'Em

Lack of exercise is one of the primary causes of osteoporosis. Using your bones keeps them strong and healthy. Weight-bearing exercise significantly increases bone density in older women, while also increasing elasticity and toughness. *Weight-bearing* means exercise that uses your bones to support the weight of your body. Brisk walking counts as weight-bearing exercise, but add some light handheld weights and it's even better. (Hold the weights with arms bent at the elbows and pumping vigorously, not dangling by your sides. Letting the weights hang puts undue stress on the rotator cuffs and can lead to injury.) Pushing a vacuum cleaner or lawn mower, gardening, dancing, and doing aerobic exercise also qualify.

Your exercise plan should include a minimum of 20 minutes of weight-bearing exercise three to four times a week. An hour is even better. In contrast to women who exercise, those who don't continue to lose bone, regardless of what else they are doing. Studies of elderly people who fall and break a bone show that these people had poor flexibility, poor leg strength, instability when first standing, and difficulty getting up and down in a chair. Exercise can help increase flexibility, strength, and coordination. A weight-lifting program of just half an hour three to four times a week can significantly improve bone density. You don't need to go to the gym to do a weight-lifting program. You can lift a can of peas or a small carton of milk. Women with advanced osteoporosis should work with a physical therapist to create a safe, effective program to reduce the risk of fracture. The Asian movement exercises such as yoga, tai chi, and qi gong can also be excellent for improving strength, flexibility, and coordination.

In a recent study on bone density and exercise, older women who did high-intensity weight training two days per week for a year were able to increase their bone density by 1 percent, while a control group of women who did not exercise had a bone density *decrease* of 1.8 to 2.5 percent. The women who exercised also had improved muscle strength and better balance, while both decreased in the nonexercising control group.

Chapter 21

Drugs for Herpes and Their Natural Alternatives

Cold sores (type 1 herpes), genital herpes (type 2 herpes), and shingles (herpes zoster) affect many millions of Americans, causing painful, burning, itchy blisters. The herpes virus is in the same strain as the chicken pox virus, and we know that shingles has its origin in chicken pox, which hides out in the nerves for decades, usually reappearing in the elderly as extremely painful blisters around the rib cage. We don't know where cold sores and genital herpes originated, but we do know that genital herpes is a highly contagious sexually transmitted disease. Some researchers have implicated cold sores with Bell's palsy, which causes facial paralysis.

Having oral sex with a partner who has a cold sore on the lips can also cause a genital herpes outbreak, and vice versa.

No herpes virus ever completely goes away that we know of; it just retreats back into the nerves.

Genital herpes is a virtual epidemic among the baby boomers, affecting an estimated 20 million people. The first outbreak of blisters is usually the most painful and lasts the longest. After that, the progression of the disease varies greatly among individuals. In a lucky 40 percent of people who are infected, it retreats completely, never appearing again. In others, it reappears only occasionally. Others are plagued by constant outbreaks that can have a negative impact on self-esteem and sexuality.

Like all sexually transmitted diseases, herpes carries with it the burden of shame, guilt, and the risk of passing it on to somebody else. The first thing you can do is drop the shame and guilt (it will reduce emotional stress, which will help prevent the next outbreak) and be extremely careful about passing it on to somebody else. This is possible by using condoms vigilantly and avoiding sex during outbreaks. Although it may be an embarrassment to pass it on to another adult, it can be dangerous when passed on to a newborn baby during a vaginal birth.

Although the virus can theoretically be present and thus contagious when there are no symptoms, if you're in touch with your body, you can usually feel it coming on. That's the time to abstain or use a condom—abstention is safer.

Examples of Drugs for Treating Herpes

Acyclovir (Zovirax)
Famciclovir (Famvir)
Penciclovir (Denavir)
Valacyclovir (Valtrex)

What Do They Do in the Body? Inhibit the herpes virus.

What Are They Prescribed For? Treatment of herpes virus infections.

What Are the Possible Side Effects? Valacyclovir is used for treating all types of herpes. It is a remarkably effective and reasonably safe drug for most people. Its most common side effect is headaches. Other side effects can include abdominal pain, nausea, missed periods, joint pain, dizziness, depression, and vomiting. In the elderly, especially those with kidney disease, this drug has been reported to cause central nervous system adverse reactions, including agitation, hallucinations, confusion, delirium, seizures, and encephalopathy.

Acyclovir has caused testicular atrophy in rats. It can cause kidney damage, liver damage, and electrolyte (mineral) balance disturbances. Adverse reactions to acyclovir have included fatigue, nausea, vomiting, headaches, dizziness, skin rash, loss of appetite, water retention, swollen lymph glands, numbness, and tingling.

Famciclovir has caused cancer, mutated cells, and impaired fertility in rodents. Adverse effects include a high incidence of headaches as well as dizziness, insomnia, fatigue, itching, fever, sinus infections, back and joint pain, numbness, nausea, diarrhea, constipation, vomiting, and appetite loss.

Penciclovir is a topical cream approved for treating cold sores. It has caused headaches, rash, and numbness.

CAUTION!
Think Twice About Taking These Drugs If . . .
You have kidney or liver disease.

Natural Alternatives for Herpes Drugs

Herpes is one of the few health problems where we would recommend a drug. For most people, Valtrex is a reasonably safe and effective drug. Now that generic versions are available, the price is also reasonable. If Valtrex gives you a headache or other side effects, try the following natural remedies. Regardless of whether you take Valtrex, these suggestions can help prevent a herpes outbreak and may eliminate the need to take any drugs.

Your best strategy for preventing a herpes outbreak is to keep your immune system strong. That means following the Six Core Principles for Optimal Health. You can also take extra vitamin A for up to two weeks (10,000 IU daily), an extra 10 to 15 mg of zinc daily for up to two weeks, and the herbs astragalus and echinacea, which both stimulate and support the immune system. Naturopath and author Michael Murray recommends thymus extracts derived from young calves and then standardized (follow the directions on the container).

You Probably Don't Need Herpes Drugs During Pregnancy

Genital herpes can be passed on to a baby when it passes through the birth canal if the mother is having an active outbreak when she gives birth. This can cause severe problems in a newborn, including blindness. So when women with herpes are told by their obstetricians that they should take Zovirax or another antiherpes drug for the last trimester of pregnancy, they may think that not doing so would be tantamount to negligence.

The truth is that it's quite rare for a woman with herpes to have active lesions when she gives birth. This may be due to high levels of estrogens and progesterone, or the simple fact that her body is marshaling its every effort to create an ideal environment for the arrival of her baby. Herpes inhibitors have definitely not been proven safe during pregnancy and have been found to cause birth defects in animal studies. No adequate, well-controlled studies have been done with pregnant women. The only time these antiviral drugs are justified during pregnancy is

if a woman has her first herpes outbreak during pregnancy. If this happens, the disease can affect the baby, and drugs may be the best course of action.

According to the Santa Barbara Midwives, a group of certified nurse midwives who have been delivering babies for two decades, herpes lesions detected during labor can be covered with special sticky bandages that prevent the baby from coming into contact with them. If worse comes to worst, a cesarean section will protect the baby from being exposed. Natural approaches to preventing herpes outbreaks will also help. Avoid foods rich in arginine such as nuts, and take supplemental lysine as directed later in this chapter. Don't use vitamin A, thymus extracts, or astragalus during pregnancy. Echinacea, elderberry, or lemon balm should be used during pregnancy only if you are under the care of a natural health practitioner. Selenium is OK to use during pregnancy in recommended doses.

With both pharmacological and natural treatments, it's important to begin treatment in the earliest possible stages of the outbreak. Shingles doesn't recur very often, but when it does, it is generally preceded by fatigue and an aching or sharp pain in the area of the first outbreak.

Most people know when an outbreak of cold sores or genital herpes is coming. The area around the mouth where cold sores occur is usually tingly or numb for a day or two before the outbreak. Genital herpes may be preceded by fatigue; sore or tired muscles; a fever; pain in the groin, hips, or legs; swollen lymph glands in the groin area; and then shortly before the outbreak, numbness and tingling in the area where the blisters will appear.

Some of the factors that we know can bring on an outbreak of cold sores or genital herpes are stress, infections, fevers, colds and flus, sun exposure, and menstruation. Women have noticed that sexual conflict or ambivalence (a form of stress) can aggravate herpes.

Arginine and Lysine

We also know that chocolate, nuts, grains, beans, and other foods containing high levels of the amino acid arginine can precipitate a herpes outbreak. (It's possible that for some people it's only peanuts that aggravate herpes—you'll have to experiment for yourself.) Too much acidic food such as tomatoes, and in some people, vitamin C, can also aggravate an outbreak.

Lysine is the amino acid that opposes arginine, so taking a lysine supplement, 500 mg three times daily between meals at the first sign of an outbreak, can help reduce symptoms. If you have chronic herpes outbreaks, you can take 500 mg of lysine daily as a preventive. Foods that are high in lysine include fish, turkey, chicken, beef, and dairy products.

The Antiviral Duo: Selenium and Elderberry

Two recent additions to your antiviral natural medicine cabinet are elderberry extracts and selenium. Both are powerful antiviral agents. See Chapter 12 on colds and flus for details on elderberry. There are anecdotal reports that a combination of elderberry and selenium at the first signs of an impending genital herpes outbreak stopped the outbreak altogether. Follow the directions on the container for elderberry dosage.

For some people, taking a preventive dose of 200 mcg of selenium daily has noticeably reduced the incidence of outbreaks. If you feel an outbreak coming on or have one, you can increase the dosage for a week. By the way, you can try this dynamic duo of elderberry and selenium for any type of viral infection.

Lemon Balm

It's nice to have lemon balm (*Melissa officinalis* L.) around the garden because it smells so good. This member of the mint family is also an herbal remedy for herpes, and a lemon balm cream is the bestselling cold sore remedy in Germany, where it has been well studied. Some reports say that when the cream is applied to cold sores regularly, eventually they don't recur. At the very least, lemon balm cream speeds up the healing process. You should be able to find it at your health food store.

Chapter 22

Drugs for Impotence and Their Natural Alternatives

J ust as women go through menopause and have a decline in the hormones estrogen and progesterone around the age of 50, men go through a more gradual but sometimes equally distressing age-related decline in hormones. In men it is the male hormones, or androgens, that decline, and for this reason the male version of menopause is sometimes called andropause.

Andropause can cause weight gain, hair loss, breast growth, and perhaps most distressing for many men, impotence or the inability to achieve and maintain an erection. Many other factors are related to impotence besides declining hormones, the most important being the same blood vessel problems that cause heart disease. Before the release of the impotence drug Viagra, erection problems in older men were not openly talked about, and most men simply resigned themselves to an old age without sex.

But Viagra has brought male impotence out into the open, and millions of the now-infamous and expensive blue pills were sold within a few months of its introduction.

Mechanics of Impotence

By age 75, more than 50 percent of men have impotence problems. The medical point of view used to be that it was caused by anxiety, but we now have scientific evidence that most impotence is caused by circulatory problems ranging from clogged arteries to high blood pressure.

The penis becomes erect through signals from the brain that cause changes in its blood vessels. The arteries that bring blood into the penis open wider, while the veins in the penis that take blood back to the heart constrict, so that more blood enters the penis than exits it. Two chambers in the penis fill with blood, causing the penis to stiffen, or become erect. The contraction of muscles surrounding the base of the penis raises the internal pressure even higher.

Impotence can be caused by a failure of the blood vessels in the penis to operate correctly, or it can be caused by a lack of libido or sex drive. Lack of libido is most often due to a decline in male hormones or by prescription drugs. If impotence is caused by clogged arteries, leaky veins, or poor blood pressure control, it may be a first sign of heart disease. Diabetics have poor circulation, and as a result as many as 50 percent of diabetic men are impotent.

Hormone Imbalance

Anything that increases estrogen levels in men will create a corresponding drop or suppression of testosterone and the male hormone androstenedione. Some ways that men may unwittingly create a rise in estrogen levels include using exces-sive alcohol, using pesticides and solvents, eating a lot of nonorganic red meat from livestock that has been fed estrogens (which includes virtually all U.S. livestock), or taking the drugs Tagamet (cimetidine), ketoconazole, or cyproterone acetate. Because fat cells make estrogen, obese men also tend to have higher estrogen levels.

Although men with low testosterone may still be able to physically achieve an erection, testosterone seems to be what drives libido in men, so a man with testosterone deficiency may have less sexual desire. See Chapter 19 for details on using supplemental testosterone and DHEA.

Are Prescription Drugs Sinking Your Sex Life?

Impotence is a known side effect of many prescription drugs, including blood pressure drugs; antidepressants; antibiotics; antihistamines; stimulant drugs; H2 blockers such as Tagamet and Zantac; heart drugs such as beta-blockers, calcium channel blockers, ACE inhibitors, and angina drugs; painkillers; sedatives; tranquilizers; sleeping pills; and prostate drugs. The SSRI antidepressants (e.g., Prozac, Zoloft, Paxil, and Effexor) tend to help maintain erections, but because they also tend to deaden the emotions and dampen the libido, they aren't good impotence drugs. In fact, because they tend to create a false sense of emotional detachment, they tend to be sex sinkers for both men and women.

Cocaine, marijuana, alcohol, and smoking can all contribute to impotence. Marijuana can cause a drop in testosterone levels.

Examples of Impotence Drugs

Sildenafil (Viagra)
Tadalafil (Cialis)
Vardenafil (Levitra, Nuviva)

Drugs That Can Cause Impotence

- Antidepressants, including monoamine oxidase inhibitors (MAOIs), Prozac and other selective serotonin reuptake inhibitors (SSRIs), and tricyclic antidepressants
- Tranquilizers, sedatives, sleeping pills, narcotics, and hypnotics, including phenothiazines, benzodiazepines, meprobamate, and barbiturates
- Estrogens and antiandrogens prescribed for prostate cancer, and drugs that can act as antiandrogens such as cimetidine (Tagamet), ketoconazole, and cyproterone acetate
- Drugs used to treat benign prostatic hypertrophy (BPH), or enlarged prostate
- Antihistamines used to treat colds and allergies
- Heart drugs, including drugs that lower blood pressure, beta-blockers, calcium channel blockers, ACE inhibitors, and angina drugs

What Do They Do in the Body? These drugs work by increasing blood flow into the penis. Cialis works for up to 36 hours and has been approved for daily use. Cialis and Viagra have also been approved for the treatment of pulmonary arterial hypertension.

What Are They Prescribed For? Erectile dysfunction (ED), or impotence—the inability to get an erection.

What Are the Possible Side Effects? The most common side effects are nausea, back pain, muscle aches, flushing, stuffy or runny nose, impaired or blurred vision, and sudden hearing loss. Other less common side effects can include photosensitivity, eye pain, facial swelling, high blood pressure, very low blood pressure, palpitations, rapid heartbeat, joint pain, muscle pain, rash, and itch. All of these drugs can cause priapism, in which the penis does not return to its flaccid state within four hours. This should be considered a medical emergency and can cause damage to the penis that can result in permanent impotence. These drugs can also cause a heart attack.

CAUTION!

- If you have any type of heart disease or blood vessel disease, do not take this drug without consulting a doctor.
- These drugs can cause vision to change, casting a blue tint over everything. Pilots aren't allowed to use them before they fly, because they can't see the numbers on the instrument panel.

Natural Remedies for Impotence

Let's find out more about natural remedies for impotence. If you'd like a great, Viagra-free sex life—for the rest of your life—the first step is good food, good vitamins, regular exercise, and remembering that a little bit of tenderness goes a long way with your partner. But we also want to let you in on a little secret, backed up by scientific studies. The herb *Ginkgo biloba* isn't just great for improving blood flow to the brain and improving memory, it improves blood flow everywhere!

Even if you haven't been diagnosed with atherosclerosis (clogged arteries), impotence is nearly always a sign that circulation in the penis isn't as good as it could be. See Chapter 10 on drugs for heart disease for natural remedies for better circulation.

Ginkgo Biloba

This herb, originally from China, is well-known for improving memory by improving circulation to the brain, but it is also known to improve erectile function in those with mild blood vessel disease. It is very gentle and safe and works best when taken daily.

Yohimbine

Made from the bark of the yohimbine tree, this product has been patented for use as a prescription drug called Yocon or Yohimbex. This is a potent stimulating substance, so a man with any type of heart disease should check with his doctor before using it.

Ginseng

This root is known as an adaptogen, which is a substance that tends to bring the body into balance. Its balancing effect increases energy and stamina. Ginseng and ginkgo together is a good herbal tonic for men to use regularly, as they both have a balancing and tonifying effect throughout the body.

Ashwagandha

This is an herb originally used in Ayurvedic medicine in India. Like ginseng, it is a tonic herb and was traditionally used to improve libido and sexual performance.

Arginine

The amino acid arginine is involved in the production of the neurotransmitter and artery-relaxing substance nitric oxide. If you remember, Viagra has its effect through relaxing the arteries in the penis. Arginine has a similar effect on some men, although it is not as potent. Try 1,200 to 1,500 mg of L-arginine on an empty stomach.

Drugs for Attention Deficit/ Hyperactivity Disorder and Their Natural Alternatives

A ttention deficit/hyperactivity disorder (ADHD) is believed to affect 1 in 20 American children. As of 2008, between 4 and 12 percent of children in the United States   depending on whose estimate you trust—were said to meet the diagnostic criteria for this disorder. About 56 percent of those children end up being prescribed medication to control their behavior. In some communities, one in five children is on Ritalin or another ADHD drug. These children are currently taking one of a class of stimulant drugs that includes Ritalin, Adderall, Concerta, Dexedrine, and Metadate.

One to two million more children are being prescribed the selective serotonin reuptake inhibitors (SSRIs), including Prozac, Zoloft, and Paxil; other antidepressants, such as Wellbutrin, Effexor, and trazodone; the antipsychotic drugs Risperdal, Zyprexa, and Haldol; anticonvulsants such as Depakote and Tegretol, used to treat mood disorders and to control anger, irritability, and aggression; and the blood pressure drug clonidine to control inattention, impulsivity, and insomnia. In many instances, kids with behavior problems end up taking a "cocktail" consisting of two or three of these drugs. In 2003, spending on psychotropic drugs for children surpassed spending on antibiotics and asthma medications.

Psychiatrists openly admit that little to nothing is known about these drugs' long-term impact when given to children. On "The Medicated Child," a PBS "Frontline" special that aired in 2007, psychiatrist Patrick Bacon said, "It's really to some extent an experiment, trying medications in these children of this age. . . . It's a gamble. And I tell parents there's no way to know what's going to work." Parents find themselves faced with a choice between giving their children potentially dangerous drugs for life or having a child who could hurt him- or herself and others and fail socially and academically. Dr. Steven Hyman, a former director of the National Institute of Mental Health, told "Frontline": "I think the real question is, are those diagnoses right? And in truth, I don't think we yet know the answer."

And ADHD isn't just for kids anymore; nor are the drugs used to treat it. According to a survey of over 3,000 randomly selected American adults between ages 18 and 44, about 4.4 percent of U.S. adults match the diagnostic criteria for ADHD. Drugmakers have made it quite easy for adults to take an ADHD "self-test" online or in magazines, which encourages them to ask their doctors about being diagnosed and treated. Both men and women are being prescribed ADHD medication at increasing rates. For both adults and children, substance abuse is a major concern with the drugs discussed in this chapter; for more on this, refer to Chapter 2.

ADHD isn't only about hyperactivity anymore, either. There is now an "inattentive" variant of attention deficit disorder (ADD), which is said to be more common in girls. If a child tends to daydream, makes careless mistakes, fails to pay attention to details, can't pay attention for a long time, is a poor listener, fails to follow through on tasks, is poorly organized, loses things, or is easily distracted or forgetful . . . he or she, too, may end up being pegged as ADD and in need of medication.

Did you know that Winston Churchill had "symptoms" of ADHD as a child? He struggled in school. How would the world be different today if he had been given Ritalin? What about John F. Kennedy, Jr.; Ludwig van Beethoven; Benjamin Franklin; or the Wright Brothers? It has been said that all of these men might have been diagnosed with ADHD if the *Diagnostic and Statistical Manual of Mental Disorders* (the diagnostic "bible" of the American Psychiatric Association) had existed in their childhood days.

The ADHD diagnosis was created in its present form in the 1980s. For decades before that time, it was recognized that some kids were more active and impulsive than others. Psychiatry called this impulsivity by various names, including "defect of moral control," "postencephalitic behavior disorder," "minimal brain dysfunction," and "hyperkinetic disorder of childhood." It took until the 1980s for psychiatry to name and describe the modern version in the *Diagnostic and Statistical Manual of Mental Disorders*. As early as the 1930s, low doses of stimulant drugs were used to try to modify the behavior of children with these diagnoses.

It was not until the 1960s that these drugs were widely used for this purpose. During that decade, the notion of biochemical psychiatry really began to catch on. Studies with drugs such as LSD showed that even tiny amounts of certain substances could cause enormous alterations in thoughts, perceptions, and behaviors. If this were so, they reasoned, abnormal behavior must be caused by alterations in the natural substances that carry information through the nervous system. From there, it was a short leap to the idea that by giving them drugs, we could "improve" anyone who seemed psychologically "abnormal." The question is who gets to define what is normal and abnormal, and what are the implications of allowing the mass medication of children, and adults, based on that definition?

In 1996, Adderall was approved by the Food and Drug Administration (FDA) for treatment of ADHD. Since then, use of these drugs has skyrocketed, and the brands and varieties available have multiplied. At this writing, over 2.5 million children are taking ADHD drugs in United States alone. Growth of ADHD drug use in girls between birth and age 19 in the years 2000 to 2005: 87 percent. Boys in the same age bracket used 48 percent more ADHD meds in 2005 than in 2000.

The double standard embraced by the medical mainstream is plain: Just say no to drugs, kids, unless a man in a white coat tells you to take them because you aren't socially acceptable without them. If you're going to take Ritalin to perform better on a test or stay up all night to study, well, that's not OK—unless you've been diagnosed with ADHD. Keep in mind that some of the drugs used to treat ADHD are identical to speed, used by recreational drug users in search of a high, and that kids can (and do) sell their Ritalin for a pretty penny in the schoolyard.

What are the long-term effects of drugging children with medicines that alter their neurotransmitter activities, carry very real potential for addiction, and overstimulate their brains? No one knows. And where did this disease come from, anyhow? Why had barely anyone heard of it 20 years ago, and why is it suddenly affecting 12 percent of American boys between the ages of 6 and 18?

Here's how it happened. In 1980, a group of psychiatrists sat down together at the American Psychiatric Convention and brainstormed a list of 18 common behavior problems seen in children, including inattention and "hyperactivity-impulsivity." They decreed that a child who had six of the problems on their list would, from that point forward, be diagnosed with attention deficit disorder. In 1987, "hyperactivity" was added to this so-called disease's name. Once the disease had a name and the diagnosis frenzy began, parents felt reassured that their children's problems had a name and a definition. And, of course, the drug companies had a new market.

Psychiatry has made a big deal out of ADHD, anxiety, and depression being caused by some sort of "biochemical imbalance" in the brain. This theory proposes to explain why neurotransmitter-tweaking drugs can control symptoms—because they "correct" this so-called imbalance. *This has not been proven.* There is no scientific proof that any biochemical imbalance is behind any psychiatric disorder. There is no proof that the brains of people who are distractible, inattentive, or hyperactive are any different from those of people who are naturally focused and grounded.

Any study that claims to show these differences can be easily refuted.

For example, a series of brain scan studies conveyed that the portion of the brain that controls ADHD symptoms is smaller in people with ADHD than that of non-ADHD people . . . but in truth, all the ADHD patients in the study had been on Ritalin for an extended period. Extended use of stimulant drugs has been shown to actually cause shrinkage of parts of the brain! In various studies, scientists have found relationships between the activity of the neurotransmitters serotonin, dopamine, and norepinephrine and behavior problems in children—but none of these studies has indicated whether these neurotransmitter levels are a cause or an effect of those behavior problems. One study found that giving Ritalin to non-ADHD adults increased dopamine levels in their brains, which made boring math tasks feel interesting and increased their motivation to perform these tasks. This is used to support the biochemical imbalance theory: because the drug calms and focuses people by raising dopamine levels, that means ADHD people must not have enough circulating dopamine in their brains. This theory has never been proven or even vaguely supported by strong scientific research.

Any diagnosis of ADHD is a subjective venture. Behaviors that to one person seem out of the ordinary in terms of attention deficit or hyperactivity may seem par for the course to another. In one telling study from McLean University, some teachers rated none of around 1,000 kids as having ADHD, while other teachers saw the potential for the disorder in almost every boy in the group. Martin Teicher, director of McLean Hospital's Developmental Biopsychiatry Research Program, told *The New York Times*'s Tara Parker-Pope that "teachers differ significantly in their sensitivity and tolerance

for certain behaviors." So do parents, and so do doctors.

We don't deny that some children and adults have big, life-altering problems with inattention, hyperactivity, impulsivity, and difficulty completing tasks. But these problems are too often diagnosed as a disease state and medicated. Although other nations are getting more keen on diagnosing and medicating children for ADHD, the United States uses by far the lion's share of the world's ADHD drugs and has by far the most diagnoses of this disorder. Is there something wrong with our brains that doesn't affect people elsewhere—or is this another example of America's tendency to turn to the wonders of pharmaceuticals to solve its problems?

Too little exercise, too much sugar and junk food, inadequate healthy food, too little sleep, and too much TV, video, and computer game time could make even the most levelheaded kid into a problem case who seems to require drugs to achieve calm self-control. Throw in exposure to toxins such as pesticides, plastics, and formaldehyde, as well as exposure to potential allergens such as air fresheners, scented laundry detergents, fabric softeners, and cheap perfumes, and you have a recipe for brain dysfunction in children.

Harvard School of Public Health researcher Philippe Grandjean, M.D., has collaborated for decades with Philip Landrigan, M.D., of New York's Mount Sinai School of Medicine to investigate the possible impact of industrial contaminants on child brain development. It's widely accepted that lead, mercury, arsenic, PCBs, and toluene can damage a child's developing nervous system, but Grandjean and Landrigan have identified a total of 202 industrial chemicals that scientific evidence indicates could be contributing to ADHD, autism, and other brain disorders in children. Half of those are commonly used today and are dramatically underinvestigated in terms of their potential harmfulness to developing brains. In their paper, Grandjean and Landrigan point out that, in the past, years—sometimes, decades—passed between the time that a neurodevelopmental threat was recognized and the time that threat's use was appropriately regulated (e.g., lead was not removed from paint or gasoline until the late 1970s and early 1980s, nearly a century after its link to childhood illness had been established). These scientists, who have long researched the neurotoxic effects of lead and mercury, don't want to see the same mistakes made with other neurotoxins. This topic is a tough one because so many children may have already been affected, perhaps irreversibly, perhaps subtly, perhaps profoundly. But we owe it to them and to their children to do all we can to reduce the toxic burden on our most vulnerable citizens: babies and children. We also owe it to them to avoid adding to their chemical burden by dosing them up on psychotropic medications with uncertain benefit and frightening risks.

Making bad behavior into a disease state and medicating it may seem like a viable alternative, but that's a road that leads only to dead ends. When we change brain function, personality, and behavior with drugs, we are not fixing anything. As soon as people with ADHD "symptoms" stop using the drugs, those symptoms return. This is not because they have an incurable disease, but because they didn't have a disease to begin with.

Drugs for Attention Deficit/ Hyperactivity Disorder

Because these drugs are used most often to treat children, we have addressed parents who are considering giving them to a child to treat ADHD. If you are considering ADHD medications for yourself, the precautions, warnings, drug interactions, and side-effect information on the medicines in this chapter apply to adults as well.

Methylphenidate HCl (Ritalin, Concerta, Methylin, Metadate CD)
Dexmethylphenidate (Focalin, Focalin XR)

What Does It Do in the Body? Drugs in this class have a mild stimulant action on the central nervous system. These drugs are thought to work much like the amphetamines, but their mechanism of action is not fully understood. In the dosages used to treat ADHD, these drugs have what's known as a paradoxical effect—calming rather than stimulating. Dexmethylphenidate is billed as a "rapid onset" version of methylphenidate, but in terms of its effects and side effects, it is very similar to methylphenidate, with some evidence that Focalin is more effective. In the rest of this section, both methylphenidate and dexmethylphenidate are referred to by the generic name, methylphenidate.

What Is It Used For? Treatment of ADHD and narcolepsy. It has also been used off-label to treat depression in the elderly, for brain injury, HIV infection, and anesthesia-related hiccups, and to treat people recovering from strokes.

What Are the Potential Side Effects? Blood pressure and pulse changes (increased and decreased), rapid heartbeat, angina, irregular heartbeat, palpitations, dizziness, headache, inability to sit still, drowsiness, Tourette's syndrome (see sidebar "Tourette's Syndrome"), growth suppression, toxic psychosis, anorexia, nausea, abdominal pain, weight loss (during prolonged therapy), hypersensitivity reactions (skin rash, itching, pain, dermatitis), rebound hyperactivity, nervousness, insomnia, abdominal pain, hallucinations, aggressive behaviors, and vision disturbances. May mask symptoms of fatigue, impair physical

Beware Adult ADHD Self-Tests

In one ad from a drug company that makes ADHD medications, there was a series of photographs of an attractive, dark-haired woman sitting in her office, adopting various poses of distractedness and worry. Over her picture appear words like DISTRACTED? FRUSTRATED? DISORGA- NIZED? Below that, there's a black box, over which is written: "Modern Life or Adult ADD?" Then there's text with a heading, "Take the Attached Test and Talk With Your Doctor."

The test was adapted from the Adult Self- Report Scale from the World Health Organization (WHO) Composite International Diagnostic Inter- view, which in its entirety contains 18 questions. Here, there are 6 questions (perhaps the drug company figured that a person with adult ADHD wouldn't be able to manage all 18 questions), along these lines:

"How often do you have trouble wrapping up the final details of a project, once the challenging parts have been done?"

"How often do you have problems remembering appointments or obligations?"

"How often do you fidget or squirm with your hands or feet when you have to sit down for a long time?"

The reader evaluates him- or herself on each question in one of five categories: *Never, Rarely, Sometimes, Often,* or *Very Often.* Four or more checkmarks in the range of *Sometimes* to *Very Often,* says the ad, "indicate that your symptoms may be consistent with adult ADD," and it recom- mends that you "give the completed questionnaire to your health care professional during your next appointment to discuss the results."

This is clearly an example of a disease being created out of thin air to create a market for a drug. Putting this kind of "diagnostic quiz" in a magazine is a great tactic for selling prescriptions directly to consumers. We love to attribute our problems in life to a disease and then get a drug to fix it all. But as many people are beginning to recognize, this is only a short-term solution, and it doesn't—in the end—improve anyone's situation other than to increase pharmaceutical company profit margins.

---

coordination, or produce dizziness or drowsiness severe enough to impair driving ability.

CAUTION!

Don't Give This Drug to Your Child If . . .

- He or she has a seizure disorder.
- He or she has hypertension.
- He or she is severely depressed.
- He or she seems chronically tired.
- He or she shows signs of psychosis or bipo- lar disorder (these drugs can make these conditions worse).

- He or she is less than 6 years of age.
- His or her symptoms are due to acute stress. The drug can make symptoms worse if this is the case.
- His or her symptoms include agitation or aggression. These symptoms can also be made worse with Ritalin and other stimulants.
- He or she is vulnerable to addiction or drug abuse.

The drug should be discontinued in children who do not appear to be growing normally.

Tourette's Syndrome

Many people think that Tourette's is a disorder that leads to uncontrollable shouting and cursing, but this is only one aspect of the disorder, and a rare one at that. People with Tourette's may suffer from mild tics, including repetitive humming or growling in the throat, sniffing, head jerking, grimacing, or blinking. It can also involve seemingly odd behaviors, such as needing to touch things with both hands to "even things out," or other habits that bear some similarity to obsessive-compulsive disorder. Sufferers can temporarily suppress tics, but they eventually have to be released, and many people with Tourette's try to hold back and then find private places where they can release tics.

Tourette's can range in severity from almost unnoticeable to almost debilitating. There is no reliable treatment; some doctors will prescribe SSRIs, but risking further damage to a child's neurotransmitter system is not a good solution. In about a third of children who develop Tourette's, symptoms fade on their own by adulthood.

Giving children methylphenidate, dexmethylphenidate, or amphetamines can cause Tourette's syndrome. Risk is especially high in children with relatives who have Tourette's. If you are considering giving these drugs to your child, consider how you will feel if the result is an incurable, socially disabling tic disorder that may never go away.

What Are the Interactions with Other Drugs? Methylphenidate can increase the effects or prolong the action of the following drugs:

Anticonvulsants (phenytoin, phenobarbitol, primidone)
Selective serotonin reuptake inhibitors (SSRIs)
Tricyclic antidepressants

Methylphenidate can decrease the effects of the following drugs:

Guanethidine and other drugs used to lower blood pressure
Antiseizure medications (phenobarbital, phenytoin, primidone)

Monoamine oxidase inhibitors (MAOIs) can increase the effects or prolong the action of methylphenidate.

Clonidine, a drug sometimes given to help children sleep when coming off of stimulant drugs for ADHD, can interact negatively with stimulants.

What Are the Interactions with Food? It is recommended that methylphenidate be taken 30 to 45 minutes before meals, with the last dose of the day taken before 6 P.M. to avoid insomnia. Extended-release versions are taken less often and early in the day.

With this class of medications—the stimulant drugs—the worst side effect may turn out to be the drug's actual "therapeutic" effects on the brain. According to a 1999 article in the *International Journal of Risk and Safety in Medicine* by psychiatrist Peter Breggin, M.D., arguably the world's foremost expert on the dangers of psychiatric drugs, the millions of North American children who are diagnosed with ADHD and treated with stimulant drugs (including Ritalin, Adderall, and Cylert) are subjected to "a continuum of central nervous system toxicity that begins with increased energy, hyper-alertness, and over-focusing on rote activities" and that may progress

. . . toward obsessive-compulsive or perseverance activities, insomnia, agitation, hypomania, mania, and sometimes seizures . . . They also commonly result in apathy, social withdrawal,

Heart Hazards and Hallucinations with Stimulant Drugs

Manufacturers of stimulant ADHD drugs have been instructed to add patient warnings about increased risks of psychiatric symptoms (hallucinations, delusions, manic or aggressive behavior) and cardiovascular problems in people who previously had not experienced any of these kinds of problems.

Between 1992 and February 2005, 27 patients 18 and younger who were on stimulant drugs for ADHD (including methylphenidate and amphetamines) suffered sudden death related to heart problems. About half of these kids were found to have underlying cardiovascular defects or ailments. It has long been well-understood that these medications increase blood pressure.

This evidence of serious cardiovascular risk has led to a call for more intensive evaluation of any patient who is considering taking these drugs, and more focused, ongoing follow-up with a physician for those who are already using them. Like two other related stimulants—phenylpropanolamine (PPA) and ephedra—methylphenidate and amphetamines have been linked to cases of heart damage that are sometimes fatal. PPA and ephedra have been banned, however; so far, there's no sign of this happening with ADHD drugs. At this writing, clinicians are considering giving heart function tests to any child who seems to merit a prescription for a stimulant medication.

An FDA advisory board recently heard from hundreds of parents about children on stimulant drugs who had terrifying visual and tactile hallucinations, often involving bugs and snakes. These hallucinations were both visual and tactile, meaning that the children both saw and felt these critters. Hallucinations stopped when the drug was stopped and began again when the meds were started again. Drugmakers fearing more requirements for labeling changes and warnings to the public suggested that their meds were not to blame for this rare but significant problem, but that the drug "brought out" underlying psychiatric problems that "emerged when their ADHD was brought under control." The FDA panel nixed this idea and insisted that labeling inserts for stimulant ADHD drugs Adderall, Focalin, Concerta, Metadate, Methylin, Ritalin, and Dexedrine mention the potential for hallucinations and aggressive behaviors in users who have never had them before and who are on the standard dosage of the medication. The drugs' makers have also added risk of heart attack, stroke, or sudden death in people with undiagnosed heart problems to their package inserts.

emotional depression, and docility. Psychostimulants also cause physical withdrawal, including rebounding and dependence. They inhibit growth, and produce various cerebral dysfunctions, some of which can become irreversible.

Breggin tells us that any

... "therapeutic" effects of stimulants are a direct expression of their toxicity. Animal and human research indicates that these drugs often suppress spontaneous and social behaviors while promoting obsessive-compulsive behaviors. These adverse drug effects make the psychostimulants seemingly useful for controlling the behavior of children, especially in highly structured environments that do not attend to their genuine needs.

Studies on rats strongly suggest that Ritalin and drugs like it could permanently alter the brain for the worse. One of the studies came from the lab of McLean Hospital in Belmont, Massachusetts, which is part of the medical school of Harvard University; the other came from the University of Texas–Southwestern. Both studies administered either Ritalin or a placebo to young rats, in doses equivalent to those that would be given to a child with ADHD. After stopping the treatment, the rats—now all grown up—were given a series of tests used to measure depression and despair. Rats exposed to Ritalin showed less interest in sugar water and sexual activity in comparison with rats who got the placebo. In a test where rats are dropped into a tank full of water to see how long they swim before giving up, the Ritalin rats gave up a full two minutes sooner than the placebo rats.

Here's an interesting snag: the rats were also given the option of consuming cocaine. Normally, rats love the stuff, but the Ritalin rats were much less interested in it than their placebo-using counterparts. This suggests that studies showing decreased risk of cocaine abuse in kids who used Ritalin may be on the mark—not because the kids who used Ritalin were happier and better adjusted because of the use of the drug, as the drug's makers might like you to believe, but because the brain pathways that are involved in pleasure (including the pleasure experienced with cocaine use) may have been permanently affected adversely by the stimulant drug.

Examples of Amphetamines

Amphetamine sulfate

Dextroamphetamine sulfate (Dexedrine, Dextrostat)

Methamphetamine HCl, also known generically as desoxyephedrine HCl (Desoxyn)

Dextroamphetamine plus amphetamine (Adderall, Adderall XR)

Lisdexamfetamine dimesylate (Vyvanse)

What Do They Do in the Body? Stimulate the central nervous system by causing the release of the neurotransmitter norepinephrine. At higher doses, the neurotransmitter dopamine is also released.

What Are They Prescribed For? Treatment of ADHD, narcolepsy, and obesity.

What Are the Potential Side Effects? Palpitations, rapid heartbeat, high blood pressure, decrease in heart rate, heart rate irregularities, overstimulation, restlessness, dizziness, insomnia, irritability, inability to sit still, euphoria, dysphoria (mild depression), tremor, headache, changes in libido, psychotic episodes, Tourette's syndrome, aggravation of pre-existing motor and vocal tics, dry mouth, unpleasant taste, diarrhea, constipation, anorexia, weight loss, elevations in serum thyroid hormone levels, itching, and impotence.

Children given stimulants have been found to have temporary slowing of growth rate—on average, they are 2 centimeters shorter and 6 pounds lighter than their same-age peers after three years of taking the drugs—but they catch up once they stop taking it.

Amphetamines can cause a significant increase in blood levels of corticosteroid hormones—"stress" hormones. For more on the hazards of this situation, refer to Chapter 19.

CAUTION!

Don't Give Your Child These Drugs If . . .

- He or she is vulnerable to drug addiction or abuse.
- He or she has a family history of Tourette's-like symptoms.

- He or she has symptoms of psychosis, mania, aggression, or bipolar illness.
- He or she is younger than 3 years of age.
- He or she is hypertensive.
- He or she is sensitive to tartrazine.

Adults with hypertension, heart disease, or glaucoma should not take stimulant drugs.

Atomoxetine (Strattera)

What Does It Do in the Body? It affects the action of the neurotransmitter dopamine in the brain.

What Is It Prescribed For? Treatment of ADHD.

What Are the Potential Side Effects? Abdominal pain, vomiting, nausea, fatigue, irritability, decreased weight, decreased appetite, anorexia, headache, sleepiness, dizziness, rash, mood swings, heart palpitations, dry mouth, constipation, insomnia. In adults, the following side effects have been found: urinary hesitation or retention, erectile dysfunction, priapism (an erection lasting four or more hours), irregular periods, sweating, and hot flashes.

CAUTION!

Don't Give Your Child This Drug If . . .

- He or she takes MAOIs or has taken them within the last two weeks.
- He or she has symptoms of psychosis, mania, aggression, or bipolar illness.

Adults with narrow-angle glaucoma should not use atomoxetine.

Sudden cardiac death has occurred in children and adults taking atomoxetine; it increases heart rate and blood pressure significantly. It should not be taken by anyone with high blood pressure, a heart condition, or atherosclerosis.

This drug has rarely been linked to suicidal thinking and suicide attempts in children. Parents are warned to look for side effects like akathisia (restlessness), agitation, anxiety, panic, insomnia, irritability, hostility, aggressiveness, impulsivity, and mania, and to use these as cautionary signs that the child may become suicidal or violent.

This drug is also linked to liver injury that, rarely, has been fatal. Itching, jaundice (yellowing of eyes and skin), dark urine, upper right abdominal tenderness, and flulike symptoms all suggest that this drug is causing damage to the liver.

Natural Alternatives for ADHD

Having a child with symptoms of ADHD can be extremely trying. Such children can be impossible to handle at times, and they can disrupt classrooms and family life with equal zest. In more extreme cases, ADHD kids may have impulsively violent tendencies that cause them to hurt others. It's understandable that teachers and parents grow desperate to control the wayward behaviors of such children in the hopes that they can weed out the bad and allow the good that they know is inside the child to come through. Please don't imagine that we are minimizing the hardships that come with ADHD when we caution against the drugs used to treat it.

Natural alternatives to these drugs can be time-consuming and trying. They can involve a good amount of trial and effort on the part of parents. By pointing out the dangers of ADHD drugs, we hope to make the point that the effort is worth it.

Commonsense Approaches

If you're a baby boomer, you likely recall kids who were "impulsive," "hyperactive," or "inattentive" from your own childhood. Perhaps you were one yourself. We remember how those kids were dealt with, and it certainly wasn't with drugs. It was with discipline. Many of today's schools are trapped in an environment of overwhelming political correctness, and educators and caregivers are unwilling to risk doing anything that could be even remotely construed as abusive to a child. Many schools of thought on teaching and parenting focus more on improving a child's self-esteem than on building the internal framework that enables that child to be disciplined and well behaved. The disease's classification information points out that ADHD disappears when a child is "under very strict control, is in a novel setting, is engaged in especially interesting activities, [or] is in a one-to-one situation."

This is not a book on parenting or teaching, and we are not claiming to be experts on either topic. This is a book about alternatives to prescription drugs. If stronger discipline is a viable alternative to the increase in the use of psychotropic drugs in children, it's certainly worth mentioning.

When a child seems to have problems behaving, focusing, or sitting still, the first thing to look at is the child's overall situation. Kids who are stressed by problems at home or with peers, difficulty sleeping, or health problems may exhibit symptoms consistent with an ADHD diagnosis. Peter Breggin, M.D., the expert mentioned earlier and author of several excellent books on the dangers of psychiatric drugs, has found that many children with ADHD symptoms would be more appropriately diagnosed with "DADD," or "Dad Attention Deficit Disorder," caused by lack of adequate attention from fathers or other male role models. Counseling for the child and parenting education for parents hold far better hope for an ADHD cure than any pharmaceutical.

If problems seem most pronounced in school, you may want to consider exploring other educational options where your child can have more one-on-one attention and can work in a way that interests him or her more. Most kids with ADHD are very bright and get bored easily in school (the tests used to diagnose ADHD and those used to gauge which children are gifted and talented are remarkably similar), and some do better with alternative approaches that allow them to be more physically active and have more engagement with teachers and other adults.

If all else fails and a child seems out of control, try exercise. Set up a specific space or course for him to go to when he feels he can't sit still, focus, or control himself. You might try a punching bag, a mini trampoline, or a course where he can run laps to release his extra energy.

Diet

Researchers on the Isle of Wight in Great Britain performed a study involving 1,873 3-year-old children. First, they were all screened for the presence of hyperactivity and of atopy (eczema)—both conditions that have been linked with consumption of additives, colorings, and preservatives in children. The children then had a week's complete elimination of artificial colorings and benzoate preservatives. Over the next three weeks, they were given drinks containing these ingredients or placebo drinks.

Parents of these children reported a significant decrease in hyperactive behaviors in the weeklong elimination period, and significant increase in those behaviors when the children were challenged with the colorings and preservatives. The children's behavior worsened when they consumed artificial colorings and benzoate preservatives—whether they had been classified as hyperactive or not.

Abundant research aside from this study points to a diet-ADHD link. Clearly, the typical American child's diet, consisting mostly of processed foods, white flour, dairy, and sugars, is nutritionally inadequate.

The more organic whole foods you can coax your children to eat, the better. Giving them a high-quality multivitamin is a must whether they have ADHD or not. (One great way to get children interested in whole foods is to grow a vegetable garden together!) For parents who don't know where to start cooking with whole foods for their families, we highly recommend *Feeding the Whole Family* by Cynthia Lair and Peggy O'Mara (Sasquatch Books, 2008) and *The Art of Simple Food: Notes, Lessons, and Recipes from a Delicious Revolution* by Alice Waters (Clarkson Potter, 2007).

Make sure a child with ADHD eats adequate protein. A diet composed mostly of sugars and refined flour along with some fruit now and then is enough to make anyone behave badly. Don't send children to school on a bowl of sugary cereal with skim milk; try slow-cooked high-protein oatmeal with fruit and yogurt, or try whole-grain toast with butter and cottage cheese or eggs. Or try unconventional foods such as turkey burgers, chicken, fish, or tofu at breakfast. Organic cheeses, nut butters, and toasted, lightly seasoned pumpkin or sunflower seeds are good lunchbox additions to keep protein intake steady throughout the day.

Other recent research has found that children who have been diagnosed with ADHD are far more likely to have inflammation in the gastrointestinal tract. This inflammation, similar to Crohn's disease (an autoimmune disorder), has also been found with greater frequency in children with autism. Gut inflammation can lead to increased gut permeability, meaning that the small-intestinal wall contains "holes" that allow food particles to move into the circulation, in turn causing an immune response that creates a state of low-grade inflammation throughout the body. This is the scenario for food allergy, also a common finding in children with ADHD.

In one study published in the *European Journal of Pediatrics*, changes in electroencephalogram (EEG) activity—a measurement of electrical activity in the brain—were seen in children with food-induced ADHD when they ate the foods known to provoke their symptoms.

The only reliable way to identify foods to which a child is sensitive is to put the child on an elimination diet. Elimination diets are hard enough for adults, and with children they can be downright frustrating. But consider that many studies have found that a significant proportion of children with ADHD show dramatic improvement when food allergens are removed from their diets. Additives, preservatives, artificial colorings, and artificial flavorings may also exacerbate ADHD symptoms—yet another reason to banish foods that contain them from your family's life. If you need help with an elimination diet for your child, refer to the work of Dr. Benjamin Feingold, the first scientist to assert that artificial colorings, flavorings, and preservatives were directly related to hyperactivity, learning disorder, and behavior or conduct disorders in children. For those who are trying to eliminate food allergens from their finicky child's diet but can't imagine what they might cook, check out *The Allergy Self-Help Cookbook* by Marjorie Hurt Jones (Rodale, 2001). You can find a lot of Feingold-friendly recipes online.

For further information, check out *Is This Your Child? Discovering and Treating Unrecognized Allergies in Children and Adults* by Doris Rapp (William Morrow & Co., 1992). Dr. Feingold has also written a classic book on this subject, which also includes recipes, entitled *Why Your Child Is Hyperactive* (Random House, 1985).

Nutritional Supplements

Several studies have found that even slight improvements in nutrient intake with low-dose multivitamins have the effect of improving concentration and academic performance, as well as reducing the incidence of antisocial and violent behavior in children.

The overuse of antibiotics in children fosters an imbalanced environment in their bodies where probiotic bacteria are depleted and never get a chance to replenish themselves. Increased gut permeability, the precursor to food allergy, can be made worse by yeast overgrowth. Children with ADHD may benefit from the regular use of a probiotic supplement to counteract the growth of yeasts. If your child is too young to swallow a pill, buy a powdered form to mix into juice or milk, or try acidophilus milk or kefir, which are available in health food stores.

Studies have shown that ADHD children tend to have low levels of the essential fat DHA. Supplementing diets of kids with ADHD with fish oil high in DHA may help even them out and foster better concentration and impulse con-

trol. Chewable children's DHA supplements are widely available; follow the dosage instructions on the container.

Supplementation with specific amino acids, the building blocks of protein, have been found to help some ADHD kids. If you'd like to try this approach, do so with the guidance of a nutritionist or alternative health practitioner.

A significant percentage of children with ADHD have low zinc levels. A good multivitamin should remedy the problem.

Parent Education and Behavioral Approaches

Any parent who seeks nondrug alternatives for ADHD will find many solutions and an active, highly engaged group of like-minded parents. As the risks of stimulants, Strattera, and other psychiatric medications become increasingly evident, more parents are "just saying no" to pharmaceutically leashing their children. They are learning new ways to parent their intense children, and teachers are learning new ways to manage classrooms that almost always contain at least one such child.

Current research shows that counseling and small adjustments in parenting style can make an enormous difference for children who might otherwise be out of control. One of the most promising nondrug interventions was created by psychologist Howard Glasser, who has developed a parenting and teaching technique he calls the Nurtured Heart Approach, a method where parents or teachers focus on the child's positive behaviors and give little energy to negative behaviors. Glasser believes that difficult children feed on the energy they receive from negative attention, and that if we give positive behavior that kind of energy and all but ignore the negatives, we can help that child to behave better without robbing them of their intensity or feeding them pills. This approach is being used in homes, schools, counseling practices, even whole schools and school systems, with huge success. His books, all published by Nurtured Heart Publications, include *Transforming the Difficult Child* (1999), *The Inner Wealth Initiative: The Nurtured Heart Approach for Educators* (2007), and *All Children Flourishing: Igniting the Greatness of Our Children* (2008).

RESOURCES AND RECOMMENDED READING

Hormone Testing

Virginia Hopkins Test Kits
(888) 438-1211
www.virginiahopkinstestkits.com

Vitamin D Testing

If you get a vitamin D test from your doctor, ask for the 25(OH) D test. You can also get a vitamin D test online that measures both vitamin D_2 and D_3 in the OH form at www.virginia hopkinstestkits.com.

Online Prescription Drug Information

Drugs.com
www.drugs.com

Drug Digest
www.drugdigest.org

FDA Index to Drug-Specific Information
www.fda.gov/cder/drug/DrugSafety/
    DrugIndex.htm

Rx List
www.rxlist.com

Online Medical Dictionaries

Medline—National Library of Medicine
www.nlm.nih.gov/medlineplus/mplus
    dictionary.html

Medicine.net
www.medterms.com

Finding a Health Care Professional Who Uses Natural Remedies

Two places to ask for a recommendation for a health care professional who uses natural remedies are your local health food store and your local compounding pharmacy. You can also write or call:

American College for Advancement
    in Medicine
P.O. Box 3427
Laguna Hills, CA 92654
(800) 532-3688
In California: (714) 583-7666

Reporting an Adverse Drug Reaction to the FDA

You can report adverse events to the FDA through their MedWatch Online Voluntary Reporting Form:

https://www.accessdata.fda.gov/scripts/med
   watch/medwatch-online.htm.

If you prefer not to make the report online, you can download and print a form at http://www .fda.gov/medwatch/getforms.htm and either mail or fax the completed 3500 Form and your attachments to:

5600 Fishers Lane
Rockville, MD 20852-9787
(800) FDA-0178 to MedWatch (fax)
(800) FDA-1088 (phone: be prepared to talk to recordings and to wait endlessly on hold)

Newsletters

Virginia Hopkins Health Watch
(888) 438-1211
www.virginiahopkinshealthwatch.com

Alternatives: Dr. David Williams
www.drdavidwilliams.com/MainSite/
   Newsletter.aspx
(888) 887-8262

Dr. Julian Whitaker's Health & Healing
www.drwhitaker.com/MainSite/Newsletter.aspx
800-219-8590

Websites and Contact Numbers

The Virginia Hopkins Health Watch
Natural Hormone & Nutrition News, Drug
   Watch and More . . .

(888) 438-1211
www.virginiahopkinstestkits.com

Harvard Health Publications
Harvard Medical School: Trusted Advice for a
   Healthier Life
www.health.harvard.edu

National Clearinghouse for Alcohol and Drug
   Abuse Information
(800) 729-6686

Narcotics Anonymous
(818) 780-3951
For referrals to local meetings, call
(212) 870-3400

People's Pharmacy with Joe and Terry Graedon
Home remedies, drug references, herb library,
   and more . . .
www.peoplespharmacy.com

Worst Pills, Best Pills
Your expert, independent second opinion for
   prescription drug information.
www.worstpills.org

Recommended Reading

Alternative Medicine

Bland, Jeffrey, Ph.D. *The 20-Day Rejuvenation Diet Program*. New Canaan, CT: Keats Publishing, 1997.
Bland, John H., M.D. *Live Long, Die Fast*. Minneapolis, MN: Fairview Press, 1997.
Galland, Leo, M.D. *The Four Pillars of Healing*. New York, NY: Random House, 1997.
Glenmullen, Joseph, M.D. *Prozac Backlash: Overcoming the Dangers of Prozac, Zoloft, Paxil, and Other Antidepressants with Safe,*

Effective Alternatives. New York, NY: Simon & Schuster, 2000.

Mindell, Earl, R.Ph., and Virginia Hopkins. *What You Should Know About: Herbs, Supplements, Trace Minerals and Homeopathic Remedies.* New Canaan, CT: Keats Publishing, 1995.

Pizzorno, Joseph N. *Total Wellness.* Berkeley, CA: Prima Publishing, 1996.

Smolensky, Michael, and Lynne Lamberg. *The Body Clock Guide to Better Health.* Owl Books, 2001.

Food

Blaylock, Russell. *Excitotoxins: The Taste That Kills.* Santa Fe, NM: Health Press, 1994.

DeVille, Nancy. *Death by Supermarket: The Fattening, Dumbing Down and Poisoning of America.* Fort Lee, NJ: Barricade, 2007.

Fallon, Sally. *Nourishing Traditions.* San Diego, CA: ProMotion Publishing, 1995.

Robbins, John. *Reclaiming Our Health.* Tiburon, CA: HJ Kramer, 1996.

Sears, Barry. *The Omega Rx Zone: The Miracle of the New High-Dose Fish Oil.* New York, NY: ReganBooks, 2002.

———. *The Zone.* New York, NY: HarperCollins, 1996.

Steinman, David. *Diet for a Poisoned Planet: How to Choose Safe Foods for You and Your Family—the Twenty-First Century Edition.* New York, NY: Running Press, 2006.

Stoll, Andrew L., M.D. *The Omega-3 Connection.* New York, NY: Simon & Schuster, 2001.

Todd, Gary Price, M.D. *Nutrition, Health, and Disease.* West Chester, PA: Whitford Press, 1985.

Hormones

Arem, Ridha, M.D. *The Thyroid Solution.* New York, NY: Ballantine Books, 1999.

Barnes, Broda. *Hypothyroidism: The Unsuspected Illness.* New York, NY: Harper and Row, 1976.

Colborn, Theo. *Our Stolen Future.* New York, NY: Penguin Books, 1997.

Crook, William, M.D. *The Yeast Connection: A Medical Breakthrough.* Jackson, TN: Professional Books, 1991.

Khalsa, Dharma Singh, M.D. *Brain Longevity.* New York, NY: Warner Books, 1997.

Klatz, Ronald, and Robert Goldman. *Stopping the Clock.* New York, NY: Bantam Books, 1996.

Lee, John R., M.D. *Hormone Balance for Men: What Your Doctor May Not Tell You About Prostate Health and Natural Hormone Supplementation.* Available online at virginiahopkinstestkits.com.

Lee, John R., M.D., and Virginia Hopkins. *Dr. John Lee's Hormone Balance Made Simple.* New York, NY: Hachette Books, 2006.

———. *What Your Doctor May Not Tell You About Menopause: The Breakthrough Book on Natural Progesterone.* New York, NY: Warner Books, 1996.

Lee, John R., M.D., Jesse Hanley, M.D., and Virginia Hopkins. *What Your Doctor May Not Tell You About Premenopause: Balance Your Hormones and Your Life From Thirty to Fifty.* New York, NY: Warner Books, 1999.

Lee, John R., M.D., David Zava, Ph.D., and Virginia Hopkins. *What Your Doctor May Not Tell You About Breast Cancer: How Hormone Balance Can Help Save Your Life.* New York, NY: Warner Books, 2002.

Randolph, C.W., M.D., and James Genie. *From Belly Fat to Belly Flat: How Your Hormones Are Adding Inches to Your Waistline and Subtracting Years from Your Life*. Deerfield Beach, FL: Health Communications Inc, 2008.

Sahelian, Ray. *DHEA: A Practical Guide*. Garden City Park, NY: Avery Publishing, 1996.

———. *Melatonin: Nature's Sleeping Pill*. Garden City Park, NY: Avery Publishing, 1995.

Drugs

Breggin, Peter. *Talking Back to Prozac*. New York, NY: St. Martin's Press, 1994.

Cohen, Suzy, R.Ph. *The 24-Hour Pharmacist: Look Younger, Feel Healthier and Save Time and Money—No Doctor Required!* New York, NY: Collins, 2007.

Gaby, Alan R., M.D. *A-Z Guide to Drug-Herb-Vitamin Interactions Revised and Expanded 2nd Edition: Improve Your Health and Avoid Side Effects When Using Common Medications and Natural Supplements Together*. New York, NY: Three Rivers Press, 2006.

Lappe, Marc. *When Antibiotics Fail: Restoring the Ecology of the Body*. Berkeley, CA: North Atlantic Books, 1995.

Schmidt, Michael, Lendon Smith, M.D., and Keith Sehnert. *Beyond Antibiotics*. Berkeley, CA: North Atlantic Books, 1994.

Wolfe, Sidney M., et al. *Worst Pills, Best Pills: A Consumer's Guide to Avoiding Drug-Induced Death or Illness*. New York, NY: Pocket Books, 2005.

Children

Feingold, Benjamin F., M.D. *Why Your Child Is Hyperactive*. New York, NY: Random House, 1985.

Lappe, Marc. *When Antibiotics Fail: Restoring the Ecology of the Body*. Berkeley, CA: North Atlantic Books, 1995.

Rapp, Doris, M.D. *Is This Your Child? Discovering and Treating Unrecognized Allergies in Children and Adults*. New York, NY: William Morrow & Company, 1992.

Rountree, Robert, M.D. *The New Breastfeeding Diet Plan: Breakthrough Ways to Reduce Toxins and Give Your Baby the Best Start in Life*. New York, NY: McGraw-Hill, 2007.

Schmidt, Michael, Lendon Smith, M.D., and Keith Sehnert. *Beyond Antibiotics*. Berkeley, CA: North Atlantic Books, 1994.

Smith, Lendon, M.D. *How to Raise a Healthy Child*. New York, NY: M. Evans & Co., 1996.

Zand, Janet, O.M.D., Rachel Walton, R.N., and Robert Roundtree, M.D. *A Parent's Guide to Medical Emergencies*. Garden City Park, NY: Avery Publishing, 1997.

Vitamins, Herbs, Supplements

Balch, Phyllis A. *Prescription for Nutritional Healing*, 4th edition. New York, NY: Avery, 2006.

Mindell, Earl, R.Ph. *Earl Mindell's New Herb Bible: A Complete Update of the Bestselling Guide to New and Traditional Herbal Remedies*. New York, NY: Pocket, 2002.

Mindell, Earl, R.Ph., and Hester Mundis. *Earl Mindell's New Vitamin Bible: 25th Anniversary Edition*. New York, NY: Grand Central Publishing, 2004.

Miscellaneous

Baillie-Hamilton, Paula, M.D., Ph.D. *Toxic Overload: A Doctor's Plan for Combating the Illnesses Caused by Chemicals in Our*

Foods, Our Homes, and Our Medicine Cabinets. New York, NY: Avery, 2005.

Brownlee, Shannon. *Overtreated: Why Too Much Medicine Is Making Us Sicker and Poorer*. New York, NY: Bloomsbury, 2007.

Doidge, Norman, M.D. *The Brain That Changes Itself: Stories of Personal Triumph from the Frontiers of Brain Science*. New York, NY: Viking, 2007.

Graedon, Joe, M.S., and Teresa Graedon, Ph.D. *Best Choices from the People's Pharmacy*. New York, NY: NAL Trade, 2008.

Lesser, Micheal, M.D., with Colleen Kapklein. *The Brain Chemistry Plan: Balancing Mood, Relieving Stress, Conquering Depression*. New York, NY: Perigree, 2002.

Moynihan, Ray, and Alan Cassels. *Selling Sickness: How the World's Biggest Pharmaceutical Companies Are Turning Us All Into Patients*. New York, NY: Nation Books, 2005.

REFERENCES

Chapter 1
Changing the Pill-Popping Mind-Set

Alberti, K. G. M. M. "Medical Errors: A Common Problem." *British Medical Journal* 322 (March 3, 2001): 501–2.

Allan, E. L., and K. N. Barker. "Fundamentals of Medication Error Research." *American Journal of Hospital Pharmacy* 47, no. 3 (March 1990): 555–71.

Bates, D. W. "Medication Errors: How Common Are They and What Can Be Done to Prevent Them?" *Drug Safety* 15, no. 5 (November 1996): 303–10.

Brennan, T. A., et al. "Incidence of Adverse Events and Negligence in Hospitalised Patients: Results of the Harvard Medical Practice Study I." *New England Journal of Medicine* 324 (1991): 370–76.

Budnitz, D. S., D. A. Pollock, et al. "National Surveillance of Emergency Department Visits for Outpatient Adverse Drug Events." *Journal of the American Medical Association* 296 (2006): 1858–66.

Classen, D. "Adverse Drug Events in Hospitalized Patients." *Journal of the American Medical Association* 1197, no. 277: 301–6.

Gurwtiz, J. H. , T. S. Field, et al. "Incidence and Preventability of Adverse Drug Events Among Older Persons in the Ambulatory Setting." *Journal of the American Medical Association* 3, no. 289: 1107–16.

Johnson, J., et al. "Drug Related Morbidity and Mortality—a Cost of Illness Model." *Archives Internal Medicine* 155 (October 9, 1996).

Lasser, K. E., et al. "Timing of New Black Box Warnings and Withdrawals for Prescription Medications." *Journal of the American Medical Association* 287, no. 17 (May 2002): 2215–20.

Leape, L. L., et al. "The Nature of Adverse Events in Hospitalised Patients: Results of the Harvard Medical Practice Study II." *New England Journal of Medicine* 324 (1991): 377–84.

Nelson, K., et al. "Drug-Related Hospital Admissions." *Pharmacotherapy* 16, no. 4 (1996): 701–7.

Nissen, S. E., and K. Wolski. "Effect of Rosiglitazone on the Risk of Myocardial Infarction and Death from Cardiovascular Causes." *New England Journal of Medicine* 356 (2007): 2457.

Soumerai, S. B., et al. "Effects of Medicaid Drug-Payment Limits on Admissions to Hospitals and Nursing Homes." *New England Journal of Medicine* 325 (1991): 1072–77.

Sox, H. C., Jr., and S. Woloshin. "How Many Deaths Are Due to Medical Error? Getting the Number Right." *Effective Clinical Practice* 3, no. 6 (November–December 2000): 277–83.

Thomas, E. J., and T. A. Brennan. "Incidence and Types of Preventable Adverse Events in Elderly Patients: Population Based Review of Medical Records." *British Medical Journal* 320 (2000): 741–45.

U.S. Government Accountability Office (2006). "Prescription Drugs: Price Trends for Frequently Used Brand and Generic Drugs from 2000 Through 2004." http://www.gao.gov/new.items/d05779.pdf.

Zoellner, T. "America's Other Drug Problem." *Men's Health* (October 2001): 118–23.

Zwillich, T. "FDA Drug Recalls Jumped in 1990s." *Reuters Health* (September 24, 2002).

Chapter 2
How to Avoid Prescription Drug Abuse

Breggin, P., M.D. "The Hazards of Treating 'Attention Deficit/Hyperactivity Disorder' with Methylphenidate (Ritalin)." *The Journal of College Student Psychotherapy* 10, no. 2 (1995): 55–72.

Office of National Drug Control Policy. "Prescription Drug Abuse Prevention." http://www.whitehousedrugpolicy.gov/drugfact/prescr_drg_abuse.html.

Tanouye, E. "Antidepressant Makers Study Kids' Market." *Wall Street Journal.* April 4, 1997.

U.S. Department of Health and Human Services, SAMHSA Health Information Network Clearinghouse for Alcohol and Drug Information. Prevention Alert: "Trouble in the Medicine Chest (I): Rx Drug Abuse Growing," 6, no. 4 (March 7, 2003).

U.S. National Library of Medicine and National Institutes of Health, "Prescription Drug Abuse." http://www.nlm.nih.gov/medlineplus/prescriptiondrugabuse.html.

Weber, T. "Tarnishing the Golden Years with Addiction." *Los Angeles Times*, December 20, 1996.

Chapter 3
Drug Interactions and How Your Body Processes Drugs

Logsdon, B. A. "Drug Use During Lactation." *Journal of the American Pharmaceutical Association* NS37, no. 4 (July–August 1997).

Merck Manual. Drug Kinetics, "Factors Affecting Response to Drugs." http://www.merck.com/mmhe/sec02/ch013/ch013a.html#sec02-ch013-ch013a-112.

Stachulski, A. V., and J. M. Lennard. "Drug Metabolism: The Body's Defense Against Chemical Attack," *Journal of Chemical Education* 2000 77: 349.

Tschanz, C., et al. "Interactions Between Drugs and Nutrients." *Advances in Pharmacology* 35 (1996).

Chapter 4
How Drugs Interact with Food, Drink, and Supplements

Kirk, J. K. "Significant Drug-Nutrient Interactions." *American Family Doctor* 51, no. 5 (April 1995): 1175–82.

Tschanz, C., et al. "Interactions Between Drugs and Nutrients." *Advances in Pharmacology* 35 (1996).

Chapter 7
Surgery, Drugs, and Nutrition: Minimizing the Damage and Maximizing Your Recovery

Baker, G. R., P. G. Norton, and V. Flintoft. "The Canadian Adverse Events Study: The Incidence of Adverse Events Among Hospital Patients in Canada." *Canadian Medical Association Journal* 170, no. 11 (May 25, 2004), doi:10.1503.

Lowenfels, A. "Adverse Events in the Hospital Setting: How Safe Is Your Operating Room? Review of De Vries EN, Ramrattan MA, Smorenburg SM, et al., *Qual Saf Health Care*." *Medscape Today* 17 (August 27, 2008): 216–23, http://www.medscape.com/viewarticle/578928.

Vincent, C., G. Neale, and M. Woloshynowych. "Adverse Events in British Hospitals: Preliminary Retrospective Record Review." *British Medical Journal* 322 (2001): 517–19.

Weissman, J. S., E. C. Schneider, S. N. Weingart, et al. "Comparing Patient-Reported Hospital Adverse Events with Medical Record Review: Do Patients Know Something That Hospitals Do Not?" *Annals of Internal Medicine*, 149, no. 215 (July 2008): 100–8.

Chapter 9
Six Core Principles for Optimal Health

Antioxidants

Aruoma, O. I., et al. "Nutrition and Health Aspects of Free Radicals and Antioxidants." *Food and Chemical Toxicology* 32, no. 7 (1994): 671–83.

Costanzo, L. L., et al. "Antioxidant Effect of Copper on Photosynthesized Lipid Peroxidation." *Journal of Inorganic Biochemistry* 57 (1995): 115–25.

Fuller, C. J., et al. "Effects of Antioxidants and Fatty Acids on Low-Density-Lipoprotein Oxidation." *American Journal of Clinical Nutrition* 60, supp. (1994): 1010S–3S.

Gaziano, J. M., et al. "Natural Antioxidants and Cardiovascular Disease: Observational Epidemiologic Studies and Randomized Trials." *Natural Antioxidants in Human Health and Disease* 13 (1994): 387–409.

Geoffroy-Perez, B., and S. Cordier. "Fluid Consumption and the Risk of Bladder Cancer: Results of a Multicenter Case-Control Study." *International Journal of Cancer* 93, no. 6 (2001): 880–87.

Gilligan, D. J., M.D., et al. "Effect of Antioxidant Vitamins on Low Density Lipoprotein Oxidation and Impaired Endothelium-Dependent Vasodilation in Patients with Hypercholesterolemia." *Journal of the American College of Cardiology* 24, no. 7 (December 1994): 1611–17.

Haas, E. M. "Cholesterol- and Tumor-Suppressive Actions of Fruits and Vegetables." *The Nutrition Report* 13, no. 4 (April 1995): 17, 24.

Hoffman, R. M., M.D., and H. S. Garewal. "Antioxidants and the Prevention of Coronary Heart Disease." *Archives of Internal Medicine* 155 (February 13, 1995): 241–46.

Kanter, M. M. "Free Radicals, Exercise, and Antioxidant Supplementation." *International Journal of Sports Nutrition* 4 (1994): 205–20.

Lee, S. H., T. Oe, and I. A. Blair. "Vitamin C–Induced Decomposition of Lipid Hydroperoxides to Endogenous Genotoxins." *Science* 292, no. 5524 (June 15, 2001): 2083–86.

Liu, M., et al. "Mixed Tocopherols Have a Stronger Inhibitory Effect on Lipid Per-oxidation Than Alpha-Tocopherol Alone." *Journal of Cardiovascular Pharmacology* 39, no. 51 (May 2002): 714–21.

Oliver, M. F. "Antioxidant Nutrients, Athero-sclerosis, and Coronary Heart Disease." *British Heart Journal* 73 (1995): 299–301.

Rautalahti, M., et al. "Antioxidants and Car-cinogenesis." *Annals of Medicine* 25 (1993): 435–41.

Regling, G., et al. "The Biological Role of Oxygen Radicals, Lipid Peroxidation and Antioxidative Therapy in Connective Tissue Regulation." *Wolff's Law and Connective Tissue Regulation* (1993): 231–41.

Singh, R., et al. "Diet, Antioxidants, Vitamins, Oxidative Stress and Risk of Coronary Artery Disease: The Purzuda Prospective Study." *Acta Cardiology* 49, no. 5 (1995): 453–67.

Stavric, B. "Role of Chemopreventers in Human Diet." *Clinical Biochemistry* 27, no. 5 (1994): 319–32.

Todd, S., et al. "An Investigation of the Rela-tionship Between Antioxidant Vitamin Intake and Coronary Heart Disease in Men and Women Using Logistic Regression Analysis." *Journal of Clinical Epidemiology* 48, no. 2 (1995): 307–16.

Tribble, D. L., Ph.D., et al. "Dietary Antioxi-dants, Cancer, and Atherosclerotic Heart Disease." *Western Journal of Medicine* 161 (1994): 605–13.

Wei, Q., et al. "Vitamin Supplementation and Reduced Risk of Basal Cell Carcinoma." *Journal of Clinical Epidemiology* 47, no. 8 (1994): 829–36.

Yogurt

Burns, A. J., and I. R. Rowland. "Anti-Carcinogenicity of Probiotics and Prebiotics." *Current Issues in Intestinal Microbiology* 1, no. 1 (March 2000): 13–24.

Elner, G. W. "Probiotics: 'Living Drugs.'" *American Journal of Health System Phar-macy: The Official Journal of the American Society of Health System Pharmacists* 58, no. 12 (June 2001): 1101–9.

Massey, L. K. "Dairy Food Consumption, Blood Pressure, and Stroke." *Journal of Nutrition* 131, no. 7 (July 2001): 1875–78.

Meydani, S. N., and W. K. Ha. "Immunologic Effects of Yogurt." *American Journal of Clinical Nutrition* 71, no. 4 (2001): 861–72.

Fish and Fish Oils

Crenson, S. L. "Levels of Mercury Reported Elevated Among Fish Eaters." *Associated Press*, October 20, 2002.

Crenson, S. L., and M. Mendoza. "There's Something Fishy About Mercury Levels." *Associated Press*, October 13, 2002.

Sears, B. *The Omega Rx Zone: The Miracle of the New High-Dose Fish Oil.* New York: ReganBooks, 2002.

Stoll, A. L., M.D. *The Omega-3 Connection.* New York: Simon & Schuster, 2001.

Grapeseed Bioflavonoids

Chang, W. C., et al. "Inhibition of Platelet Aggregation and Arachidonate Metabolism in Platelets by Procyanidins." *Prostaglan-dins, Leukotrienes & Essential Fatty Acids* 38 (1989): 181–88.

Frankel, E. N., et al. "Inhibition of Oxidation of Human Low-Density Lipoprotein by Phenolic Substances in Red Wine." *The Lancet* 341 (1993): 454–57.

Gomez Trillo, J. T. "Varicose Veins of the Lower Extremities: Symptomatic Treatment with a New Vasculotrophic Agent." *La Prensa Medica Mexicana* 38 (1973): 293–96.

Harmand, M. F., et al. "The Fate of Total Flavonolic Oligomers (OFT) Extracted from 'Vitis vinifera L.' in the Rat." *European Journal of Drug Metabolism and Pharmacokinetics* 1 (1978): 15–30.

Henriet, J. P. "Veno-Lymphatic Insufficiency: 4,729 Patients Undergoing Hormonal and Procyanidol Oligomer Therapy." *Phlebolgie* 46 (1993): 313–25.

Hertog, M. G., et al. "Dietary Antioxidant Flavonoids and Risk of Coronary Heart Disease: The Zutphen Elderly Study." *The Lancet* 342 (1993): 1007–11.

Kilham, C., and J. Masquelier. *OPC: The Miracle Antioxidant*. New Canaan, CT: Keats Publishing Company, 1997.

Lagrue, G., et al. "A Study of the Effects of Procyanidol Oligomers on Capillary Resistance in Hypertension and in Certain Nephropathies." *La Semaine des Hospitaux de Paris* (Paris) 57 (1981): 1399–401.

Masquelier, J., et al. "Flavonoids et Pycnogenols." *International Journal of Vitamin and Nutrition Research* (1979): 307–11.

———. "Stabilization of Collagen by Procyanidolic Oligomers." *Acta Therapeutica* 7 (1981): 101–5.

Meunier, M. T., et al. "Inhibition of Angiotensin I Converting Enzyme by Flavenolic Compounds: In Vitro and In Vivo Studies." *Planta Medica* 54 (1987): 12–15.

Schwitters, B., et al. "OPC in Practice: Bioflavanols and Their Application." *Alfa Omega* (Rome), 1993.

Tixier, J. M., et al. "Evidence by In Vivo and In Vitro Studies That Binding of Pycnegols to Elastin Affects Its Rate of Degradation by Elastases." *Biochemical Pharmacology* 3 (1984): 3933–39.

Wegrowski, J., et al. "The Effect of Procyanidolic Oligomers on the Composition of Normal and Hypercholesterolemic Rabbit Aortas." *Biochemical Pharmacology* 33 (1984): 3491–97.

Green Tea Bioflavonoids

Apostolides, Z., et al. "Screening of Tea Clones for Inhibition of PhIP Mutagenicity." *Mutation Research* 326, no. 2 (February 1995): 219–25.

Bu-Abbas, A., et al. "Marked Antimutagenic Potential of Aqueous Green Tea Extracts: Mechanism of Action." *Mutagenesis* 9, no. 4 (July 1994): 325–31.

Burr, M. L., et al. "Antioxidants and Cancer." *Journal of Human Nutrition and Dietetics* 7 (1994): 409–16.

"Foods That May Prevent Breast Cancer: Studies Are Investigating Soybeans, Whole Wheat and Green Tea Among Others." *Primary Care and Cancer* 14, no. 2 (February 1994): 10–11.

Gao, F. M., et al. "Studies on Mechanisms and Blockade of Carcinogenic Action of Female Sex Hormones." *Science in China*, Series B 37, no. 4 (April 1994): 418–29.

Graham, H. N. "Green Tea Composition, Consumption, and Polyphenol Chemistry." *Preventive Medicine* 21, no. 3 (May 1992): 334–50.

Hirose, M., et al. "Inhibition of Mammary Gland Carcinogenesis by Green Tea Catechins and Other Naturally Occurring Antioxidants in Female Sprague-Dawley Rats Pretreated with 7,12-demethylbenz[alpha] anthracene." *Cancer Letters* 83, nos. 1–2 (1994): 149–56.

Ikigai, H., et al. "Bactericidal Catechins Damage the Lipid Biolayer." *Biochimica et Biophysica Acta* 1147, no. 1 (April 8, 1993): 132–36.

Imai, K., et al. "Cross-Sectional Effects of Drinking Tea on Cardiovascular and Liver Diseases." *British Medical Journal* 310, no. 6981 (March 18, 1995): 693–96.

Katiyar, S. K., et al. "Inhibition of Spontaneous and Photo-Enhanced Lipid Peroxidation in Mouse Epidermal Microsomes by Epicatechin Derivatives from Green Tea." *Cancer Letters* 79, no. 1 (April 29, 1994): 61–66.

———. "Protection Against Malignant Conversion of Chemically Induced Benign Skin Papillomas to Squamous Cell Carcinomas in SENCAR Mice by a Polyphenolic Fraction Isolated from Green Tea." *Cancer Research* 53, no. 22 (November 15, 1993): 5409–12.

———. "Protective Effects of Green Tea Polyphenols Administered by Oral Intubation Against Chemical Carcinogen-Induced Forestomach and Pulmonary Neoplasia in A/J Mice." *Cancer Letters* 73, nos. 2–3 (September 30, 1993): 167–72.

Kawaguchi, M., et al. "Three Month Oral Repeated Administration Toxicity Study of Seed Saponins of *Thea Sinensis* L. (Ryokucha Saponin) in Rats." *Food and Chemical Toxicology* 32, no. 5 (May 1994): 431–42.

Kimura, R., et al. "Effect of Theanine on Norepinephrine and Serotonin Levels in Rat Brain." *Chemical and Pharmaceutical Bulletin* 34, no. 7 (July 1986): 3053–57.

Kubo, I., et al. "Antimicrobial Activity of Green Tea Flavor Components and Their Combination Effects." *Journal of Agricultural and Food Chemistry* 40 (1992): 245–48.

Makimura, M., et al. "Inhibitory Effect of Tea Catechins on Collagenase Activity." *Journal of Periodontal Research* 64, no. 7 (July 1993): 630–36.

Mukhtar, H., et al. "Green Tea and Skin-Anticarcinogenic Effects." *The Journal of Investigative Dermatology* 102, no. 1 (January 1994): 3–7.

———. "Green Tea Components: Antimugenic and Anticarcinogenic Effects." *Preventive Medicine* 21, no. 3 (May 1, 1992): 351–60.

Nagata, T., et al. "Differences in Caffeine, Flavonols and Amino Acid Contents in Leaves of Cultivated Species of Camellia." *Japanese Journal of Breeding* 34, no. 4 (1984): 459–67.

Narisawa, T., et al. "A Very Low Dose of Green Tea Polyphenols in Drinking Water Prevents N-methyl-N-nitrosourea-Induced Colon Carcinogenesis in F344 Rats." *Japanese Journal of Cancer Research*, Gann 84, no. 10 (October 1993): 1007–9.

Nishida, H., et al. "Inhibitory Effects of (-)-epigallocatechin Gallate on Spontaneous Hepatoma in C3H/HeNCrj Mice and Human Hepatoma-derived PLC/PRF/5 Cells." *Japanese Journal of Cancer Research*, Gann 85, no. 3 (March 1994): 221–25.

Shetty, M., et al. "Antibacterial Activity of Tea (*Camillia sinensis*) and Coffee (*Coffee arabica*) with Special Reference to *Salmonella typhimurium*." *The Journal of Communicable Diseases* 26, no. 3 (September 1994): 147–50.

Tao, P. "The Inhibitory Effects of Catechin Derivatives on the Activities of Human

Immunodeficiency Virus Reverse Transcriptase and DNA Polymerases." *Chung Kuo I Huo I Hsueh Yuan Hsueh Pao* 14, no. 5 (October 1992): 334–38.

Tsushida, T., et al. "An Enzyme Hydrolyzing L-theanine in Tea Leaves." *Agricultural and Biological Chemistry* 49, no. 10 (1985): 2913–17.

Valstar, E. "Nutrition and Cancer: A Review of Preventive and Therapeutic Abilities of Single Nutrients." *Journal of Nutritional Medicine* 4 (1994): 176–78.

Wang, Z. Y., et al. "Inhibitory Effects of Black Tea, Green Tea, Decaffeinated Black Tea, and Decaffeinated Green Tea on Ultraviolet Light-Induced Skin Carcinogenesis in 7, 12-dimethylbenz[a]anthracene-initiated SKH-1 Mice." *Cancer Research* 54, no. 13 (July 1, 1994): 3428–35.

Weisburger, J. H., et al. "Prevention of Heterocyclic Amine Formation by Tea and Tea Polyphenols." *Cancer Letters* 83, nos. 1–2 (August 15, 1994): 143–47.

Yang, C. S., et al. "Tea and Cancer." *Journal of the National Cancer Institute* 85, no. 13 (July 7, 1993): 1038–49.

Yen, G. C., et al. "Antioxidant Activity of Various Tea Extracts in Relation to Their Antimutagenicity." *Journal of Agricultural and Food Chemistry* 43 (1995): 27–32.

Yin, P., et al. "Experimental Studies of the Inhibitory Effects of Green Tea Catechin on Mice Large Intestinal Cancers Induced by 1, 2-Dimethylhydrazine." *Cancer Letters* 79, no. 1 (April 29, 1994): 33–38.

Yokogoshi, H., et al. "Reduction Effect of Theanine on Blood Pressure and Brain 5-Hydroxyindoles in Spontaneously Hypertensive Rats." *Bioscience, Biotechnology,* and *Biochemistry* 59, no. 4 (April 1995): 615–18.

Yoshino, K., et al. "Antioxidative Effects of Black Tea Theaflavins and Thearubigin on Lipid Peroxidation of Rat Liver Homogenates Induced by Tert-butyl Hydroperoxide." *Biological and Pharmaceutical Bulletin* 17, no. 1 (January 1994): 146–49.

Protein

Dawson-Hughes, B., and S. S. Harris. "Calcium Intake Influences the Association of Protein Intake with Rates of Bone Loss in Elderly Men and Women." *American Journal of Clinical Nutrition* 75, no. 4 (April 2002): 773–79.

Water

Geoffroy-Perez, B., and S. Cordier. "Fluid Consumption and the Risk of Bladder Cancer: Results of a Multicenter Case-Control Study." *International Journal of Cancer* 93, no. 6 (September 15, 2001): 880–87.

Kahn, H. A., et al. "Association Between Reported Diet and All-Cause Mortality: Twenty-One-Year Follow-Up on 27,530 Adult Seventh-Day Adventists." *American Journal of Epidemiology* 119, no. 5 (May 1984): 775–87.

Chapter 10
Drugs for Heart Disease and Their Natural Alternatives

Abbott, L., et al. "Magnesium Deficiency in Alcoholism: Possible Contribution to Osteoporosis and Cardiovascular Disease in Alcoholics." *Alcoholism: Clinical and Experimental Research* 18, no. 5 (September–October 1994): 1076–82.

Albert, C. M., et al. "Prospective Study of C-Reactive Protein, Homocysteine, and Plasma Lipid Levels as Predictors of Sudden Cardiac Death." *Circulation* 105, no. 22 (June 4, 2002): 2595–99.

Alfthan, G., A. Aro, and K. F. Gey. "Plasma Homocysteine and Cardiovascular Disease Mortality." *The Lancet* 349 (1997): 397.

al-Ghamdi, S. M., et al. "Magnesium Deficiency: Pathophysiologic and Clinical Overview." *American Journal of Kidney Disease* 24, no. 5 (November 1994): 737–52.

Altura, B. M., et al. "Role of Magnesium in the Pathogenesis of Hypertension Updated: Relationship to Its Action on Cardiac, Vascular Smooth Muscle and Endothelial Cells." *Hypertension: Pathophysiology, Diagnosis, and Management* 72 (1995): 1213–42.

Aw, T. Y., et al. "Intestinal Absorption and Lymphatic Transport of Peroxidized Lipids in Rats: Effects of Exogenous GSH." *American Journal of Physiology* (November 1992): 263.

Bermudez, E. A., and P. M. Ridker. "C-Reactive Protein, Statins, and the Primary Prevention of Atherosclerotic Cardiovascular Disease." *Preventive Cardiology* 5, no. 1 (Winter 2002): 42–46.

Blake, G. J., and P. M. Ridker. "Inflammatory Mechanisms in Atherosclerosis: From Laboratory Evidence to Clinical Application." *Italian Heart Journal* 2, no. 11 (November 2001): 796–800.

Booth, G. L., and E. L. Wang, with the Canadian Task Force on Preventive Health Care. "Preventive Health Care, 2000 Update: Screening and Management of Hypohomocysteinemia for the Prevention of Coronary Artery Disease Events." *Canadian Medical Association Journal* 163 (2000): 21–29.

Ceconi, C., et al. "The Role of Glutathione Status in the Protection Against Ischaemic and Reperfusion Damage: Effects of N-Acetyl Cysteine." *Journal of Molecular and Cellular Cardiology* 20, no. 1 (January 1988): 5–13.

Chan F. K., J. Y. Ching, L. C. Hung, et al. "Clopidogrel Versus Aspirin and Esomeprazole to Prevent Recurrent Ulcer Bleeding." *New England Journal of Medicine* 352, no. 3 (January 20, 2005): 238–44.

Classen, U. G. "Influence of High and Low Dietary Magnesium Levels on Functional, Chemical and Morphological Parameters of 'Old' Rats." *Magnesium Research* 7, nos. 3–4 (December 1994): 233–43.

Decensi, A., et al. "Effect of Transdermal Estradiol and Oral Conjugated Estrogen on C-Reactive Protein in Retinoid-Placebo Trial in Healthy Women." *Circulation* 106, no. 10 (September 2002): 1224–28.

Durlach, J. "Primary Mitral Valve Prolapse: A Clinical Form of Primary Magnesium Deficit." *Magnesium Research* 7, nos. 3–4 (December 1994): 339–40.

———. "Magnesium and Therapeutics." *Magnesium Research* 7, nos. 3–4 (December 1994): 313–28.

Elin, R. "Magnesium: The 5th But Forgotten Electrolyte." *American Journal of Clinical Pathology* 102, no. 5 (1994): 616–22.

"Final Report on the Aspirin Component of the Ongoing Physicians' Health Study." *New England Journal of Medicine* 321, no. 3 (July 20, 1989): 129–35.

Flagg, E. W., et al. "Plasma Total Glutathione in Humans and Its Association with Demographic and Health-Related Factors."

The British Journal of Nutrition 70, no. 3 (November 1993): 797–808.

Gardner, C. D., et al. "The Effect of Plant-based Diet on Plasma Lipids in Hypercholesterolemic Adults." *Annals of Internal Medicine* 142, no. 9 (May 3, 2005): 725–33.

Giovannucci, E., et al. "Alcohol, Low-Methionine-Low Folate Diets and the Risk of Colon Cancer in Men." *Journal of the National Cancer Institute* 87, no. 4 (February 15, 1995): 265–73.

Hackam, D. G., et al. "What Level of Plasma Homocyst(E)Ine Should Be Treated? Effects of Vitamin Therapy on Progression of Carotid Atherosclerosis in Patients with Homocyst(E)Ine Levels Above and Below 14 Micromol/L." *American Journal of Hypertension* 13 (2000): 100–105.

Igawa, A., et al. "Comparison of Frequency of Magnesium Deficiency in Patients with Vasospastic Angina and Fixed Coronary Artery Disease." *American Journal of Cardiology* 75 (April 1, 1995): 728–31.

Jialal. I., and S. Devaraj. "Inflammation and Atherosclerosis: The Value of the High-Sensitivity C-Reactive Protein Assay as a Risk Marker." *American Journal of Clinical Pathology* 116, supp. (December 2001): S108–15.

Julius, M., et al. "Glutathione and Morbidity in a Community-Based Sample of Elderly." *Journal of Clinical Epidemiology* 47, no. 9 (September 1994): 1021–26.

Kang, S. S., et al. "Hyperhomocyst(E)Inemia as a Risk Factor for Occlusive Vascular Disease." *Annual Review of Nutrition* 12 (1992): 279–98.

Kinscherf, R., et al. "Effect of Glutathione Depletion and Oral N-Acetyl-Cysteine Treatment on CD4+ and CD8+ Cells."

The FASEB Journal: Official Publication of the Federation of American Societies for Experimental Biology 8, no. 6 (April 1, 1994): 448–51.

Lanza, F. L. "A Review of Gastric Ulcer and Gastroduodenal Injury in Normal Volunteers Receiving Aspirin and Other Non-Steroidal Anti-Inflammatory Drugs." *Scandinavian Journal of Gastroenterology* 24, no. 163 (supp.) (1989): 24–31.

Loralie, J., et al. "Hyperhomocyst(e)inemia and the Increased Risk of Venous Thromboembolism." *Archives of Internal Medicine* 160 (2000): 961–64.

Malinow, M. R., et al. "Homocyst(E)Ine, Diet, and Cardiovascular Diseases: A Statement for Healthcare Professionals from the Nutrition Committee, American Heart Association." *Circulation* 99 (1999): 178–82.

Miura, K., et al. "Cystine Uptake and Glutathione Level in Endothelial Cells Exposed to Oxidative Stress." *American Journal of Physiology* (January 1992): 262.

Mizui, T., et al. "Depletion of Brain Glutathione by Buthionine Sulfoximine Enhances Cerebral Ischemic Injury in Rats." *American Journal of Physiology* (February 1992): 262.

Nozue, T., et al. "Magnesium Status, Serum HDL Cholesterol, and Apolipoprotein A-1 Levels." *Journal of Pediatric Gastroenterology and Nutrition* 20 (1995): 316–18.

Nygård, O., et al. "Plasma Homocysteine and Mortality in Patients with Coronary Artery Disease." *New England Journal of Medicine* 337 (1997): 230–36.

Paolisso, G., et al. "Plasma GSH/GSSG Affects Glucose Homeostasis in Healthy Subjects and Non-Insulin-Dependent Diabetics."

American Journal of Physiology (September 1992): 263.

Peterson, J. C., and J. D. Spence. "Vitamins and Progression of Atherosclerosis in Hyper-Homocyst(E)Inaemia." *The Lancet* 351 (1998): 263.

Pittler, M. H., R. Guo, E. Ernst, et al. "Hawthorn Extract May Benefit Patients with Chronic Heart Failure." *Cochrane Database of Systematic Reviews*, no. 1 (2008); Issue 1, Art. no.: CD005312. DOI: 10.1002/14651858.CD005312.pub2.

Pradhan, A. D., et al. "Inflammatory Biomarkers, Hormone Replacement Therapy, and Incident Coronary Heart Disease: Prospective Analysis from the Women's Health Initiative Observational Study." *Journal of the American Medical Association* 288, no. 8 (August 28, 2002): 980–87.

Ridker, P. M., et al. "Homocysteine and Risk of Cardiovascular Disease Among Postmenopausal Women." *Journal of the American Medical Association* 281 (1999): 1817–21.

———. "Inflammation, Aspirin, and the Risk of Cardiovascular Disease in Apparently Healthy Men." *New England Journal of Medicine* 336, no. 14 (April 3, 1997): 973–79.

Rifai, N., and P. M. Ridker. "Inflammatory Markers and Coronary Heart Disease." *Current Opinion in Lipidology* 13, no. 4 (August 2002): 383–89.

Rifai, N., et al. "C-Reactive Protein and Coronary Heart Disease." *Cardiovascular Toxicology* 1, no. 2 (2001): 153–57.

Sastre, J., et al. "Exhaustive Physical Exercise Causes Oxidation of Glutathione Status in Blood: Prevention by Antioxidant Administration." *American Journal of Physiology* 263 (5Pt2) (November 1992): R992–95.

Schulman, S. P., L. C. Becker, D. A. Kass, et al. "L-arginine Therapy in Acute Myocardial Infarction: The Vascular Interaction with Age in Myocardial Infarction (VINTAGE MI) Randomized Clinical Trial." *Journal of the American Medical Association*. 295, no. 1 (January 4, 2006): 58–64.

Selhub, J., et al. "Vitamin Status and Intake as Primary Determinants of Homocysteinaemia in an Elderly Population." *Journal of the American Medical Association* 270 (1993): 2693–98.

Toto, K. H., et al. "Magnesium: Homeostasis, Imbalances, and Therapeutic Uses." *Critical Care Nursing Clinics of North America* 6, no. 4 (December 1994): 767–83.

Van Zandwijk, N. "N-Acetylcysteine for Lung Cancer Prevention." *Chest* 107, no. 5 (May 1995): 1437–41.

Wang, T. J., et al. "C-Reactive Protein Is Associated with Subclinical Epicardial Coronary Calcification in Men and Women: The Framingham Heart Study." *Circulation* 106, no. 10 (September 3, 2002): 1189–91.

Wang, T. J., M. J. Pencina, S. L. Booth, et al. "Vitamin D Deficiency and Risk of Cardiovascular Disease." *Circulation* 117, no. 4 (January 2008): 503–11.

Zairis, M., et al. "C-Reactive Protein and Multiple Complex Coronary Artery Plaques in Patients with Primary Unstable Angina." *Atherosclerosis* 164, no. 2 (October 2002): 355.

High Blood Pressure/Hypertension Drugs

Beckett, N. S., R. Peters, A. E. Fletcher, et al. (HYVET Study Group). "Treatment of Hypertension in Patients 80 Years of Age or Older." *New England Journal of Medicine* 358, no. 18 (May 1, 2008): 1887–98.

Borok, G. "Nutritional Aspects of Hypertension." *South African Medical Journal* 76 (August 5, 1989): 125–26.

Devereaux P. J., H. Yang, S. Yusuf, et al. (POISE Study Group). "Effects of Extended-Release Metoprolol Succinate in Patients Undergoing Non-Cardiac Surgery (POISE trial): A Randomised Controlled Trial." *Lancet* 371, no. 1926 (May 2008): 1839–47.

Gale, C. R., et al. "Vitamin C and Risk of Death from Stroke and Coronary Heart Disease in Cohorts of Elderly People." *British Medical Journal* 310 (1995): 1563–66.

Kisters, K., et al. "Plasma Magnesium and Total Intracellular Magnesium Ion Content of Lymphocytes in Untreated Normotensive and Hypertensive Patients." *Trace Elements and Electrolytes* 13, no. 4 (1996): 163–66.

Levy, D. "Hypertension from Framingham to ALLHAT: Translating Clinical Trials into Practice." *Cleveland Clinic Journal of Medicine* 74, no. 9 (September 2007): 672–78.

Lindberg, G., U. Lindblad, L. Bent, et al. "Use of Calcium Channel Blockers as Antihypertensives in Relation to Mortality and Cancer Incidence: A Population-Based Observational Study." *Pharmacoepidemiology and Drug Safety* 11 (2002): 493–97.

Nicolson, D. J., et al. "Lifestyle Interventions for Drugs for Patients with Essential Hypertension: A Systematic Review." *Journal of Hypertension* 22, no. 11 (November 2004): 2043–48.

Oates, D. J., D. R. Berlowitz, M. E. Glickman, et al. "Blood Pressure and Survival in the Oldest Old." *Journal of the American Geriatrics Society* 55 (2007): 383–88.

Romero-Alvira, D., et al. "High Blood Pressure, Oxygen Radicals and Antioxidants: Etiological Relationships." *Medical Hypotheses* 46 (1996): 414–20.

Sanjuliani, A. F., et al. "Effects of Magnesium on Blood Pressure and Intracellular Ion Levels of Brazilian Hypertensive Patients." *International Journal of Cardiology* 56 (1996): 177–83.

Stoschitzky, K., A. Sakotnik, et al. "Influence of Beta-Blockers on Melatonin Release." *European Journal of Clinical Pharmacology* 55, no. 2 (1999): 111–15.

Yoshida, M., T. Matsumoto, T. Suzuki, et al. "Effect of Concomitant Treatment with a CYP3A4 Inhibitor and a Calcium Channel Blocker." *Pharmacoepidemiology and Drug Safety* 17, no. 1 (January 2008): 70–75.

Cholesterol-Lowering Drugs

Aleman, C. L., et al. "A 12-Month Study of Policosanol Oral Toxicity in Sprague Dawley Rats." *Toxicology Letters* 70 (1994): 77–87.

Araghiniknam, M., et al. "Antioxidant Activity of Dioscorea and Dehydroepiandrosterone (DHEA) in Older Humans." *Life Sciences* 59, no. 11 (1996): 147–57.

Barnard, J. R., Ph.D., et al. "Effects of Diet and Exercise on Qualitative and Quantitative Measures of LDL and Its Susceptibility to Oxidation." *Arteriosclerosis, Thrombosis, and Vascular Biology* 16, no. 2 (February 1996): 201–7.

Batista, J., et al. "Effect of Policosanol on Hyperlipidemia and Coronary Heart Disease in Middle-Aged Patients: A 14-Month Pilot Study." *International Journal of Clinical Pharmacology, Therapy and Toxicology* 34, no. 3 (1996): 134–37.

Boston, P. F., et al. "Serum Cholesterol and Treatment-Resistance in Schizophrenia." *Biological Psychiatry* 40 (1996): 542–43.

Brown, D. "Hyperlipidemia and Prevention of Coronary Heart Disease." *Quarterly Review of Natural Medicine* (Spring 1997): 61–71.

Canetti, M., et al. "A Two-Year Study on the Efficacy and Tolerability of Policosanol in Patients with Type II Hyperlipoprotein-aemia." *International Journal of Clinical Pharmacology Research* 15, no. 4 (1995): 159–65.

Carbajal, D., et al. "Effect of Policosanol on Platelet Aggregation and Serum Levels of Arachidonic Acid Metabolites in Healthy Volunteers." *Prostaglandins, Leukotrienes, & Essential Fatty Acids* 58 (1998): 61–64.

Chang, A. K., et al. "Low Plasma Cholesterol Predicts an Increased Risk of Lung Cancer in Elderly Women." *Preventive Medicine* 24 (1995): 557–62.

Gardner, C. D., et al. "The Effect of Plant-Based Diet on Plasma Lipids in Hypercholesterolemic Adults." *Annals of Internal Medicine* 142, no. 9 (May 3, 2005): 725–33.

Gatto, L. M., et al. "Ascorbic Acid Induces a Favorable Lipoprotein Profile in Women." *Journal of the American College of Nutrition* 15, no. 2 (1996): 154–58.

Gigleux, I., et al. "Comparison of a Dietary Portfolio of Cholesterol-Lowering Foods and a Statin on LDL Particle Size Phenotype in Hypercholesterolaemic Participants," *British Journal of Nutrition* 98, no. 6 (December 2007): 1229–36.

Gotto, A. M., et al. "The Cholesterol Facts: A Summary of the Evidence Relating Dietary Fats, Serum Cholesterol and Coronary Heart Disease." *Circulation* 81 (1990): 1721–33.

Harris, W. S. "N-3 Fatty Acids and Lipoproteins: Comparison of Results from Human and Animal Studies." *Lipids* 31, no. 3 (1996): 243–52.

Heber, D. "Dietary Supplement or Drug? The Case for Cholestin." *American Journal of Clinical Nutrition* 70, no. 1 (July 1999): 106–8.

Heber, D., et al. "Cholesterol-Lowering Effects of a Proprietary Chinese Red-Yeast-Rice Dietary Supplement." *American Journal of Clinical Nutrition* 69, no. 2 (February 1999): 231–36.

Jancin, B. "Psyllium Adds to Diet for Lowering Cholesterol." *Family Practice News* (November 1, 1996): 13.

Jenkins, D. A., C. C. Kendell, and A. Marchie. "Diet and Cholesterol Reduction." *Annals of Internal Medicine* 142, no. 9 (May 3, 2005): 793–94.

Keys, A. "Coronary Heart Disease in Seven Countries." *Circulation* 41, supp. 1 (1970): 1–211.

Kondo, K., et al. "Inhibition of LDL Oxidation by Cocoa." *The Lancet* 348 (November 30, 1996): 1514.

Kraus, W. E., et al. "Effects of the Amount and Intensity of Exercise on Plasma Lipoproteins." *New England Journal of Medicine* 347, no. 19 (November 7, 2002): 1483–92.

Lien, W. P., M.D., et al. "Low Serum, High-Density Lipoprotein Cholesterol Concentration Is an Important Coronary Risk Factor in Chinese Patients with Low Serum Levels of Total Cholesterol and Triglyceride." *American Journal of Cardiology* 77 (May 15, 1996): 1112–15.

Link, E., S. Parish, J. Armitage, et al. "SLCO1B1 Variants and Statin-Induced Myopathy—A Genomewide Study." *New*

England Journal of Medicine 359, no. 8 (August 21, 2008): 789–99.

"Lipid-Lowering Effects of Red Yeast Rice." *Medical Sciences Bulletin*, no. 244 (January 1999).

Malhotra, S. C., M. M. S. Ahuja, and K. R. Sundarum. "Long-Term Clinical Studies on the Hypolipidemic Effect of Commiphora Mukul (Guggul) and Clofibrate." *Indian Journal of Medical Research* 65 (1977): 390–95.

Mas, R., et al. "Effects of Policosanol in Patients with Type II Hypercholesterolemia and Additional Coronary Risk Factors." *Clinical Pharmacology and Therapeutics* 65, no. 4 (1999): 439–47.

Nestel, P., et al. "The N-3 Fatty Acids Eicosapentaenoid Acid and Docosahexaenoic Acid Increase Systemic Arterial Compliance in Humans." *American Journal of Clinical Nutrition* 76, no. 2 (August 2002): 326–30.

Newman, T. B., et al. "Carcinogenicity of Lipid-Lowering Drugs." *Journal of the American Medical Association* 275, no. 1 (1996): 55–60.

Prat, H., O. Roman, and E. Pino. "Comparative Effects of Policosanol and Two HMG-CoA Reductase Inhibitors on Type II Hypercholesterolemia." *Revista Medica de Chile* 127, no. 3 (1999): 286–94.

Ravnskov, U., M.D. *The Cholesterol Myths*. Washington, D.C.: New Trends Publishing, 2000.

Ridker, P. M., N. Rifai, L. Rose, et al. "Comparison of C-Reactive Protein and Low-Density Lipoprotein Cholesterol Levels in the Prediction of First Cardiovascular Events." *New England Journal of Medicine* 347 (November 14, 2002): 1557–65.

Simons, L. A., et al. "What Dose of Vitamin E Is Required to Reduce Susceptibility of LDL to Oxidation?" *Australian New Zealand Journal of Medicine* 26 (1996): 496–503.

Steiner, M., et al. "A Double-Blind Crossover Study in Moderately Hypercholesterolemic Men That Compared the Effect of Aged Garlic Extract and Placebo Administration on Blood Lipids." *American Journal of Clinical Nutrition* 64 (1996): 866–70.

Stusser, R., et al. "Long-Term Therapy with Policosanol Improves Treadmill Exercise-ECG Testing Performance of Coronary Heart Disease Patients." *International Journal of Clinical Pharmacology, Therapy and Toxicology* 36 (1998): 469–73.

Temple, N. J. "Dietary Fats and Coronary Heart Disease." *Biomedicine and Pharmacotherapy* 50 (1996): 261–68.

Wander, R. C., et al. "Effects of Interaction of RRR-Alpha-Tocopheryl Acetate and Fish Oil on Low Density Lipoprotein Oxidation in Postmenopausal Women With and Without Hormone-Replacement Therapy." *American Journal of Clinical Nutrition* 63 (1996): 193–94.

Chapter 11
Drugs for the Digestive Tract and Their Natural Alternatives

Al-Somal. N., et al. "Susceptibility of *Helicobacter pylori* to the Antimicrobial Activity of Manuka Honey." *Journal of the Royal Society of Medicine* 87 (January, 1994): 9–12.

Bachman, A. "Glutamine: Is It a Conditionally Required Nutrient for the Human Gastrointestinal System?" *Journal of the Ameri-*

can *College of Nutrition* 15, no. 3 (1996): 199–205.

Batchelder, H. J., and R. Scalzo. "Naturopathic Specific Condition Review: Constipation." *Protocol Journal of Botanical Medicine* 1, no. 1 (Summer 1995): 52–55.

———. "Allopathic Specific Condition Review: Peptic Ulcer." *Protocol Journal of Botanical Medicine* 1, no. 3 (Winter 1996): 191–96.

Beil, W., C. Birkholz, and K. F. Sewing. "Effects of Flavonoids on Parietal Cell Acid Secretion, Gastric Mucosal Prostaglandin Production and *Helicobacter pylori* Growth." *Arzneim-Forsch Drug Research* 45 (1995): 697–700.

Buddington, R. K., et al. "Dietary Supplement of Neosugar Alters the Fecal Flora and Decreases Activities of Some Reductive Enzymes in Human Subjects." *American Journal of Clinical Nutrition* 63 (1996): 709–16.

Dunjic, B. S., et al. "Green Banana Protection of Gastric Mucosa Against Experimentally Induced Injuries in Rats." *Scandinavian Journal of Gastroenterology* 28 (1993): 894–98.

Goso, Y., et al. "Effects of Traditional Herbal Medicine on Gastric Mucin Against Ethanol-Induced Gastric Injury in Rats." *Comparative Biochemistry and Physiology* 113C (1996): 17–21.

Ianoco, G., et al. "Chronic Constipation as a Symptom of Cow Milk Allergy." *Journal of Pediatrics* 126 (1995): 34–39.

Laheij, R. J. F., M. C. J. M. Sturkenboom, R.-J. Hassing, et al. "Risk of Community-Acquired Pneumonia and Use of Gastric Acid-Suppressive Drugs." *Journal of the American Medical Association* 292, no. 16 (2004): 1955–60.

LeVan, B. "New Therapy for Irritable Bowel Syndrome." *Life Extension* 59 (November 2002): 57–60.

Liva, R., N.D. "Naturopathic Specific Condition Review: Peptic Ulcer." *Protocol Journal of Botanical Medicine* 1, no. 3 (winter 1996): 197–202.

Salminen, S., E. Isolauri, and T. Onnela. "Gut Flora in Normal and Disordered States." *Chemotherapy* 41, supp. 1 (1995): 5–15.

Seppa, N. "Bad to the Bone: Acid Stoppers Appear to Have a Downside." *Science News* 171, no. 1 (January 7, 2007): 3.

Yang, Y. X., J. D. Lewis, S. Epstein, and D. C. Metz. "Long-Term Proton Pump Inhibitor Therapy and Risk of Hip Fracture." *Journal of the American Medical Association* 296, no. 24: 2947–53.

Walker, A. F., R. W. Middleton, and O. Petrowicz. "Artichoke Leaf Extract Reduces Symptoms of Irritable Bowel Syndrome in a Post-Marketing Surveillance Study." *Phytotherapy Research* 15 (2001): 58–61.

Chapter 12
Cold, Cough, Asthma, and Allergy Drugs and Their Natural Alternatives

Abulhosn, R. A., M.D., et al. "Passive Smoke Exposure Impairs Recovery After Hospitalization for Acute Asthma." *Archives of Pediatric and Adolescent Medicine* 151 (February 1997): 135–39.

Aggarwal, B. B., and S. Shishodia. "Suppression of the Nuclear Factor-KappaB Activation Pathways by Spice-Derived Phytochemicals: Reasoning for Seasoning." *Annals of the New York Academy of Sciences* 1030 (December 2004): 434–41.

Associated Press/Reuters, "FDA Wants Warnings on Flu Drugs for Kids: Tamiflu and Relenza Linked to Abnormal Behavior in Some Patients." *MSNBC News Services*, updated 3:00 P.M. PT, November 23, 2007.

Baker, B. "Patient History Often Fails to Uncover Allergies." *Skin & Allergy News*, April 1997, 11.

Ben-Yehuda, A., et al. "The Influence of Sequential Annual Vaccination and of DHEA Administration on the Efficacy of the Immune Response to Influenza Vaccine in the Elderly." *Mechanisms of Ageing and Development* 102, nos. 2–3 (May 15, 1998): 299–306.

Bogden, J. D. "Micronutrient Nutrition and Immunity." *Nutrition Report* 13, no. 2 (February 1995): 1.

Braun-Fahrlander, C., et al. "Environmental Exposure to Endotoxin and Its Relation to Asthma in School-Age Children." *New England Journal of Medicine* 347, no. 12 (September 19, 2002): 869–77.

Broughton, K. S., et al. "Reduced Asthma Symptoms with n-3 Fatty Acid Ingestion Are Related to 5-Series Leukotriene Production." *American Journal of Clinical Nutrition* 65 (1997): 1011–17.

Cairns, C. B., M.D., and M. Kraft, M.D. "Magnesium Attenuates the Neutrophil Respiratory Burst in Adult Asthmatic Patients." *Academy of Emergency Medicine* 3 (1996): 1093–97.

Carroll, L. "Leukotriene Inhibitors Represent Important Class of Asthma Drugs." *Medical Tribune*, March 6, 1997, 4.

Centers for Disease Control and Prevention. Leads from the *Morbidity and Mortality Weekly Report*. "Pneumonia and Influenza Death Rates—United States, 1979–1994." *Journal of the American Medical Association* 274, no. 7 (August 16, 1995): 532.

Chatzi, L, et al. "Protective Effect of Fruits, Vegetables and the Mediterranean Diet on Asthma and Allergies Among Children in Crete." *Thorax*, 2007.

Dang, Devra K., "Inhaled Corticosteroids in Asthma: Less Is Better." *AphA Drug Info-Line* (July 2005): 4.

Derry S., and Y. K. Loke. "Risk of Gastrointestinal Haemorrhage with Long Term Use of Aspirin: Meta-Analysis." *British Medical Journal* 321 (2000): 1183–87.

Donahue, J., D.V.M., Ph.D. "Inhaled Steroids and the Risk of Hospitalization for Asthma." *Journal of the American Medical Association* 277, no. 11 (March 19, 1997): 887–91.

Donn, J. "Exposure to Germs Now and Then May Be Healthy." *Associated Press*, September 19, 2002.

Dowling, C. G., and A. Hollister. "An Epidemic of Sneezing and Wheezing." *Life*, May 1997, 76–92.

Eby, G. A. "Zinc Lozenges as Cure for Common Colds." *Annals of Pharmacotherapy* 30 (November 1996): 1336–38.

———. "Linearity in Dose-Response from Zinc Lozenges in Treatment of Common Colds." *Journal of Pharmacy Technology* 22 (May/June 1995): 110–22.

Fantidis, P., et al. "Intracellular (Polymorphonuclear) Magnesium Content in Patients with Bronchial Asthma Between Attacks." *Journal of the Royal Society of Medicine* 88, no. 8 (August 1995): 441–45.

Gilliland, F. D., et al. "Dietary Magnesium, Potassium, Sodium, and Children's Lung Function." *American Journal of Epidemiology* 155, no. 2 (January 2002): 125–31.

Govaert, T., et al. "The Efficacy of Influenza Vaccination in Elderly Individuals: A Randomized, Double-Blind, Placebo-Controlled Trial." *Journal of the American Medical Association* 272 (December 7, 1994): 1661–65.

Hill, D. J., et al. "The Melbourne House Dust Mite Study: Eliminating House Dust Mites in the Domestic Environment." *Journal of Allergy and Clinical Immunology* 99 (March 1997): 323–29.

Holloway, E. A., and R. J. West. "Integrated Breathing and Relaxation Training (the Papworth Method) for Adults with Asthma in Primary Care: A Randomized Controlled Trial." *Thorax* 62 (2007):1039–42.

Hurst, D. S., M.D. "The Association of Otitis Media with Effusion and Allergy as Demonstrated by Intradermal Skin Testing and Eosinophil Cationic Protein Levels in Both Middle Ear Effusions and Mucosal Biopsies." *Laryngoscope* 106 (September 1996): 1128–37.

Hurst, D. S., M.D., and P. Venge, M.D., Ph.D. "Levels of Eosinophil Cationic Protein and Myeloperoxidase from Chronic Middle Ear Effusion in Patients with Allergy and/or Acute Infection." *Otalaryngology—Head and Neck Surgery* 114 (1996): 531–44.

Jackson, B., et al. "Does Harboring Hostility Hurt? Associations Between Hostility and Pulmonary Function in the Coronary Artery Risk Development in Young Adults (CARDIA) Study." *Health Psychology* 26, no. 3 (2007): 333–40.

Jefferson, T. "Influenza Vaccine: Policy Versus Evidence." *British Medical Journal* (October 28, 2006): 912–15.

Knutsen, R., T. Bohmer, and J. Falch. "Intravenous Theophylline-Induced Excretion of Calcium, Magnesium and Sodium in Patients with Recurrent Asthmatic Attacks." *Scandinavian Journal of Clinical and Laboratory Investigation* 54, no. 2 (April 1994): 119–25.

Kummeling, I., et al. "Early Life Exposure to Antibiotics and the Subsequent Development of Eczema, Wheeze, and Allergic Sensitization in the First Two Years of Life: The KOALA Birth Cohort Study." *Pediatrics* 119, no. 1 (January 2007): e225–31.

Little, P., et al. "Predictors of Poor Outcome and Benefits from Antibiotics in Children with Acute Otitis Media: Pragmatic Randomised Trial." *British Medical Journal* 325, no. 7354 (July 6, 2002): 22.

Majamaa, H., M.D., and E. Isolauri, M.D. "Probiotics: A Novel Approach in the Management of Food Allergy." *Journal of Allergy and Clinical Immunology* 99 (1997): 179–85.

Margolis, K. L., et al. "Frequency of Adverse Reactions After Influenza Vaccination." *American Journal of Medicine* (University of Minnesota) 88, no. 1 (January 1990): 27–30.

Martin, M. "Flu Vaccine Shortage May Not Be a Real Crisis," *Health Care News*, January 1, 2005, http://www.newcoalition.org/Article.cfm?artId=16132.

McCann, J. "Conjugated Flu Vaccine Boosts Response in Elderly: Binding a Diphtheria Toxoid to the Standard Influenza Vaccine May Make Flu Shots More Effective for This Group." *Medical World News* 29, no. 15 (August 8, 1988): 16(1).

Mendell, J. J., et al. "Elevated Symptom Prevalence Associated with Ventilation Type in Office Buildings." *Epidemiology* 7 (1996): 583–89.

Millqvist, E., and O. Lowhagen. "Placebo-Controlled Challenges with Perfume in Patients with Asthma-Like Symptoms." *Allergy* 51 (1996): 434–39.

Moneret-Vautrin, D. A., and G. Kanny. "Food and Drug Additives: Hypersensitivity and Intolerance." *Human Toxicology*, Amsterdam: Elsevier, 1996.

Nemecz, G. "Hyssop." *U.S. Pharmacist* 34 (July 2001).

Peters, A., et al. "Acute Health Effects of Exposure to High Levels of Air Pollution in Eastern Europe." *American Journal of Epidemiology* 144, no. 6 (1996): 570–81.

Rubin, R. N., L. Navon, and P. A. Cassano, "Relationship of Serum Antioxidants to Asthma Prevalence in Youth." *American Journal of Respiratory and Critical Care Medicine* 169 (2004): 398.

Rumchev, K., et al. "Association of Domestic Exposure to Volatile Organic Compounds with Asthma in Young Children." *Thorax* 59 (2004): 746–51.

Scaglione, F., et al. "Efficacy and Safety of the Standardized Ginseng Extract G 115 for Potentiating Vaccination Against Common Cold and/or Influenza Syndrome." *Drugs in Experimental and Clinical Research* 22, no. 2 (1996): 65–72.

Seelig, M. S. "Consequences of Magnesium Deficiency on the Enhancement of Stress Reactions: Preventive and Therapeutic Implications." *Journal of the American College of Nutrition* 13, no. 5 (October 1994): 429–46.

Suissa, S., Ph.D., and P. Ernst, M.D. "Albuterol in Mild Asthma." *New England Journal of Medicine* 336, no. 10 (March 6, 1997): 729.

Thijs, C., W. E. Beyer, P. M. Govaert, et al. "Mortality Benefits of Influenza Vaccination in Elderly People." *The Lancet* 8 (August 8, 2008): 460–61; author reply, 463–65.

Trenga, C. A., J. K. Koenig, and P. V. Williams. "Dietary Antioxidants and Ozone-Induced Bronchial Hyperresponsiveness in Adults with Asthma." *Archives of Environmental and Occupational Health* 56, no. 3 (May/June 2001): 242–49.

U.S. Centers for Disease Control. "Crude Percentages (with Standard Errors) of Selected Respiratory Diseases Among Persons 18 Years of Age and Over, by Selected Characteristics: United States, 2004." *Summary Health Statistics for U.S. Adults: National Health Interview Survey*, May 2006, http://www.cdc.gov/nchs/data/series/sr_10/sr10_228.pdf.

Vlaski, E., et al. "Acetaminophen Intake and Risk of Asthma, Hay Fever and Eczema in Early Adolescence." *Iranian Journal of Allergy, Asthma and Immunology* 6, no. 3 (September 2007): 143–49.

Weiss, S. T. "Eat Dirt—the Hygiene Hypothesis and Allergic Diseases." *New England Journal of Medicine* 347, no. 12 (September 19, 2002): 930–31.

Weitzberg, E., and Jon Lundberg. "Humming Greatly Increases Nitric Oxide." *American Journal of Respiratory and Critical Care Medicine* 166 (July 2002): 144–45.

Wjst, M., et al. "Early Antibiotic Therapy and Later Asthma." *European Journal of Medical Research* 6, no. 6 (June 28, 2001): 263–71.

Zakay-Rones, Z., et al. "Randomized Study of the Efficacy and Safety of Oral Elderberry Extract in the Treatment of Influenza A and

B Virus Infections." *Journal of International Medical Research* 32, no. 2 (March/April 2004): 132–40.

Chapter 13
Drugs for Pain Relief and Their Natural Alternatives

Altman, R. D., and K. C. Marcussen. "Effects of a Ginger Extract on Knee Pain in Patients with Osteoarthritis." *Arthritis and Rheumatism* 44, no. 11 (November 2001): 2531–38.

Associated Press. "Pediatricians Warn of Acetaminophen Overdose." *Los Angeles Times*, October 1, 2001.

Brater, D. C. "Effects of Nonsteroidal Antiinflammatory Drugs on Renal Function: Focus on Cyclooxygenase-2-selective Inhibition." *American Journal of Medicine* 107, no. 6A (December 13, 1999): 65S–70S; discussion 70S–71S.

Brown, S. J., et al. "Panel OKs Alternative Therapy for Chronic Pain." *Family Practice News* (December 15, 1995): 4.

Felson, D. T. "Weight and Osteoarthritis." *American Journal of Clinical Nutrition* 63, supp. (1996): 430S–32S.

Ferris, D. G., et al. "Over-the-Counter Antifungal Drug Misuse Associated with Patient-Diagnosed Vaginal Candidiasis." *Obstetrics and Gynecology* 99, no. 3 (March 2002): 41–49.

Harris, G. "Study Finds Celebrex as Likely to Cause Ulcers as Older Drugs." *Los Angeles Times*, June 10, 2002, B3.

Hubner, W. D., and T. Kirste. "Experience with St. John's Wort (*Hypericum perforatum*) in Children Under 12 Years with Symptoms of Depression and Psychovegetative Disturbances." *Phytotherapy Research* 15 (2001): 367–70.

Kjeldsen-Kragh, J. et al. "Changes in Laboratory Variables in Rheumatoid Arthritis Patients During a Trial of Fasting and One-Year Vegetarian Diet." *Scandinavian Journal of Rheumatology* 24, no. 2 (1995): 85–93.

Kremer, J. M., M.D. "Effects of Modulation of Inflammatory and Immune Parameters in Patients with Rheumatic and Inflammatory Disease Receiving Dietary Supplementation of N-3 and N-6 Fatty Acids." *Lipids* 31, supp. (1996): S-243–S-47.

McAlindon, T. E., et al. "Do Antioxidant Micronutrients Protect Against the Development and Progression of Knee Osteoarthritis?" *Arthritis and Rheumatism* 39, no. 4 (April 1996): 648–56.

Messier, S. P., et al. "Exercise and Dietary Weight Loss in Overweight and Obese Older Adults with Knee Osteoarthritis: The Arthritis, Diet, and Activity Promotion Trial." *Arthritis and Rheumatism* 50, no. 5 (May 2004): 1501–10.

Miller, G. D., et al. "Intensive Weight Loss Program Improves Physical Functions in Older Obese Adults with Knee Osteoarthritis." *Obesity* 14, no. 7 (July 2006): 1219–30.

Pavelka, K., et al. "Glucosamine Sulfate Use and Delay of Progression of Knee Osteoarthritis: A 3-Year, Randomized, Placebo-Controlled, Double-Blind Study." *Archives of Internal Medicine* 162, no. 18 (October 14, 2002): 2113–23.

Peikert, A., et al. "Prophylaxis of Migraine with Oral Magnesium: Results from a Prospective, Multi-Center, Placebo-Controlled and Double-Blind Randomized Study." *Cephalalgia* 16 (1996): 257–63.

Ruane, R., and P. Griffiths. "Glucosamine Therapy Compared to Ibuprofen for Joint Pain." *British Journal of Community Nursing*, no. 3 (March 2002): 148–52.

Rubin, R. "FDA Sends a Warning Letter to Maker of Vioxx Painkiller." *USA Today* (September 25, 2001): 7D.

Shapiro, J. A., M.D., et al. "Diet and Rheumatoid Arthritis in Women: A Possible Protective Effect of Fish Consumption." *Epidemiology* 7 (1996): 256–63.

Silman, A. J., et al. "Cigarette Smoking Increases the Risk of Rheumatoid Arthritis." *Arthritis and Rheumatism* 39, no. 5 (May 1996): 732–35.

Stevinson, C., and E. Ernst. "A Pilot Study of *Hypericum perforatum* for the Treatment of Premenstrual Syndrome." *British Journal of Obstetrics and Gynaecology* 107 (2000): 870–76.

Whitaker, J. "Prolotherapy: End Chronic Pain." *Health & Healing* 11, no. 3 (March 2001): 1–3.

Wilder, R. L. "Adrenal and Gonadal Steroid Hormone Deficiency in the Etiopathogenesis of Rheumatoid Arthritis." *Journal of Rheumatology* 23, supp. 44 (1996): 10–12.

Chapter 14
Antibiotics, Antifungals, and Their Natural Alternatives

Bergus, G. R., M.D., et al. "Antibiotic Use During the First 200 Days of Life." *Archives of Family Medicine* 5 (October 1996): 523–26.

Goldman, E., et al. "Otitis Accounts for Bulk of Antibiotic Overuse." *Family Practice News* (June 15, 1996): 43.

Hansen, B. L., and K. Andersen. "Fungal Arthritis." *Scandinavian Journal of Rheumatology* 24 (1995): 248–50.

Hoel, D., and D. N. Williams. "Antibiotics: Past, Present, and Future: Unearthing Nature's Magic Bullets." *Postgraduate Medicine* 101, no. 1 (January 1997): 114–22.

Hooten, T. M., M.D., and S. B. Levy, M.D., "Confronting the Antibiotic Resistance Crisis: Making Appropriate Therapeutic Decisions in Community Medical Practice." January 25, 2001. www.medscape.com/ viewprogram/618

Kaiser, L., et al. "Effects of Antibiotic Treatment in the Subset of Common-Cold Patients Who Have Bacteria in Nasopharyngeal Secretions." *The Lancet* 347 (June 1, 1996): 1507–10.

Mainous, A. G., III, Ph.D., et al. "Antibiotics and Upper Respiratory Infection: Do Some Folks Think There Is a Cure for the Common Cold?" *Journal of Family Practice* 42, no. 4 (April 1996): 357–61.

Nidecker, A. "Antibiotic Use Linked to Resistant Organism." *Family Practice News*, October 15, 1996, 55.

Norrby, S. R. "Antibiotic Resistance: A Self-Inflicted Problem." *Journal of Internal Medicine* 239 (1996): 373–75.

Roos, K., E. G. Hakansson, and S. Holm. "Effect of Recolonisation with 'Interfering' Streptococci on Recurrences of Acute and Secretory Otitis Media in Children: A Randomized, Placebo Controlled Trial." *British Medical Journal* 322, no. 7280 (January 27, 2001): 210–12.

Saadia, R., and J. Lipman. "Antibiotics and the Gut." *European Journal of Surgery* supp. 576 (1996): 39–41.

Zajicek, G., M.D. "Antibiotic Resistance and the Intestinal Flora." *Cancer Journal* 9, no. 5 (September/October 1996): 214.

Zittell, N. K. "Is Antibiotic Use Coming Back to Haunt Us?" *Medical Tribune*, October 24, 1996, 18.

Chapter 15
Drugs for Insomnia, Anxiety, and Depression and Their Natural Alternatives

Adams, P. B., et al. "Arachidonic Acid to Eicosapentaenoic Acid Ratio in Blood Correlates Positively with Clinical Symptoms of Depression." *Lipids* 31, supp. (1996): S-157–S-161.

AHRQ Publications, "S-Adenosyl-L-Methionine for Treatment of Depression, Osteoarthritis, and Liver Disease: Summary." *AHRQ Publication* no. 02-E033 (August 2002), http://www.ncbi.nlm.nih.gov/books/bv.fcgi?rid=hstat1.chapter.88067.

Aldhous, P. "Antidepressants May Harm Male Fertility." *New Scientist* (September 24, 2008).

Assisi A. et al. "Fish Oil and Mental Health: The Role of Omega-3 Long-Chain Polyunsaturated Fatty Acids in Cognitive Development and Neurological Disorders." *International Clinical Psychopharmacology* 21, no. 6 (November 2006); 319–36.

Borok, G., et al. "Atopy: The Incidence in Chronic Recurrent Maladies." *XVI European Congress of Allergology and Clinical Immunology*, June 24–25, 1995.

Cincipirini, P. M., Ph.D. "Depression and Cholesterol-Lowering Chemotherapy: Potential Influence of Smoking Cessation, Depression History, and Dietary Change." *Behavioral Medicine* (1996): 85–86.

Clouatre D. L. "Kava-kava: Examining New Reports of Toxicity." *Toxicology Letters* 150, no. 1 (April 15, 2004): 85–96.

Corkeron, M. A. "Serotonin Syndrome—a Potentially Fatal Complication of Antidepressant Therapy." *Medical Journal of Australia* 163 (November 6, 1995): 481–82.

Driver, H. S., and S. R. Taylor. "Sleep Disturbances and Exercise." *Sports Medicine* 21, no. 1 (January 1996): 1–6.

Glenmullen, J., M.D. *Prozac Backlash*. New York: Simon & Schuster, 2000.

Helin-Salmivaara, A., T. Huttunen, J. M. Grönroos, et al. "Risk of Serious Upper Gastrointestinal Events with Concurrent Use of NSAIDs and SSRIs: A Case-Control Study in the General Population." *European Journal of Clinical Pharmacology* 63, no. 4 (April 2007): 403–8.

Herber, K. W. "The Influence of Kava-Special Extract WS 1490 on Safety-Relevant Performance Alone and in Combination with Ethylalcohol." *Blutalkohol* 30 (1993): 96–105.

King, A. C., Ph.D., et al. "Moderate-Intensity Exercise and Self-Rated Quality of Sleep in Older Adults: A Randomized Controlled Trial." *Journal of the American Medical Association* 277, no. 1 (January 1, 1997): 32–37.

Kinzler, E., J. Kromer, and E. Lehmann. "Clinical Efficacy of a Kava Extract in Patients with Anxiety Syndrome: Double-Blind Placebo Controlled Study over 4 Weeks." *Arzneim Forsch* 41 (1991): 584–88.

Lacasse, Jeffrey R., and Jonathan Leo, "Serotonin and Depression: A Disconnect Between the Advertisements and the Scientific Literature." *PLOS Medicine* 2, no. 12 (December 5, 2005). http://medicine .plosjournals.org/archive/1549-1676/2/12/ pdf/10.1371_journal.pmed.0020392-L.pdf.

Lawson, Willow. "Omega-3s for Boosting Mood." *Psychology Today,* http://www .psychologytoday.com/articles/pto-20030103 000005.html.

Lebot, V., M. Merlin, and L. Lindstrom. *Kava—The Pacific Drug.* New Haven, CT: Yale University Press, 1992.

Lictha, R., M.D. "Neuropsychiatric Disorders Associated with Folate Deficiency in the Presence of Elevated Serum and Erythrocyte Folate: A Preliminary Report." *Journal of Nutritional Medicine* 4 (1994): 441–47.

Loke, Y. K., A. N. Trivedi, and S. Singh. "Meta-analysis: Gastrointestinal Bleeding Due to Interaction Between Selective Serotonin Uptake Inhibitors and Non-steroidal Anti-inflammatory Drugs." *Alimentary Pharmacology and Therapeutics* 27, no. 1 (January 1, 2008): 31–40.

Maes, M., et al. "Lower Serum L Tryptophan Availability in Depression as a Marker of a More Generalized Disorder in Protein Metabolism." *Neuropsychopharmacology* 15, no. 3 (1996): 243–51.

———. "Fatty Acid Composition in Major Depression: Decreased Omega-3 Fractions in Cholesterol Esters and Increased C20:406/C20:503 Ratio in Cholesterol Esters and Phospholipids." *Journal of Affective Disorders* 38 (1996): 35–46.

Martinez, B., et al. "Hypericum in the Treatment of Seasonal Affective Disorders." *Journal of Geriatric Psychiatry and Neurology* 7, supp. 1 (1994): S29–S33.

Meyer, T., and A. Brooks. "Therapeutic Impact of Exercise on Psychiatric Diseases: Guidelines for Exercise Testing and Prescription." *Sports Medicine* 30, no. 4 (October 2000): 269–79.

Munte, T. F., et al. "Effects of Oxazepam and an Extract of Kava Roots on Event-Related Potentials in a Word Recognition Task." *Neuropsychobiology* 27 (1993): 46–53.

Neumeister, A., M.D., et al. "Effects of Tryptophan Depletion on Drug-Free Patients with Seasonal Affective Disorder During a Stable Response to Bright Light Therapy." *Archives of General Psychiatry* 54 (1997): 133–38.

Pilar, S., M.D. "Amelioration of Premenstrual Depressive Symptomatology with L-Tryptophan." *Journal of Psychiatry and Neuroscience* 19, no. 2 (1994): 114–19.

Ploeckinger, B., et al. "Rapid Decrease of Serum Cholesterol Concentration and Postpartum Depression." *British Medical Journal* 313 (September 14, 1996): 664.

Poulos, C. X., and M. Zack. "Low-Dose Diazepam Primes Motivation for Alcohol and Alcohol Related Semantic Networks in Problem Drinkers." *Behavioral Pharmacology* 15, no. 7 (November 2004): 503–12.

Reichert, R. G., N.D. "St. John's Wort Extract as a Tricyclic Medication Substitute for Mild to Moderate Depression." *Quarterly Review of Natural Medicine* (winter 1995): 275–78.

Reid, K., et al. "Day-Time Melatonin Administration: Effects on Core Temperature and Sleep Onset Latency." *Journal of Sleep Research* 5 (1996): 150–54.

Scholing, W. E., and H. D. Clausen. "On the Effect of D, L-Kavain: Experience with Neuronika." *Medizinische Klinik* 72 (1977): 1301–6.

Singh, Y. N. "Kava: An Overview." *Journal of Ethnopharmacology* 37 (1992): 13–45.

———. "Potential for Interaction of Kava and St. John's Wort with Drugs." *Journal of Ethnopharmacology* 100, nos. 1–2 (August 22, 2005): 108–13.

Stagnitti, M. "Antidepressant Use in the U.S. Civilian Non-institutionalized Population, 2002." Statistical brief #77. Rockville, MD: Medical Expenditure Panel, Agency for Healthcare Research and Quality.

Szabadi, E. "St. John's Wort and Its Active Principles in Depression and Anxiety." *British Journal of Clinical Pharmacology* 62, no. 3 (September 2006): 377–78.

Thachil, A. F., R. Mohan, and D. Bhugra. "The Evidence Base of Complementary and Alternative Therapies in Depression." *Journal of Affective Disorders* 97, no. 1–3 (January 2007): 23–35.

Volz, H. P., and M. Kieser. "Kava-Kava Extract WS 1490 Versus Placebo in Anxiety Disorders—a Randomized Placebo-Controlled 25-Week Outpatient Trial." *Pharmacopsychiatry* 30 (1997): 1–5.

White, H. L., et al. "Extracts of Ginkgo Biloba Leaves Inhibit Monoamine Oxidase." *Life Sciences* 58, no. 16 (1996): 1315–21.

Wiley, T. S., with Bent Formby, Ph.D. *Lights Out: Sleep, Sugar, and Survival.* New York, NY: Simon & Schuster, 2000.

"Working off depression." *Harvard Mental Health Letter* 22, no. 6 (December 2005): 6–7.

Wright, K. P., Jr., et al. "Caffeine and Light Effects on Nighttime Melatonin and Temperature Levels in Sleep-Deprived Humans." *Brain Research* 747 (1997): 78–84.

Zal, H. M. "Seasonal Affective Disorder: How to Lighten the Burden of Winter Depression." *Consultant* (March 1997): 641–49.

Chapter 16
Diabetes Drugs, Obesity Drugs, and Their Natural Alternatives

Arivazhagan, P., K. Ramanathan, and C. Panneerselvam. "Effect of DL-Alpha-Lipoic Acid on Mitochondrial Enzymes in Aged Rats." *Chemical and Biological Interactions* 138, no. 2 (November 28, 2001): 189–98.

Aron, D. C., and T. Hornick. "Managing Diabetes in the Elderly: Go Easy, Individualize." *Cleveland Clinic Journal of Medicine* 75, no. 1 (January 2008): 70–78.

Assan, R., et al. "Dehydroepiandrosterone (DHEA) for Diabetic Patients?" *European Journal of Endocrinology* 135 (1996): 37–38.

Basualdo, C. G., M.Sc., R.D., et al. "Vitamin A (Retinol) Status of First Nation Adults with Non-Insulin Dependent Diabetes Mellitus." *Journal of the American College of Nutrition* 16, no. 1 (1997): 38–45.

Bode, A. M. "Metabolism of Vitamin C in Health and Disease." *Advances in Pharmacology* 40 (1997): 334–44.

Boldyrev, A., et al. "Carnosine Protects Against Excitotoxic Cell Death Independently of Effects on Reactive Oxygen Species." *Neuroscience* 94, no. 2 (1999): 571–77.

Cameron, N. E., A. M. Jack, and M. A. Cotter. "Effect of Alpha-Lipoic Acid on Vascular Responses and Nociception in Diabetic Rats." *Free Radical Biology Medicine* 31, no. 1 (July 1, 2001): 125–35.

Cao, H., I. Hininger-Favier, M. A. Kelly, et al. "Green Tea Polyphenol Extract Regulates the Expression of Genes Involved in Glucose Uptake and Insulin Signaling in Rats Fed a High Fructose Diet." *Journal of Agricultural and Food Chemistry* 55, no. 15 (July 25, 2007): 6372–78.

Ceriello, A., M.D., et al. "Vitamin E Reduction of Protein Glycosylation in Diabetes: New Prospect for Prevention of Diabetic Complications?" *Diabetes Care* 14, no. 1 (January 1991): 68–72.

Challem, J. "Antioxidants Might Ease Diabetic Complications." *Medical Tribune*, December 12, 1996, 18.

Dela, F. "On the Influence of Physical Training on Glucose Homeostasis." *Acta Physiologica Scandinavica* (1996): 5–33.

Gillies, C. L., et al. "Pharmacological and Lifestyle Interventions to Prevent or Delay Type 2 Diabetes in People with Impaired Glucose Tolerance: Systematic Review and Meta-Analysis." *British Medical Journal*, doi: 10.1136/bmj.39063.689375.55.

Greenwood-Robinson, M. "Start Your Fat-Burning Engine." *Let's Live* (December 2001).

Heitzer, T., et al. "Beneficial Effects of Alpha-Lipoic Acid and Ascorbic Acid on Endothelium-Dependent, Nitric Oxide-Mediated Vasodilation in Diabetic Patients: Relation to Parameters of Oxidative Stress." *Free Radical Biology Medicine* 31, no. 1 (July 1, 2001): 53–61.

Holliday, R., and G. A. McFarland. "A Role for Carnosine in Cellular Maintenance." *Biochemistry* (Moscow) 65, no. 7 (July 2000): 843–48.

Houstis, N., E. D. Rosen, and E. S. Lander. "Reactive Oxygen Species Have a Causal Role in Multiple Forms of Insulin Resistance." *Nature* 440, no. 7086 (April 2006): 944–48.

Ishihara, K., et al. "Chronic (-)-Hydroxycitrate Administration Spares Carbohydrate Utilization and Promotes Lipid Oxidation During Exercise in Mice." *Journal of Nutrition* 130, no. 12 (December 2000): 2990–95.

Jain, S. K., Ph.D., et al. "Effect of Modest Vitamin E Supplementation on Blood Glycated Hemoglobin and Triglyceride Levels and Red Cell Indices in Type I Diabetic Patients." *Journal of the American College of Nutrition* 15, no. 5 (1996): 458–61.

———. "Hyperglycemia Can Cause Membrane Lipid Peroxidation and Osmotic Fragility in Human Red Blood Cells." *Journal of Biological Chemistry* 264, no. 35 (December 15, 1989): 21340–45.

Kakkar, R., et al. "Antioxidant Defense System in Diabetic Kidney: A Time Course Study." *Life Sciences* 60, no. 9 (1997): 667–79.

Lee, H. A., and D. A. Hughes. "Alpha-Lipoic Acid Modulates NF-Kappab Activity in Human Monocytic Cells by Direct Interaction with DNA." *Experimental Gerontology* 37, nos. 2–3 (January 3, 2002): 401–10.

Lincoff, M. A., K. Wolski, and S. J. Nicholls. "Pioglitazone and Risk of Cardiovascular Events in Patients with Type 2 Diabetes Mellitus: A Meta-analysis of Randomized Trials." *Journal of the American Medical Association* 298, no. 10 (2007): 1180–88.

Liu, F., et al. "An Extract of *Lagerstroemia speciosa* L. Has Insulin-Like Glucose Uptake-Stimulatory and Adipocyte Differentiation-Inhibitory Activities in 3T3-L1 Cells." *Journal of Nutrition* 131, no. 9 (September 2001): 2242–47.

Lutsey, P. L., L. M. Steffen, and J. Stevens. "Dietary Intake and the Development of the Metabolic Syndrome: The Atherosclerosis Risk in Communities Study." *Circulation* 117, no. 6 (February 2008): 754–61.

Mahendran, P., A. J. Vanisree, and C. S. Shyamala Devi. "The Antiulcer Activity of Garcinia Cambogia Extract Against Indomethacin-Induced Gastric Ulcer in Rats." *Phytotherapy Research* 16, no. 1 (February 2002): 80–83.

Matsukura, T., and H. Tanaka. "Applicability of Zinc Complex of L-Carnosine for Medical Use." *Biochemistry* (Moscow) 65, no. 7 (July 2000): 817–23.

McFarland, G. A., and R. Holliday. "Further Evidence for the Rejuvenating Effects of the Dipeptide L-Carnosine on Cultured Human Diploid Fibroblasts." *Experimental Gerontology* 34, no. 1 (January 1999): 35–45.

Melhem, M. F., P. A Craven, J. Liachenko, and F. R. DeRubertis. "Alpha-Lipoic Acid Attenuates Hyperglycemia and Prevents Glomerular Mesangial Matrix Expansion in Diabetes." *Journal of the American Society of Nephrology* 13, no. 1 (January 2002): 108–16.

Nissen, S. E., and K. Wolski. "Effect of Rosiglitazone on the Risk of Myocardial Infarction and Death from Cardiovascular Causes." *New England Journal of Medicine* 356, no. 24 (June 14, 2007): 2457–71.

Ohia, S. E., et al. "Effect of Hydroxycitric Acid on Serotonin Release from Isolated Rat Brain Cortex." *Research Communications in Molecular Pathology and Pharmacology* 109, nos. 3–4 (March–April 2001): 210–16.

Osterode, W., et al. "Nutritional Antioxidants, Red Cell Membrane Fluidity and Blood Viscosity in Type I (Insulin Dependent) Diabetes Mellitus." *Diabetic Medicine* 13 (1996): 1044–50.

Persson, H. L., A. I. Svensson, and U. T. Brunk. "Alpha-Lipoic Acid and Alpha-Lipoamide Prevent Oxidant-Induced Lysosomal Rupture and Apoptosis." *Redox Report: Communications in Free Radical Research* 6, no. 5 (2001): 327–34.

Pick, M. E., M.Sc., R.D., et al. "Oat Bran Concentrate Bread Products Improve Long-Term Control of Diabetes: A Pilot Study." *Journal of the American Dietetic Association* 96, no. 12 (December 1996): 1254–61.

Preuss, H. G., S. Montamarry, and B. Echard, et al. "Long-Term Effects of Chromium, Grape Seed Extract, and Zinc on Various Metabolic Parameters of Rats." *Molecular and Cellular Biochemistry* 223, nos. 1–2 (July 2001): 95–102.

Schlosser, E. *Fast Food Nation: The Dark Side of the All-American Meal*. New York: Harper-Collins, Inc., 2002.

Seo, K. I., M. S. Choi, U. J. Jung, et al. "Effect of Curcumin Supplementation on Blood Glucose, Plasma Insulin, and Glucose Homeostasis Related Enzyme Activities in Diabetic Db/Db Mice." *Molecular Nutrition and Food Research*, 52, no. 9 (April 2008): 995–1004.

Serisier, S., V. Leray, and W. Poudroux, et al. "Effects of Green Tea on Insulin Sensitivity, Lipid Profile and Expression of PPA-Ralpha and PPARgamma and Their Target Genes in Obese Dogs." *British Journal of Nutrition* 99, no. 6 (June 2008): 1208–16.

Shi, H., D. Dirienzo, and M. B. Zemel. "Effects of Dietary Calcium on Adipocyte Lipid Metabolism and Body Weight Regulation in Energy-Restricted Ap2-Agouti Transgenic Mice." *The FASEB Journal: Official Publication of the Federation of American Societies for Experimental Biology* 15, no. 2 (February 2001): 291–93.

Sigal, R. J., et al. "Physical Activity/Exercise and Type 2 Diabetes: A Consensus

Statement from the American Diabetes Association." *Diabetes Care* (2006): 1433–38.

Solomon, D. H., and W. C. Winkelmayer. "Cardiovascular Risk and the Thiazolidinediones: Déjà Vu All Over Again?" *Journal of the American Medical Association* 298, no. 10 (2007): 1216–18.

Suzuki, Y., et al. "Antiobesity Activity of Extracts from *Lagerstroemia speciosa* L. Leaves on Female KK-Ay Mice." *Journal of Nutritional Science and Vitaminology* (Tokyo) 45, no. 6 (1999): 791–95.

Trehan, S., M.D., et al. "Magnesium Disorders: What to Do When Homeostasis Goes Awry." *Consultant* (November 1996): 2485–97.

Tsuda, T., "Regulation of Adipocyte Function by Anthocyanins; Possibility of Preventing the Metabolic Syndrome." *Journal of Agricultural and Food Chemistry* 56, no. 3 (February 2008): 642–46.

Tuominen, J. A., et al. "Exercise Increases Insulin Clearance in Healthy Men and Insulin-Dependent Diabetes Mellitus Patients." *Clinical Physiology* 17 (1997): 19–30.

Vaccaro, O., et al. "Moderate Hyperhomocysteinaemia and Retinopathy in Insulin-Dependent Diabetes." *The Lancet* 349 (April 12, 1997): 1102–103.

Zhang, W. J., and B. Frei. "Alpha-Lipoic Acid Inhibits TNF-Alpha-Induced NF-Kappab Activation and Adhesion Molecule Expression in Human Aortic Endothelial Cells." *The FASEB Journal: Official Publication of the Federation of American Societies for Experimental Biology* 15, no. 13 (November 2001): 2423–32.

Chapter 17
Drugs for Eye Diseases and Their Natural Alternatives

Albert, D., M.D., et al. *Principles and Practice of Ophthalmology: Basic Sciences.* Philadelphia, PA: W. B. Saunders, 1994.

Baudoin, C., et al. "Expression of Inflammatory Membrane Markers by Conjunctival Cells in Chronically Treated Patients with Glaucoma." *Ophthalmology* 101 (1994): 454–60.

Boulton, M., et al. "Lipofuscin Is a Photoinducible Free Radical Generator." *Journal of Photochemistry and Photobiology, B-Biology* 19, no. 3 (August 1993): 201–4.

Caprioli J., M. Sears, L. Bausher, et al. Forskolin Lowers Intraocular Pressure by Reducing Aqueous Inflow." *Investigative Ophthalmology & Visual Science* 25 (1984): 268–277.

Caprioli, J., and M. Sears. "Forskolin Lowers Intraocular Pressure in Rabbits, Monkeys, and Man." *The Lancet* 1 (1983): 958-960.

Connor, W. E., et al. "Essential Fatty Acids: The Importance of N-3 Fatty Acids in the Retina and Brain." *Nutrition Reviews* 50 (1992): 21–29.

Czernin, J., et al. "Effect of Short-Term Cardiovascular Conditioning and Low-Fat Diet on Myocardial Blood Flow and Flow Reserve." *Circulation* 92, no. 2 (July 15, 1995): 192–204.

Ferris, F. L. "Senile Macular Degeneration: Review of Epidemiologic Features." *American Journal of Epidemiology* 118 (1983): 132–50.

Gottsch, J., et al. "Light-Induced Deposits in Bruch's Membrane of Protoporhyric Mice." *Archives of Ophthalmology* 111, no. 1 (January 1993): 126–29.

Head, K. A. "Natural Therapies for Ocular Disorders, Part Two: Cataracts and Glaucoma." *Alternative Medicine Review* 6, no. 2 (April 2001): 141–66.

Jacob, S., et al. "The Antioxidant Alpha-Lipoic Acid Enhances Insulin-Stimulated Glucose Metabolism in Insulin-Resistant Rat Skeletal Muscle." *Diabetes* 45, no. 8 (August 1996): 1024–29.

Jonas, J., et al. "Parapapillary Retinal Diameter in Normal and Glaucomatous Eyes." *Investigative Ophthalmology* 30 (1989): 1599–1603.

Kilic, F., et al. "Modelling Cortical Cataractogenesis 17: In Vitro Effect of A-Lipoic Acid on Glucose-Induced Lens Membrane Damage: A Model of Diabetic Cataracto-Genesis." *Biochemistry & Molecular Biology International* 37, No. 2 (October 1995): 361–70.

Leibowitz, H., D. Krueger, and L. Mauder. "The Framingham Eye Study Monograph." *Survey of Ophthalmology* 24, supp. (1980).

Li, J., R. C. Tripathi, and B. J. Tripathi. "Drug-Induced Ocular Disorders." *Drug Safety* 31, no. 2 (2008): 127–41(15).

McDougall, J., et al. "Rapid Reduction of Serum Cholesterol and Blood Pressure by a Twelve-Day, Very Low Fat, Strictly Vegetarian Diet." *Journal of the American College of Nutrition* 14, no. 5 (October 1995): 491–96.

Meyer, B. H., A. A. Stulting, F. O. Muller, et al. "The Effects of Forskolin Eye Drops on Intra-Ocular Pressure." *South African Medical Journal* 71 (198): 570–571.

Mozaffarieh, M., and J. Flammer. "Is There More to Glaucoma Treatment than Lowering IOP?" *Survey of Ophthalmology* 52, supp. 2 (November, 2007): S174–79.

Nordoy, A. "Fish Consumption and Cardiovascular Disease: A Reappraisal." *Nutrition and Metabolism in Cardiovascular Disease* 6 (1996): 103–9.

Ritch, R. "Natural Compounds: Evidence for a Protective Role in Eye Disease." *Canadian Journal of Ophthalmology* 42, no. 3 (June 2007): 425–38.

Rozanowska, M., et al. "Blue Light-Induced Reactivity of Retinal Age Pigment: In Vitro Generation of Oxygen-Reactive Species." *Journal of Biological Chemistry* 270, no. 32 (August 11, 1995): 18825–30.

Sakai, T., M. Murata, and T. Amemiya. "Effects of Long-Term Treatment of Glaucoma with Vitamin B_{12}." *Glaucoma* 14 (1992): 167–70.

Seddon, J. M., et al. "Dietary Carotenoids, Vitamins A, C, and E, and Advanced Age-Related Macular Degeneration." *Journal of the American Medical Association* 272 (1994): 1413–20.

Seto, C., S. Eguchi, M. Araie, et al. "Acute Effects of Topical Forskolin on Aqueous Humor Dynamics in Man." *Japanese Journal of Ophthalmology* 30 (1986): 238–44.

Snodderly, D. M. "Evidence for Protection Against Age-Related Macular Degeneration by Carotenoids and Antioxidant Vitamins." *American Journal of Clinical Nutrition* 63, no. 6 supp. (December 1995): 1448S–61S.

Tsai, J. C., B. J. Song, L. Wu, and M. Forbes. "Erythropoietin: A Candidate Neuroprotective Agent in the Treatment of Glaucoma." *Journal of Glaucoma* 16, no. 6 (September 2007): 567–71.

Williams, D. E., et al. "Effects of Timolol, Betaxolol, and Levobunolol on Human Tendon's Fibroblasts in Tissue Culture." *Investigative Ophthalmology and Visual Sciences* 33 (1992): 2233–41.

Ziegler, D., et al. "Treatment of Symptomatic Diabetic Peripheral Neuropathy with the Antioxidant Alpha-Lipoic Acid: A 3-Week Multicentre Randomized Controlled Trial (ALADIN Study)." *Diabetologica* 38, no. 12 (December 1995): 1425–33.

Chapter 18
Drugs for the Prostate and Their Natural Alternatives

Giovannucci, E., et al. "A Prospective Study of Dietary Fat and the Risk of Prostate Cancer." *Journal of the National Cancer Institute* 85, no. 19 (October 6, 1993): 1571–79.

Klein, L. A., and J. S. Stoff. "Prostaglandins and the Prostate: An Hypothesis on the Etiology of Benign Prostatic Hyperplasia." *Prostate* 4, no. 3 (1983): 247–51.

Milne, D. B., Ph.D., and P. E. Johnson, Ph.D. "Effect of Changes in Short-Term Dietary Zinc Intake on Ethanol Metabolism and Zinc Status Indices in Young Men." *Nutrition Research* 13 (1993): 511–21.

Morrison, H., et al. "Herbicides and Cancer." *Journal of the National Cancer Institute* 84 (1992): 1866–74.

———. "Farming and Prostate Cancer Mortality." *American Journal of Epidemiology* 137, no. 3 (1993): 270–80.

Rose, D. P. "Diet, Hormones and Cancer." *Annual Review of Public Health* 14 (1993): 1017.

Scaglione, F., V. Lucini, and M. Pannacci, et al. "Comparison of the Potency of Different Brands of Serenoa Repens Extract on 5alpha-Reductase Types I and II in Prostatic Co-Cultured Epithelial and Fibroblast Cells." *Pharmacology* 82, no. 4 (October 10, 2008): 270–75.

Talamini, R., et al. "Diet and Prostatic Cancer: A Case-Controlled Study in Northern Italy." *Nutrition and Cancer* 18 (1992): 277–86.

Chapter 19
Synthetic Hormones and Their Natural Alternatives

Conventional Hormone Replacement Therapy

McDonough, P., et al. "The Randomized World Is Not Without Its Imperfections: Reflections on the Women's Health Initiative Study." *Fertility and Sterility* 78, no. 5 (May 2002): 951–56.

Nelson, H. D., et al. "Postmenopausal Hormone Replacement Therapy: Scientific Review." *Journal of the American Medical Association* 288, no. 7 (August 21, 2002): 872–81.

Pradhan, A. D., et al. "Inflammatory Biomarkers, Hormone Replacement Therapy, and Incident Coronary Heart Disease: Prospective Analysis from the Women's Health Initiative Observational Study." *Journal of the American Medical Association* 288, no. 8 (August 28, 2002): 980–87.

Writing Group for the Women's Health Initiative Investigators. "Risks and Benefits of Estrogen and Progestin in Healthy Postmenopausal Women." *Journal of the American Medical Association* 288 (2002): 321–33.

Pregnenolone

Akwa, Y., et al. "Neurosteroids: Biosynthesis, Metabolism and Function of Pregnenolone and Dehydroepiandrosterone in the Brain." *Journal of Steroid Biochemistry, and Molecular Biology* 40, nos. 1–3 (1991): 71–81.

De Wied, D. "Hormone Influences on Motivation, Learning and Memory Processes." *Hospital Practices* 11, no. 1 (1976): 123–31.

———. "Pituitary Adrenal System Hormones and Behavior." *Acta Endocrinologica* 85, supp. 214 (1977): 9–18.

Flood, J. F., J. E. Morley, and E. Roberts. "Memory-Enhancing Effects in Male Mice of Pregnenolone and Steroids Metabolically Derived from It." *Proceedings of the National Academy of Sciences* USA 89 (1992): 1567–71.

Morfin, R., et al. "Neurosteroids: Pregnenolone in Human Sciatic Nerves." *Proceedings of the National Academy of Sciences* USA 9, no. 15 (1992): 6790–93.

Paul, S. M., and R. H. Purdy. "Neuroactive Steroids." *The FASEB Journal: Official Publication of the Federation of American Societies for Experimental Biology* 6, no. 6 (1992): 2311–22.

Weidenfeld, J., R. A. Siegel, and I. Chowers. "In Vitro Conversion of Pregnenolone to Progesterone by Discrete Brain Areas of the Male Rat." *The Journal of Steroid Biochemisty and Molecular Biology* 13, no. 8 (1980): 961–63.

Wu, F. S., et al. "Pregnenolone Sulfate: A Positive Allosteric Modulator at the N-Methyl-D-Aspartate Receptor." *Molecular Pharmacology* 40, no. 3 (1991): 333–36.

Progesterone

Cundy, T., et al. "Bone Density in Women Receiving a Depot Medroxyprogesterone Acetate for Contraception." *British Medical Journal* 303 (1991): 13–16.

Ellison, P. T., et al. "The Ecological Context of Human Ovarian Function." *Human Reproduction* 8 (1993): 2248–58.

Hargrove, J. T., et al. "Menopausal Hormone Replacement Therapy with Continuous Daily Oral Micronized Estradiol and Progesterone." *Obstetrics & Gynecology* 71 (1989): 606–12.

Lee, J. R., M.D. "Is Natural Progesterone the Missing Link in Osteoporosis Prevention and Treatment?" *Medical Hypotheses* 35 (1991): 316–18.

———. "Osteoporosis Reversal: The Role of Progesterone." *International Clinical Nutrition Review* 10 (1990): 384–91.

———. "Osteoporosis Reversal with Transdermal Progesterone." (letter) *The Lancet* 336 (1990): 1327.

Prior, J. C., and V. M. Vigna. "Spinal Bone Loss and Ovulatory Disturbances." *New England Journal of Medicine* 323 (1990): 1221–27.

Prior, J. C., V. Vigna, and N. Alojado. "Progesterone and the Prevention of Osteoporosis." *Canadian Journal of Obstetrics/Gynecology & Women's Health Care* 3 (1991): 178–84.

———. "Progesterone as a Bone-Trophic Hormone." *Endocrine Reviews* 11 (1990): 386–98.

Reyes, F. L., J. S. Winter, and C. Paiman. "Pituitary Ovarian Relationships Preceding the Menopause: A Cross-Sectional Study of Serum Follicle-Stimulating Hormone, Luteinizing Hormone, Prolactin, Estradiol and Progesterone Levels." *American Journal of Obstetrics and Gynecology* 129 (1977): 557–64.

DHEA

Araneo, B., and R. Daynes. "Dehydroepiandrosterone Functions as More than an Antigluco-corticoid in Preserving Immunocompetence After Thermal Injury."

Endocrinology 136, no. 2 (February 1995): 393–401.

Assan, R., et al. "Dehydroepiandrosterone (DHEA) for Diabetic Patients?" *European Journal of Endocrinology* 135 (1996): 37–38.

Barrett-Connor, E., and A. Ferrara. "Dehydroepiandrosterone, Dehydroepiandrosterone Sulfate, Obesity, Waist-Hip Ratio, and Noninsulin-Dependent Diabetes in Postmenopausal Women: The Rancho Bernardo Study." *Journal of Clinical Endocrinology and Metabolism* 81, no. 1 (January 1996): 59–64.

Baulieu, E. E. "Dehydroepiandrosterone (DHEA): A Fountain of Youth?" *Journal of Clinical Endocrinology and Metabolism* 81, no. 9 (1996): 3147–51.

Beer, N. A., et al. "Dehydroepiandrosterone Reduces Plasma Plasminogen Activator Inhibitor Type 1 and Tissue Plasminogen Activator Antigen in Man." *The American Journal of the Medical Sciences* 311, no. 5 (May 1996): 205–10.

Daynes, R. A., and B. A. Araneo. "The Development of Effective Vaccine Adjuvants Employing Natural Regulators of T-Cell Lymphokine Production In Vivo." *Annals of the New York Academy of Sciences* 730 (August 15, 1994): 144–61.

Eich, D. M., et al. "Inhibition of Accelerated Coronary Atheroslerosis with Dehydroepiandrosterone in the Heterotropic Rabbit Model of Cardiac Transplantation." *Circulation* 87, no. 1 (January 1993): 261–69.

Freiss, E., et al. "DHEA Administration Increases Rapid Eye Movement Sleep and EEG Power and Sigma Frequency Range." *American Journal of Physiology* 268 (1995): E107–E113.

Haffner, S. M., and R. A. Valdez. "Endogenous Sex Hormones: Impact on Lipids, Lipo-proteins, and Insulin." *American Journal of Medicine* 98, no. 1A (January 16, 1995): 40S–47S.

Herbert, J., et al. "The Age of Dehydroepiandrosterone." *The Lancet* 345 (May 13, 1995): 1193–94.

McLachlan, J. A., C. D. Serkin, and O. Bakouche. "Dehydroepiandrosterone Modulation of Lipopolysaccharide-Stimulated Monocyte Cytotoxicity." *Journal of Immunology* 156, no. 1 (January 1, 1996): 328–35.

Morales, A. J., et al. "Effects of Replacement Dose of Dehydroepiandrosterone in Men and Women of Advancing Age." *Journal of Clinical Endocrinology and Metabolism* 78 (1994): P1360–67.

Padgett, D. A., and R. M. Loria. "In Vitro Potentiation of Lymphocyte Activation by Dehydroepiandrosterone, Androstenediol, and Androstenetriol." *Journal of Immunology* 153, no. 4 (August 15, 1994): 1544–52.

Skolnick, A. A. "Scientific Verdict Still Out on DHEA." *Journal of the American Medical Association* 276, no. 17 (November 6, 1996).

Toshiyuki, H., M.D., Ph.D., et al. "Effect of Dehydroepiandrosterone Sulfate on Ophthalmic Artery Flow Velocity Wave Forms in Full-Term Pregnant Women." *American Journal of Perinatology* 12, no. 2 (March 1995): 135–37.

Yen, S. S., A. J. Morales, and O. Khorram. "Replacement of DHEA in Aging Men and Women: Potential Remedial Effects." *Annual Report of the New York Academy of Science* 774 (1995): 128–42.

Testosterone

Rako, S. *The Hormone of Desire*. New York: Three Rivers Press, 1996.

Tenover, J. S. "Effects of Testosterone Supplementation in the Aging Male." *Journal of Clinical Endocrinology and Metabolism* 75, no. 4 (October 1992): 1092–98.

Growth Hormone

Etherton, T., et al. "Mechanisms by Which Somatotropin Decreases Adipose Tissue Growth." *American Journal of Clinical Nutrition* 58, supp. (1993): 287S–95S.

Feldman, E. "Aspects of the Interrelations of Nutrition and Aging—1993." *American Journal of Clinical Nutrition* 58, no. 1 (July 1993): 1–3.

Hartman, M., et al. "Pulsatile Growth Hormone Secretion in Older Persons Is Enhanced by Fasting Without Relationship to Sleep Stages." *Journal of Clinical Endocrinology and Metabolism* 81, no. 7 (July 1996): 2694–701.

Jorgensen, J. O., and J. S. Christiansen. "Brave New Senescence: GH in Adults." *The Lancet* 341 (May 15, 1993): 1247.

Kraemer, W. J., et al. "Hormonal and Growth Factor Responses to Heavy Resistance Exercise Protocols." *Journal of Applied Physiology* 69 (1990): 1442–50.

Meling, T., and E. Nylen. "Growth Hormone Deficiency in Adults: A Review." *American Journal of the Medical Sciences* 311, no. 4 (1996): 153–66.

Rubin, C., M.D., FACP. "Southwestern Internal Medicine Conference: Growth Hormone-Aging and Osteoporosis." *American Journal of the Medical Sciences* 305, no. 2 (1993): 120–29.

Rudman, D., M.D. "Effects of Human Growth Hormone in Men Over 60 Years Old." *New England Journal of Medicine* 323, no. 1 (July 5, 1990): 1–6.

Schwartz, R. "Trophic Factor Supplementation: Effect on the Age-Associated Changes in Body Composition." *Journals of Gerontology: Series A, Biological Sciences and Medical Sciences* 50, spec. no. (November 1995): 151–56.

Toogood, A., P. O'Neill, and S. Shalet. "Beyond the Somatopause: Growth Hormone Deficiency in Adults Over the Age of 60 Years." *Journal of Clinical Endocrinology and Metabolism* 81, no. 2 (February 1996): 460–65.

Weltman, A., et al. "Endurance Training Amplifies the Pulsatile Release of Growth Hormone: Effects of Training Intensity." *Journal of Applied Physiology* 72, no. 6 (1992): 2188–96.

Wiswell, R., and R. Marcus. "Age-Dependent Effect of Resistance Exercise on Growth Hormone Secretion in People." *Journal of Clinical Endocrinology and Metabolism* 75, no. 2 (August 1992): 404–7.

Yarasheski, K., and J. Zachwieja. "Growth Hormone for the Elderly: The Fountain of Youth Proves Toxic." (letter) *Journal of the American Medical Association* 270, no. 14 (October 13, 1993): 1694.

Melatonin

Reiter, R. J. "Oxygen Radical Detoxification Processes During Aging: The Functional Importance of Melatonin." *Aging* 7, no. 5 (October 1995): 340–51.

———. "The Aging Pineal Gland and Its Physiological Consequences." *Bioessays* 14, no. 3 (March 1992): 169–75.

———. "The Role of the Neurohormone Melatonin as a Buffer Against Macromolecular Oxidative Damage." *Neurochemistry*

International 27, no. 6 (December 1995): 453–60.

———. "Functional Pleiotropy of the Neurohormone Melatonin: Antioxidant Protection and Neuroendocrine Regulation." *Frontiers in Neuroendocrinology* 16, no. 4 (October 1995): 383–415.

Thyroid Hormone

Arem, R. *The Thyroid Solution.* New York: Ballantine Books, 1999.

Chapter 20
Drugs for Osteoporosis and Their Natural Alternatives

Alonso-Coello, P., A. L. Garcia-Franco, G. Guyatt, et al. "Drugs for Pre-osteoporosis: Prevention or Disease Mongering?" *British Medical Journal* 336 (January 19, 2008): 126–29.

Black, D. M., A. V. Schwartz, K. E. Ensrud, et al. "Effects of Continuing or Stopping Alendronate After 5 Years of Treatment: The Fracture Intervention Trial Long-Term Extension (FLEX): A Randomized Trial." *Journal of the American Medical Association* 296, no. 24 (2006): 2927–38.

Chilibeck, P. D., et al. "Exercise and Bone Mineral Density." *Sports Medicine* 19, no. 2 (1995): 103–22.

Cooper, C., et al. "Water Fluoridation and Hip Fracture." (letter) *Journal of the American Medical Association* 266 (1991): 513–14.

Danielson, C., et al. "Hip Fractures and Fluoridation in Utah's Elderly Population." *Journal of the American Medical Association* 268 (1992): 746–47.

Hedlund, L. R., and J. C. Gallagher. "Increased Incidence of Hip Fracture in Osteoporotic Women Treated with Sodium Fluoride." *Journal of Bone and Mineral Research* (1989): 223–25.

Jacobsen, S. J., et al. "Regional Variation in the Incidence of Hip Fractures: U.S. White Women Aged 65 Years and Older." *Journal of the American Medical Association* 264 (1990): 500–502.

Jacqmin-Gadda, H., D. Commenges, and J. F. Dartigues. "Fluorine Concentrations in Drinking Water and Fracture in the Elderly." *Journal of the American Medical Association* 273 (1995): 775–76.

Kleerekoper, M. E., et al. "Continuous Sodium Fluoride Therapy Does Not Reduce Vertebral Fracture Rate in Postmenopausal Osteoporosis." *Journal of Bone and Mineral Research* 4, supp. 1 (1989): S376.

Kritz-Silverstein, D., and D. L. Goodman-Gruen. "Usual Dietary Isoflavone Intake, Bone Mineral Density, and Bone Metabolism in Postmenopausal Women." *Journal of Women's Health and Gender-Based Medicine* 11, no. 1 (January/February, 2002): 69–78.

Lindsay, R., M.D., Ph.D. "The Burden of Osteoporosis: Cost." *American Journal of Medicine* 98, supp. 2A (February 27, 1995): 2A-9S–11S.

Lin, J. T., and J. M. Lane. "Nonpharmacologic Management of Osteoporosis to Minimize Fracture Risk." *Nature Clinical Practice Rheumatology* 4, no. 1 (January 2008): 20–25.

Martyn-St. James, M., and S. Carroll. "High-Intensity Resistance Training and Postmenopausal Bone Loss: A Meta-Analysis." *Osteoporosis International* 17 (2006): 1225–40.

Odvina, C. V., J. E. Zerweky, S. Rao, et al. "Severely Suppressed Bone Turnover: A Potential Complication of Alendronate Therapy." *Journal of Clinical Endocrinology & Metabolism* 90, no. 3 (2004): 1294–1301.

Ott, S. "Editorial: Long-Term Safety of Bisphosphonates." *The Journal of Clinical Endocrinology & Metabolism* 90, no. 3: 1897–99.

Richards, J. B., Papaioannou, A., et al. "Effect of Selective Serotonin Reuptake Inhibitors on the Risk of Fracture." *Archives of Internal Medicine* 167, no. 2 (January 22, 2007): 188–94.

Riggs, B. L., et al. "Effect of Fluoride Treatment on the Fracture Rate in Postmenopausal Women with Osteoporosis." *New England Journal of Medicine* 322 (1990): 802–9.

Scarbeck, K. "Strength Training May Reduce the Risk of Osteoporotic Fractures." *Family Practice News* (February 15, 1995): 10.

Sowers, M. F. R., et al. "A Prospective Study of Bone Mineral Content and Fracture in Communities with Differential Fluoride Exposure." *American Journal of Epidemiology* 134 (1991): 649–60.

Yang, Y. X., and J. D. Lewis, et al. "Long-Term Proton Pump Inhibitor Therapy and Risk of Hip Fracture." *Journal of the American Medical Association* 296, no. 24 (December 27, 2006): 2947–53.

Chapter 23
Drugs for Attention Deficit/Hyperactivity Disorder and Their Natural Alternatives

Alonzo-Zaldivar, R. "FDA Calls for Improved Warnings for ADD Drugs." *Washington Times*, March 22, 2006.

Bateman, B. "The Effects of a Double-Blind, Placebo Controlled, Artificial Food Colorings and Benzoate Preservative Challenge on Hyperactivity in a General Population Sample of Preschool Children." *Archives of Disease in Childhood* 89 (2004): 506–11.

Bellanti J., W. G. Crook, and R. E. Layton. "Attention Deficit Hyperactivity Disorder: Causes and Possible Solutions." From Conference of Georgetown University, the International Center for Interdisciplinary Studies of Immunology, and the International Health Foundation at Key Bridge Marriot Hotel, Arlington, VA, November 4–7, 1999.

Boris, M., and F. S. Mandel. "Foods and Additives Are Common Causes of the Attention Deficit Hyperactive Disorder in Children." *Annals of Allergy* 72, no. 5 (May 1994): 462–68.

Breggin, Peter, "Psychostimulants in the Treatment of Children Diagnosed with ADHD: Risks and Mechanism of Action." *International Journal of Risk & Safety in Medicine* 12 (1999): 3–35.

Burgess, J. R., et al. "Long-Chain Polyunsaturated Fatty Acids in Children with Attention-Deficit Hyperactivity Disorder." *American Journal of Clinical Nutrition* 71, supp. 1 (January 2000): 327S–30S.

Carter, C. M., et al. "Effects of a Few Food Diet in Attention Deficit Disorder." *Archives of Disease in Childhood* 69, no. 5 (November 1993): 564–68.

Crook, W. G. "Sugar and Children's Behavior." *New England Journal of Medicine* 330, no. 26 (June 30, 1994): 1901–2.

DeNoon, Daniel. "Ritalin for Preschoolers? Study Shows Drug Provides 'Moderate'

Help for Preschool Kids with ADHD." *WebMD Medical News*, October 19, 2006.

Grandjean P., and P. J. Landrigan. "Developmental Neurotoxicity of Industrial Chemicals." *The Lancet* 368, no. 9553 (November 8, 2006): 2167–78.

Greenhill, L. "Efficacy and Safety of Immediate-Release Methylphenidate Treatment for Preschoolers with ADHD." *Journal of the American Academy of Child and Adolescent Psychiatry* 45 (November 2006: 1284–93.

Parker-Pope, Tara. "Studies Linking Ritalin and Depression Highlight Risk of Overdiagnosing ADHD." *Wall Street Journal* (January 25, 2005): D1.

Price, J. H. "FDA Orders Drug Warnings for ADHD Patients." *Washington Times* (February 22, 2007).

Rubin, R. "FDA Panel: ADHD Drugs for Kids Need Hallucination Warning." *USA Today* (March 23, 2006): 6D.

Sabra, A., J. A. Bellanti, and A. R. Colon. "Ileal-Lymphoid-Nodular Hyperplasia, Non-Specific Colitis, and Pervasive Developmental Disorder in Children." *The Lancet* 352, no. 9123 (July 18, 1998): 234–35.

Schoenthaler, S. J., and I. D. Bier. "The Effect of Vitamin-Mineral Supplementation on Juvenile Delinquency Among American Schoolchildren: A Randomized, Double-Blind Placebo-Controlled Trial." *Journal of Alternative and Complementary Medicine* 6, no. 1 (February 2000): 7–17.

Science News Daily. "Many Children Discontinuing Use of ADHD Medication." December 17, 2006. http://www.science daily.com/releases/2006/12/061216104616 .htm.

Stagnitti, M. N. "Trends in the Use and Expenditures for the Therapeutic Class Prescribed Psychotherapeutic Agents and All Subclasses, 1997 and 2004." *Medical Expenditure Panel Survey* (February 2007): Statistical Brief #163.

Uhlig, T., et al. "Topographic Mapping of Brain Electrical Activity in Children with Food-Induced Attention Deficit Hyperkinetic Disorder." *European Journal of Pediatrics* 156, no. 7 (July 1997): 557–61.

Vedantam, Shankar. "Warning Urged for ADHD Drugs." *The Washington Post*, February 10, 2006: A1.

Wakefield, A. J. "The Gut-Brain Axis in Childhood Developmental Disorders." *Journal of Pediatrics Gastroenterology and Nutrition* 34, supp. 1 (May/June 2002): S14–7.

Reference Books

Bosker, G., M.D., FACEP. *Pharmatecture: Minimizing Medications to Maximize Results.* St. Louis, MO: Facts & Comparisons, 1996.

Colvin, R. *Prescription Drug Abuse: The Hidden Epidemic.* Omaha, NE: Addicus Books, 1995.

Drug Facts & Comparisons. St. Louis, MO: Facts & Comparisons, 2002.

Ganong, W. F. *Review of Medical Physiology.* 16th ed. Norwalk, CT: Appleton & Lange, 1993.

Gradeon, J., and T. Gradeon, Ph.D. *The People's Guide to Deadly Drug Interactions.* New York: St. Martin's Press, 1995.

———. *The People's Pharmacy.* New York: St. Martin's Griffin, 1996.

Grahame-Smith, D. G., and J. K. Aronson. *Oxford Textbook of Clinical Pharmacology and Drug Therapy*. Oxford, England: Oxford University Press, 1992.

Handbook of Nonprescription Drugs. 11th ed. Washington, DC: American Pharmaceutical Association, 1996.

Hansten, P. D., and J. R. Horn. *Hansten and Horn's Drug Interactions Analysis and Management*. Vancouver, WA: Applied Therapeutics, Inc., 1997.

Harness, R. H. *Drug Interactions Guide Book*. Englewood Cliffs, NJ: Prentice Hall, 1991.

Holt, G. *Food and Drug Interactions: A Health Care Professional's Guide*. Chicago: Precept Press, Inc., 1992.

The Merck Manual of Diagnosis and Therapy. Rahway, NJ: Merck & Co., 1992.

Physicians' Desk Reference. Montvale, NJ: Medical Economics Data Production Company, 1997.

The PDR Family Guide to Prescription Drugs. New York: Crown, 1996.

Thomas, J. H., and B. Gillham. *Wills' Biochemical Basis of Medicine*. Oxford, England: Butterworth-Heineman Ltd., 1992.

INDEX